ACUTE MYOCARDIAL INFARCTION

This volume comprises
the Proceedings of a Symposium
held in the Pfizer Postgraduate Institute, Edinburgh,
under the auspices of the University of Edinburgh
and the Edinburgh Post-Graduate Board for Medicine
in September 1967

©

E. & S. LIVINGSTONE LTD

1968

SBN 443 00587 7

PRINTED IN GREAT BRITAIN

ACUTE MYOCARDIAL INFARCTION

Proceedings of a Symposium
sponsored by the University of Edinburgh
in September 1967

Edited by

D. G. JULIAN

M.A., M.D.Cantab., M.R.C.P.Ed., M.R.C.P.Lond., M.R.A.C.P.

and

M. F. OLIVER

M.D.Ed., F.R.C.P.Ed., M.R.C.P.Lond.

E. & S. LIVINGSTONE LTD

EDINBURGH AND LONDON
1968

' Where, however, the cessation of vital action is very complete, and continues long, we ought to inflate the lungs, and pass electric shocks through the chest: the practitioner ought never, if the death has been sudden, and the person not very far advanced in life, to despair of success, till he has unequivocal signs of real death.'

From pages 147–148 of the Chapter entitled ' Observation on disease of the coronary arteries and on syncope anginosa ' in *Observations on Some of the Most Frequent and Important Diseases of the Heart* by Allan Burns, published in Edinburgh in 1809.

FOREWORD

ACUTE myocardial infarction has for some years been the chief cause of death in middle-aged adults in developed countries. Recognising the contribution which the application of intensive care might make towards reducing the mortality from this condition, the World Health Organization sponsored its first training course on coronary care in Edinburgh from 4th to 16th September 1967. During the last three days of this course, a symposium was held on several aspects of acute myocardial infarction and this was attended by many leaders in the field.

In the last five years, there has been a fantastic rate of progress in the treatment of acute myocardial infarction and there is an insatiable demand for special intensive coronary care units throughout the world. Intensive coronary care means intensive professional preoccupation with this dangerous disease, and new discoveries, attitudes and therapies arise almost daily. We in Edinburgh felt that such a symposium, attended by so many eminent pioneers and workers in this field, would allow fruitful discussion concerning not only the present state of knowledge but also important areas where research is urgently required.

The Proceedings of this Symposium covers six major aspects of management and research related to acute myocardial infarction. First of all, a brief account is given of the results of treating patients in coronary care units together with the problems of staffing and equipping such units. Second, the nature and management of the principal arrhythmias which arise immediately after acute myocardial infarction are considered. Third, the indications and limitations of pacing are outlined. Fourth, the consequences and management of cardiogenic shock and the treatment of cardiac failure are described. Fifth, the metabolic consequences of acute myocardial infarction receive attention. Finally, the relationship of intensive coronary care to the community and the future of coronary care units are reviewed. During this Symposium, much recent work was reported and the ensuing discussions resulted in a stimulating diversity of opinions. It is hoped that this book gives some impression both of the extent and of the limitations of our knowledge with regard to acute myocardial infarction.

Notwithstanding their divergent views on a number of subjects, the participants were unanimous in regarding the development of intensive care as a milestone in the history of the management of acute myocardial infarction. Our knowledge of the prognostic significance of the various cardiac arrhythmias and conduction defects and how best to treat them, has grown remarkably. Physicians no longer accept their occurrence as fortuitous but seek more specific causes such as site of infarction, degree of failure and endocrine and metabolic disturbances. More attention is being paid to the patient as an individual and his psychological response to this life-threatening event. His reaction to the unique environment and staff of the coronary care unit is also being studied.

Again, the logistics of intensive coronary care are being considered more carefully. How much effort and experience is really necessary and how much can be afforded by various communities?

Finally, it was recognised that a formidable challenge remained in applying the techniques of coronary care to a wider community, and above all in preventing the development of this still fatal disorder.

K. W. DONALD,

Professor of Medicine and Dean of the Faculty of Medicine

ACKNOWLEDGEMENTS

THIS Symposium would not have been held were it not for the establishment of the first course on intensive coronary care in Edinburgh by the World Health Organization, and we are particularly grateful to Dr Z. Pisa of the European Office in Copenhagen and Dr Z. Fejfar of the Cardiovascular Diseases section in Geneva for their sponsorship and interest in this course and in the subsequent Symposium.

The University of Edinburgh and the Edinburgh Post-graduate Board jointly sponsored this Symposium and we would like to thank Professor Michael Swann, F.R.S., the Principal and Vice-Chancellor of the University, Professor K. W. Donald, the Dean of the Faculty of Medicine, and Professor Eric Mekie, the Director of Post-graduate Studies. We are grateful also to Professor Mekie and his staff for providing the Pfizer Post-graduate Institute as the meeting place for this Symposium. We would also like to thank Mr Bruce Millan, M.P., the Joint Parliamentary Under-Secretary at the Scottish Home and Health Department, Dr J. H. F. Brotherston and Dr John Smith of the Scottish Home and Health Department for their support on this occasion. Dr Christopher Clayson, the President, and the Councillor of Royal College of Physicians of Edinburgh kindly permitted the use of the College for one of the receptions.

We wish to express our gratitude to Messrs Hewlett Packard Ltd, the Glaxo Group and the Pharmaceuticals Division of Imperial Chemical Industries Ltd for generous financial support, and to Messrs Geigy Ltd for providing tape recordings and transcriptions of the proceedings.

We also wish to record our appreciation of the unflagging efforts of Mrs Wilson of E. & S. Livingstone Ltd in helping us to prepare and correct the proofs.

LIST OF PARTICIPANTS

ARMSTRONG, A. *Coronary Disease Community Study, 12 George Square, Edinburgh 8, U.K.*

*ASKANAS, A. *Institute of Cardiology, Lindley'a, 4, Warsaw, Poland*

*BENSAID, J. *Clinique Cardiologique, Hôpital Boucicaut, 78 Rue de la Convention, Paris 15e, France*

*BERNARD, R. *Hôpital Universitaire St Pierre, Dept au Cardiologie, 322 Rue Haute, Bruxelles 1, Belgium*

*BJERKELUND, C. *Rikshospitalet, Medisinsk Ardeling B, Universitetsklinik, Pilestredet 32, Oslo, Norway*

BOUVRAIN, Y. *Hôpital Lariboisière, rue Ambroise Paré, Paris 10e, France*

*BRUSCHKE, A. V. G. *Van Hogendorkstraat 12, Utrecht, Netherlands*

CAMERON, A. J. V. *Western Infirmary, Glasgow, U.K.*

CARLSON, L. A. *King Gustav V Research Institute, Karolinska Sjukhuset, Stockholm, Sweden*

CHAZOV, E. I. *Institute of Therapy, Petroverigsky per 10, Moscow, U.S.S.R.*

COOPER. T. *National Heart Institute, Bethesda, Maryland 20014, U.S.A.*

CROSS, E. B. *Coronary Heart Diseases Section, Heart Disease Control Program, Public Health Service, 4040 N. Fairfax Drive, Arlington, Virginia 22203, U.S.A.*

DALLE, X. *Coronaire Eenheid, St Elisabethgasthuis, 45 Lange Gasthuisstraat, Antwerp, Belgium*

DONALD, K. W. *Department of Medicine, Royal Infirmary, Edinburgh 3, U.K.*

FEJFAR, Z. *Cardiovascular Diseases Section, W.H.O., Ave. Appia, 1211 Geneva, Switzerland*

FOX, S. M. *Heart Disease Control Program, Dept. of Health, Education and Welfare, Public Health Service, 4040 Fairfax Drive, Arlington, Virginia 22203, U.S.A.*

FROMMER, P. L. *Department of Health, Education and Welfare, National Institutes of Health, Bethesda, Maryland 20014, U.S.A.*

FRY, J. *36 Croydon Road, Beckenham, Kent, U.K.*

*GEARTY, G. F. *Royal City of Dublin Hospital, Upper Baggot Street, Dublin 4, Ireland*

GEORGE, M. *Department of Cardiology, Royal Infirmary, Edinburgh, U.K.*

HAMMER, J. *Institute of Cardiovascular Research, 809 Budejovicka, Prague 4, Czechoslovakia*

HARRIS, P. C. *Institute of Cardiology, 35 Wimpole Street, London W.1, U.K.*

HEASMAN, M. A. *Scottish Department of Home and Health, St Andrew's House, Edinburgh, U.K.*

JULIAN, D. G. *Department of Cardiology, Royal Infirmary, Edinburgh 3, U.K.*

KILLIP, T. *Department of Medicine, N.Y. Hospital, Cornell Medical Center, 525 East 68th Street, New York, N.Y. 10021, U.S.A.*

KIRBY, B. J. *Central Middlesex Hospital, Park Royal, London N.W. 10, U.K.*

*KREUZER, H. *Universitat Dusseldorf, 1 Medizinische Klinik, Moorenstrasse 5, Dusseldorf, W. Germany*

LASSERS, B. W. *Department of Cardiology, Royal Infirmary, Edinburgh 3, U.K.*

LAWRIE, D. M. *Department of Medicine, Royal Infirmary, Edinburgh 3, U.K.*

LEATHAM, A. G. *St George's Hospital, Hyde Park Corner, London, U.K.*

*LETAC, B. *Centre de Réanimation, Hôpital Boucicaut, 78 Rue de la Convention, Paris 15e, France*

LOWN, B. *Peter Bent Brigham Hospital, Boston, Massachusetts, U.S.A.*

McDONALD, E. L. *Cardiac Department, The London Hospital, London, U.K.*

McKENDRICK, C. S. *Regional Cardiac Centre, Sefton General Hospital, Liverpool, U.K.*

McNICOL, M. W. *Central Middlesex Hospital, Park Royal, London, N.W.10, U.K.*

MARQUIS, R. M. *Department of Cardiology, Royal Infirmary, Edinburgh, U.K.*

MATTHEWS, J. D. *Royal Infirmary, Edinburgh, U.K.*

MATTHEWS, M. B. *Cardiac Department, Western General Hospital, Edinburgh, U.K.*

MELTZER, L. E. *Presbyterian University of Pennsylvania Medical Center, 51 North 39th Street, Philadelphia, Pennsylvania 19104, U.S.A.*

MOUNSEY, J. P. D. *Royal Postgraduate School of Medicine, Hammersmith Hospital, Ducane Road, London W.12, U.K.*

MUIR, A. L.   *Department of Medicine, Royal Infirmary, Edinburgh 3, U.K.*

NIXON, P. G. F.   *Charing Cross Hospital, London W.C.2, U.K.*

OLIVER, M. F.   *Department of Cardiology, Royal Infirmary, Edinburgh 3, U.K.*

ORINIUS, E.   *Serafimmerlasarettet, Hantverkargatan 2, Stockholm, Sweden*

PANTRIDGE, J. F.   *Royal Victoria Hospital, Belfast, U.K.*

PISA, Z.   *Regional Office for Chronic Diseases, W.H.O., 8 Scherfigsvej, Copenhagen, Denmark*

*RANZI, C. L. B.   *Department of Cardiology, Maggiore Niguarda Hospital, Milan, Italy*

*RISS, E.   *Department of Cardiology, Rambam Government Hospital, Haifa, Israel*

*ROSSI, P.   *Divisione Cardiologica A. Cesalpino 5, Camillo Hospital Cir. Gianicolense 87, Oo152—Rome, Italy*

*RUDA, M.   *Institute of Therapy, Petroverigsky per 10, Moscow, U.S.S.R.*

*SANDØE, E.   *Coronary Care Unit, Medical Dept. B, University Hospital, Copenhagen, Denmark*

SAMUEL, E.   *Department of Radiodiagnosis, Royal Infirmary, Edinburgh, U.K.*

SCHWEIZER, W.   *Burgerspital, Basel, Switzerland*

SEMPLE, T.   *Victoria Infirmary, Glasgow, U.K.*

SHILLINGFORD, J. P.   *Royal Postgraduate Medical School, Hammersmith Hospital, Ducane Road, London W.12, U.K.*

*SILTANEN, P.   *1st Department of Medicine, Meilahti Hospital, University of Helsinki, Helsinki, Finland*

SLOMAN, G.   *Cardiology Department, Royal Melbourne Hospital, Royal Parade, Parkville, Victoria, Australia*

SOWTON, G. E.   *Institute of Cardiology, 35 Wimpole Street, London W.1, U.K.*

WALLACE, A. G.   *Department of Medicine, Duke University Medical Center, Durham, North Carolina, U.S.A.*

WHITBY, L. G.   *Department of Clinical Chemistry, Royal Infirmary, Edinburgh 3, U.K.*

WILSON, J. M. G.   *Alexander Fleming House, Ministry of Health, Elephant and Castle, London S.E.1, U.K.*

*ZAVODNY, F.   *State Sanatorium, U. Malvayinsky 5, Prague 5, Czechoslovakia*

CONTENTS

CONTENTS

xiv

CONTENTS

xvi

CORONARY CARE UNITS

CURRENT POLICIES AND RESULTS

Chairman: Dr. D. G. JULIAN

PRESBYTERIAN-UNIVERSITY OF PENNSYLVANIA MEDICAL CENTER, PHILADELPHIA

Lawrence E. Meltzer

THERE have been very few medical advances that have been accepted as readily or with as much enthusiasm as the system of intensive coronary care. Within a 5-year period since the first two coronary units were established in the United States, at least 350 similar units have been developed and it has been recommended that probably all hospitals with 100 beds or more will require such facilities in the near future. This extraordinary acceptance is remarkable in view of the fact that there have been no definitive studies reported to date which actually define the true benefit of this system of care. Recognising the need for a controlled study early in the course of our work, we conducted a careful trial that was designed (among other purposes) to assess the specific effectiveness of intensive coronary care compared to usual hospital care. I should like to summarise these data at this time. In that it would be difficult to conduct a similar trial in the United States because of the moral and legal issues that have evolved, I trust this study has accomplished its aims.

The method of study was as follows: all patients with suspected acute myocardial infarction admitted to the Presbyterian-University of Pennsylvania Medical Center during a 20-month period beginning in 1964 were included in the study. When the patient presented himself at the Admissions Office (at the request of his own physician) or in the Receiving Ward (usually as an emergency) a clerk called the CCU to ascertain the availability of an unoccupied bed. If such vacancy existed, the patient was admitted directly to this research facility and was designated as a *study* subject. If the three beds in the unit were occupied at the time, the patient was assigned to regular hospital quarters and was categorised as a control subject.

Patients admitted to the CCU were treated by a well-organised team consisting of three physicians and eight cardiac nurse specialists. The control patients received the customary good care offered in a university-affiliated hospital.

At the end of 96 hours, patients in the CCU were transferred to

3

regular hospital facilities (if their condition permitted); their care
thereafter was not influenced by the research team. Those patients
originally admitted to regular facilities remained there throughout
their hospital stay and were not moved to the unit for any
reason.

It was felt that this method of sampling was equitable and would
permit a valid assessment of the value of intensive coronary care
as of 96 hours after admission.

Obviously the trial would have very limited meaning unless true
randomisation existed, and the study and control groups statistically
resembled each other. From the opinion of two groups of statis-
ticians who have studied these data, it is fair to conclude that the
groups were indeed comparable and that there were no major
areas of statistical departure.

Tables I, II and III show the distribution and some of the
characteristics of the 441 patients who entered the study. You will
note that 27 per cent. of the group were eventually excluded because
we were either unable to confirm electrocardiographically the admitting diagnosis of acute myocardial infarction, or because another
diagnosis was established. These patients were separated into a
third category (' excluded ') for statistical purposes.

Table I. *The effectiveness of intensive coronary care*
Comparability of groups

(441 Randomly Admitted Patients)

	Study %	Control %	Excluded %
Time between attack and admission:			
Less than 8 hours	50·3	43·1	56·0
Within 24 hours	24·1	26·0	20·7
More than 24 hours. . . .	18·8	26·9	13·8
Undeterminable	6·8	10·0	9·5
Clinical condition on admission:			
Good	45·5	42·3	49·6
Fair	32·5	33·8	34·8
Poor/critical	22·0	23·9	15·6

The age and sex distribution of the study and control groups
were the same. There were more Negroes in the control group.

Regarding the major determinants of in-hospital mortality, the

4

Table II. *The effectiveness of intensive coronary care*
A controlled study

Physical Examination on Admission

	Study %	Control %	Excluded %
Chest pain:			
None	38·2	34·6	42·6
Mild/moderate	40·3	38·5	42·6
Severe	21·5	26·9	14·8
Blood pressure:			
Systolic < 100 mm.	16·7	14·6	10·3
Systolic > 170 mm.	22·3	24·6	16·2
Diastolic < 60 mm.	17·3	16·5	10·3
Diastolic > 100 mm.	23·0	24·6	24·1
Pulse:			
< 60 per min.	17·3	16·5	12·9
> 120 per min.	23·0	24·6	24·1
Overt circulatory failure . . .	29·8	24·6	30·1

Table III. *The effectiveness of intensive coronary care*

The Incidence of Arrhythmias One Hour after Admission

	Study Alive (143)	Study Dead (48)	Control Alive (83)	Control Dead (47)
Premature beats	34%	52%	10%	17%
Minor arrhythmias	35%	42%	10%	30%
Major arrhythmias	21%	21%	05%	36%
Conduction disturbances . . .	14%	27%	13%	30%

time between the onset of the attack and admission, and the presence of overt circulatory failure and the overall clinical condition, it is evident that the groups were divided evenly.

If the equality of the two groups can be accepted, the respective mortality becomes meaningful. At the end of 24 hours, those

5

patients in the CCU had a death rate of 8·4 per cent. compared to a 12·8 per cent. rate for the control group. At 96 hours the respective rates were 12·0 per cent. and 20·8 per cent. This difference represents a relative reduction of 40 per cent. that can be directly attributed to the system of Intensive Coronary Care. Between 96 hours and hospital discharge, the mortality was similar in both groups. The ultimate mortality of the study patients was 19·9 per cent. versus 30·8 per cent. for the control group. The latter incidence is identical to the anticipated death rate in most hospitals, and is 35 per cent. higher than that achieved with Intensive Coronary Care.

This reduction in mortality was almost wholly the result of the prevention of arrhythmic deaths. The mortality from power failure was not lowered in any way.

DISCUSSION

Dr. Julian. I take it that although you had this particular study of randomisation, the figures you presented at the end were in fact not randomised?

Dr. Meltzer. Yes, they were. They stayed that way throughout. We selected none of them.

Dr Julian. Supposing a patient comes into your hospital and dies in the outpatient department, where does he figure?

Dr. Meltzer. He is not considered as a death in either group, because he has not reached a hospital room.

Dr Cross. Does your mortality at the end reflect a 96-hour mortality?

Dr Meltzer. No, that is total mortality at discharge. The death rate due to arrhythmias is self-limiting, as is coronary care. If one wants to improve mortality further something must be done about congestive heart failure. We have reduced the mortality recently to 14 per cent. by controlling congestive heart failure.

Professor Donald. If one of your control group developed increasing block, would they have a pacemaker inserted which would be operated automatically, if necessary?

Dr Meltzer. I would say it was up to the discretion of the physician in charge. If the patient was in the unit he would have a pacemaker. If he was in the control group he may or may not.

Dr. McKendrick (Liverpool). Did I hear you correctly when you said you had no arrhythmic deaths in two years?

Dr Meltzer. Yes.

Dr McKendrick. Some people differentiate between first-day ventricular fibrillation and ventricular fibrillation occurring in the patient in advanced failure or with hypotension. Are you including these or not?

Dr Meltzer. No, I divided them into primary and secondary—primary being those which occurred without deaths, and secondary being terminal.

Dr Bjerkelund. I would like to ask a question concerning the numbers of patients you excluded. Were they excluded after the primary randomisation and, if so, how was this exclusion done?

Dr Meltzer. Those excluded were removed after the end of 96 hours because we could not find electrocardiographic evidence of a myocardial infarction or because there was evidence of another illness, for instance, a ruptured viscus or pulmonary embolism. This excluded group represented 27 per cent. of the sample and there were as many excluded from the control group as there were from the unit group.

Dr Leatham (London). One of the problems of coronary care is the need for skilled physicians in charge of the patient. It would be interesting to establish a study where the cardiologist in the hospital looked after the control patients and the non-cardiologists looked after the unit patients. Coronary care is an expensive business and we have got to have a good excuse for doing it. I personally believe in it but to impress our politicians we have got to make it quite clear that it is not only the responsibility of skilled cardiologists.

Dr Meltzer. I think the 19 per cent. mortality could be achieved without physicians. Nursing services would be quite adequate so long as the nurses were well trained. I think you can get results whether you have physicians present or not. In two hospitals in the U.S. where there are no physicians at all and no house doctors, the mortality rate is still about 20 per cent. although there is nobody for the nurses to call. The major thing is that one person has to make all the decisions in the coronary care unit if you want to get the mortality below that.

Dr Julian. Did you match your cases from the onset of symptoms to admission to the unit or to a regular hospital bed?

Dr Meltzer. Yes.

Dr Wallace. A third of your deaths were in patients after 96 hours. What were the deaths due to?

Dr Meltzer. About half of them were due to congestive failure which developed after 96 hours, and the others were due to ventricular fibrillation, which developed spontaneously later.

ROYAL MELBOURNE HOSPITAL, MELBOURNE

Graeme Sloman

The Coronary Care Unit at The Royal Melbourne Hospital was established in 1963 with the assistance of a grant from The National Heart Foundation of Australia. By July 1967 the Unit had cared for 350 patients with suspected or proven acute myocardial infarction. Patients were admitted to the two-bed Unit on a bed-available basis and remained in the Coronary Care Unit for at least three days or until any major complication had been controlled —the average time of stay for those who survived was 6·3 days. The average age of the 350 patients was 57 years.

Patients were admitted to the Unit from the Casualty Department or from hospital wards. They were immediately examined by the Cardiology Registrar who instituted emergency therapy. Recently, the policy has been to insert an intravenous cannula to enable immediate administration of anti-arrhythmic and other drugs. Following the initial clinical examination, patients were classified into ' mild ', ' severe ' or ' cardiogenic shock ' according to the criteria of Robinson et al. (1964). This classification has enabled international comparison of results.

Patients were monitored during their stay in the Unit and ECG records were taken every 30 minutes or when an arrhythmia was noted on the monitoring oscilloscope. A serious primary arrhythmia was recorded in 42·3 per cent. of the 350 patients (Table I). With increasing experience and a wider range of anti-arrhythmic drugs, a more aggressive policy was adopted towards the suppression of arrhythmias. Procaine amide, lignocaine, phenytoin sodium and propranolol were used in the management of arrhythmias. These drugs were given by the intravenous route until the arrhythmia was controlled. Bradycardia, heart block and heart failure were treated immediately.

Trained nursing sisters staffed the Unit for 24 hours a day reporting changes in the patients' clinical condition and electro-cardiograms. The Cardiology Registrar was on immediate call to the Unit. The nursing staff were trained in cardio-pulmonary resuscitation including the use of direct current counter shock and the management of the Bird respirator. There were standing orders for the use of atropine sulphate and isoprenaline to be administered immediately in an emergency.

8

Table I. *'Serious' primary arrhythmias in 350 patients with acute myocardial infarction*

Arrhythmia	Classification on admission				
	Mild	Severe	Cardiogenic shock		Total
			a.	b.	
Atrial fibrillation . . .	13	12	0	5	30
Supraventricular tachycardia .	3	8	0	3	14
Nodal tachycardia . .	10	5	0	1	16
Ventricular tachycardia and flutter	10	11	1	3	25
2nd degree A.V. block . .	2	6	0	0	8
Complete heart block and A.V. dissociation . . .	5	8	0	1	14
Idioventricular rhythm . .	0	3	0	0	3
Ventricular standstill . .	2	8	3	1	14
Ventricular fibrillation . .	5	13	2	4	24
				Total	148
				42·3 per cent.	

Each arrhythmia recorded *once* only in each patient.

During the period under review, 91 patients of the 350 passing through the Unit died in hospital (26 per cent.). The clinical classification and the mortality in each group is detailed in Table II. Sixty-three patients died in the Unit, while 28 patients died after transfer to a general ward.

Cardiac arrest occurred in 72 patients while they were in the Unit. Twenty-eight were in ventricular fibrillation, 17 in ventricular standstill, 3 had an arrest associated with congestive cardiac failure, 21 were in cardiogenic shock and 3 sustained ruptured hearts. Although there were many short-term successful resuscitations, there were only 9 long-term survivors. All the survivors were in the group of 28 who developed ventricular fibrillation. Since arrhythmias have been treated more aggressively, fewer patients have developed primary ventricular fibrillation.

Despite the general acceptance of the Coronary Care Unit concept as part of the normal hospital service, the Unit has remained small—only two beds for a hospital bed state of over 657 and, consequently, only about half of the patients with acute myocardial infarction being admitted to the hospital are cared for in the Unit.

Table II. *Coronary Care Unit Patients*

Serial Nos.	1–50	51–100	101–150	151–200	201–250	251–300	301–350	Total series
Group I. Mild	23	25	27	28	20	22	21	166
Deaths	1	1	1	5	2	3	3	16 (9%)
Group II. Severe	17	18	17	15	16	20	23	126
Deaths	8	10	7	5	2	4	4	36 (29%)
Group III. Cardiogenic shock . .	10	7	6	7	14	8	6	53 (29%)
Deaths . . .	6	6	5	5	11	4	2	39 (67%)
Percentage mortality of each 50 patients .	30	34	26	30	30	22	18	91 (26%)

The Unit is staffed by specialist cardiologists. While the patient remains in the Unit he is managed by the Unit medical staff with consultant visits from his own physician. After transfer to the general ward, the physician manages the patient with additional consultations as required. At six weeks, all survivors are fully reviewed in the Cardiac Clinic.

The establishment of a Coronary Care Unit has improved the overall management of cardiac arrest and myocardial infarction throughout the hospital. Review of the time of admission after the onset of symptoms showed that 86 (25 per cent.) patients were admitted under four hours, 62 (18 per cent.) from four to six hours, 71 (20 per cent.) from 6–12 hours and 113 (32 per cent.) more than 12 hours after the onset of their symptoms. In 18 (5 per cent.), it was impossible to document the commencement of the acute episode. Thus, many patients arrived in hospital at a time when serious primary arrhythmias might have subsided. Notwithstanding this, the mortality of patients with ' mild ' and ' severe ' infarction admitted to the Unit was 18 per cent. compared with a hospital ward mortality of 29·8 per cent. from a group of 231 similar patients with ' mild ' and ' severe ' infarction. This difference in mortality, 18 per cent. in the Unit, compared to 29·8 per cent. outside the Unit, suggests that the reduction in the mortality might be due to earlier recognition of arrhythmias or more efficient treatment of the complications of myocardial infarction.

When the Unit was established, various anti-arrhythmic drugs were employed. Subsequently, a search has been made for a suitable prophylactic anti-arrhythmic drug. Propranolol and phenytoin sodium were shown, in a small pilot study, to lack the ability to prevent serious primary cardiac arrhythmias. More recently, lignocaine has been used in the management of arrhythmias. However, it has not been universally successful and, at the moment, no routine prophylactic regime is employed. When a significant primary arrhythmia develops, an anti-arrhythmic drug is administered by the intravenous route.

In our Unit, we have attempted to correlate the basic clinical signs with haemodynamic parameters measured at the bedside. Certain patients with ' severe ' infarction develop a degree of pulmonary hypertension. However, it is not possible to predict from clinical observation which one will have the higher pulmonary artery pressure. We have shown that the cardiac output may be reduced in both ' mild ' and ' severe ' infarcts. However, we have not felt justified in delaying treatment in order to measure output in patients with cardiogenic shock.

11

We have demonstrated a reduction in the arterial oxygen tension in most patients with infarction. This occurs without any abnormality in the carbon dioxide tension. Our findings point to this reduction in arterial tension as being due to an abnormal venoarterial shunt in the lung with an associated disturbance in the matching of pulmonary ventilation and pulmonary blood flow. Frusemide given intravenously in a dose of 80 mg. produced an improvement in the oxygen tension breathing air when a diuresis occurred. However, there was no reduction in the amount of venoarterial shunting. Oxygen therapy was shown to correct the degree of hypoxaemia.

Catecholamine metabolism and its possible relationship to cardiac arrhythmias has been studied. Daily pooled urine samples were examined for both catecholamine and for V.M.A. level. We have found levels of both increased above the upper limit of normal. The increase in V.M.A. tends to lag behind by about 24 hours. However, the incidence of arrhythmias has been so low in the 10 patients studied that no statement can be made regarding the relationship of catecholamine level and arrhythmias.

Our experience supports the opinion that patient care can be improved with the establishment of coronary care units in all acute hospitals. While the main benefit appears to lie in the management of patients with ' mild ' and ' severe ' myocardial infarction, some progress is being made in the management of cardiogenic shock.

REFERENCE

ROBINSON, J. S., SLOMAN, G. & McRAE, C. (1964). Continuous electrocardiographic monitoring in the early stages after acute myocardial infarction. *Med. J. Aust.* **1**, 427.

DISCUSSION

Dr Marquis (Edinburgh). Would you briefly define what you regard as heart failure requiring immediate treatment?

Dr Sloman. If a patient has crepitations at the lung bases which do not clear after two or three deep breaths and bouts of coughing, and if the patient hasn't a clear past history of chronic bronchitis, we give intravenous diuretics—frusemide 80 mg. In this respect we differ from a number of other units who favour the early use of digitalis, but right from the beginning in our hospital we have always treated heart failure initially with diuretics rather than digitalis.

Dr J. D. Matthews (Edinburgh). You mentioned that the average age of your patients admitted was 57. Do you think there should

12

be any selection of age for admission to your beds if you have a bed available? Has this entered into your calculations?

Dr Sloman. I get upset when a patient of 80 or 90 gets sent up to us, but I suppose if we are providing care for our population we should accept people who are sent up to us irrespective of age. From an economic point of view, probably we ought to have an upper age limit but this is a personal view and at the moment if we have a bed available and the person who is the admitting officer at that time cares to send us a patient, we have to take that patient.

PETER BENT BRIGHAM HOSPITAL, BOSTON

BERNARD LOWN

THE Coronary Care Unit of the Peter Bent Brigham Hospital was opened in February 1965. It has four beds with private rooms for each patient. The organisation and outlook of the Unit has been described previously (Lown *et al.*, 1967). All patients suspected of acute myocardial infarction arriving in the Emergency Ward or sent in by private physicians are admitted to Coronary Care. There are no restrictions as to age or sex.

Approximately 90 per cent. of patients with myocardial infarction exhibit rhythm disorders during the initial 72 hours after hospitalisation. The benefit from the Coronary Care Unit (CCU) resides primarily in early detection and control of these arrhythmias, thereby permitting the prevention of fatal derangements in the heart beat. Incidence of death from myocardial infarction declines sharply with the lapse of time from the onset of the coronary episode. These observations lead to the view that the CCU must serve as a diagnostic unit for the earliest detection of acute infarction. Of 546 admissions, 300 (54·9 per cent.) were proved to have sustained an acute myocardial infarction.

Diagnosis of myocardial infarction

In 300 patients admitted to the CCU with acute myocardial infarction, 186 (62 per cent.) showed classical changes (Table I); 26 per cent. developed depression in ST segment and/or symmetrical T-wave inversions which persisted for more than 24 hours and which were interpreted as subendocardial and intramural infarctions

13

respectively. Thus 88 per cent. of patients who are characterised
as having had infarction had electrocardiographic changes. The

Table I. *Distribution of electrocardiographic pattern of
myocardial infarction in 300 consecutive patients*

	No.	Per Cent.
Classical		
Anterior	78	26·0
Anterior-diaphragmatic	18	6·0
Diaphragmatic	50	16·7
Posterior-diaphragmatic	25	8·3
Posterior	7	2·3
High Lateral	8	2·7
ST-T Changes		
Intramural	50	16·7
Subendocardial	29	9·7
Fixed Changes	24	8·0
No Changes	11	3·7

electrocardiogram remained normal in 4 per cent. and in 8 per cent.
the stigmata of old infarction persisted unchanged. In these 12
per cent. of the patients, lacking electrocardiographic support,
a typical story and characteristic enzyme changes left little doubt
as to the diagnosis.

Clinical severity

Of the 300 patients studied, 193 were males with a mean age of 61;
107 were females with a mean age of 69. A history of coronary
artery disease was obtained from 68 per cent. of patients. Angina
pectoris had been present in 60 per cent. and previous myocardial
infarction in 39 per cent. Twenty-two per cent. had been treated
for chronic congestive failure. Left ventricular failure was diagnosed
in 63 per cent.

Diagnosis of arrhythmias

The frequent complications of acute myocardial infarction relate
to electrical instability of the heart, manifested by diverse arrhythmias, and to pump failure, manifested by either left ventricular
failure, shock or both. To date, the important contribution of the
CCU is the control of rhythm disorders. From the very opening
of our Unit in February of 1965, the philosophy has been that in
the control of minor rhythm disorders resided the possibility of
abolishing all major electrical catastrophes requiring cardiac
resuscitation. In order to implement this policy, a new classification

14

of arrhythmias in the patient with acute myocardial infarction is in order. The present classification of arrhythmias based on anatomical site of origin—namely atrial, junctional or ventricular—does not indicate the response which the CCU team should display when certain arrhythmias are detected, nor does it provide physiological insight as to their genesis. More appropriate is a physiological classification which relates the different arrhythmias to the under-lying clinical situation and thereby provides guide lines as to therapy. The disorders of the heart beat in the patient with acute myocardial infarction can be classified into three categories: those relating to electrical instability, to potential electrical instability, and those due to pump failure (Table II). The incidence of these disorders in 300 consecutive patients with acute myocardial infarction is shown in Table III.

Arrhythmias of electrical instability

Arrhythmias of electrical instability include ventricular ectopic beats and ventricular tachycardia. These disorders are treated with anti-arrhythmic drugs. Ventricular extrasystoles are the single most important rhythm abnormality in the coronary patient by virtue of frequency and possibility of precipitating ventricular fibrillation. We have introduced the use of lidocaine for the management of these arrhythmias. If treatment is prompt the prognosis is nearly the same as in the control population.

Arrhythmias of potential electrical instability

These arrhythmias have in common a slow ventricular rate. The most important abnormality in this category is sinus bradycardia, which was noted in 25 per cent. of 300 patients. The hazard from slow rates is the predisposition to ventricular ectopic mechanisms as well as a reduction in cardiac output and systemic pressure. If these disorders are treated by accelerating the rate either with atropine or isoproterenol and rarely by means of pacemakers, the prognosis is remarkably good. Bradycardia represents the lowest mortality of any group, with 4·4 per cent. dying during hospital stay. The reason probably is that a reflex from injured myocardium predisposes to bradycardia, which is overcome with larger infarction which compromises cardiac function.

Arrhythmias of pump failure

These arrhythmias generally develop in patients with left ventricular failure; digitalis drugs are presently employed in our Unit for initial therapy of any sustained arrhythmia in this group. It may

15

Table II. *Classification of arrhythmias in patients with acute myocardial infarction*

Arrhythmia Category	Specific Disorder	Prognosis	Treatment	Complications
Electrical Instability	Ventricular Extrasystoles Ventricular Tachycardia	Good	Anti-arrhythmic (lidocaine, procaine amide)	Ventricular Fibrillation
Potential Electrical Instability	Sinus Bradycardia Nodal Extrasystoles Nodal Rhythm Heart Block	Excellent*	Increase Rate (atropine, isoproterenol, pacemaker)	Asystole Ventricular Fibrillation
Pump Failure	Sinus Tachycardia Atrial Extrasystoles Atrial and Nodal Tachycardia Atrial Flutter Atrial Fibrillation	Poor	Digitalisation (ouabain, also quinidine, cardioversion)	Congestive Failure Hypotension Shock

* Except for patients with advanced degrees of heart block.

Table III. *Incidence of arrhythmias in 300 consecutive
patients with acute myocardial infarction*

Arrhythmia Category	No. of Patients		Per Cent.
1. *Electrical Instability*			
Ventricular Extrasystoles	240		80·0
Rate (2–10 per min.)		95	
Frequent		145	
Ventricular Tachycardia	83		27·6
2. *Potential Electrical Instability*			
Sinus Bradycardia	78		26·0
Transient		33	
Sustained		45	
Nodal Premature	49		16·3
Nodal Rhythm	14		4·7
Heart Block			
1°	32		10·7
2°	18		6·0
3°	21		7·0
3. *Pump Failure*			
Sinus Tachycardia	106		35·3
Atrial Extrasystoles (frequent) . . .	137		52·3
Atrial or Nodal Tachycardia . . .	34		11·3
Atrial Flutter	16		5·3
Atrial Fibrillation	39		13·0

be that increased left ventricular end-diastolic pressure with the
ensuing rise in left atrial pressure with accompanying stretch of the
atrial wall is the precipitating factor. No doubt in some the
occurrence of atrial flutter and atrial fibrillation may be due to
infarction of the atrium rather than heart failure. In the arrhythmias
of pump failure, in addition to digitalis the use of anti-arrhythmic
drugs is individualised with quinidine being used for prevention
of recurrence of atrial flutter and fibrillation. The mortality in
sinus tachycardia is 33·9 per cent. The occurrence of atrial flutter
and atrial fibrillation carries a similar bad prognosis.

Overall Results

Of the 300 patients admitted to the CCU, 53 died during the
course of their hospitalisation—a mortality of 17·7 per cent. Of

17

this number 39 patients died while in CCU during an average stay of six days. This constitutes 72 per cent. of the total deaths. Of the 39 patients who died while in CCU, 19 (49 per cent.) were admitted within less than six hours after the onset of pain, while in four this interval exceeded 24 hours. Only three of the deaths among the 300 patients were due to a primary electrical derangement, namely ventricular fibrillation. In these three patients severe congestive heart failure was present. Pump failure accounted for 32 of the deaths and miscellaneous mechanisms were responsible in the remaining four patients (Table IV).

Table IV. *Causes of death among 39 patients dying within CCU*

(300 Patients Studied)

		No.
1. Primary Electrical		
Heart Failure—Absent		0
Present		3
2. Pump Failure		
Shock and/or CHF		26
CPF*		6
3. Miscellaneous Mechanisms		4

* Complete Pump Failure

Thus the incidence of electrical failure causing death was 1 per cent. It is our view that even this figure is excessive and could have been reduced with more proper attention to details. The ability to control and prevent electrical derangements of heart rhythm is the great promise of the CCU, for it may teach us also how to deal with the larger problem of sudden death in the ambulatory coronary patient.

REFERENCE

LOWN, B., FAKHRO, A. M., HOOD, W. B., Jr. & THORN, G. W. (1967). The coronary care unit. New perspectives and directions. *J. Am. med. Ass.* **199,** 188.

DISCUSSION

Dr Meltzer. Did you say that 60 per cent. of the patients had congestive failure on admission or was that before discharge from hospital?

Dr Lown. No, 60 per cent. had failure while in the hospital.

Dr Oliver. I wonder if Dr Lown could enlarge a little on the complete pump failure group and perhaps tell us one or two details about the four who died of miscellaneous arrhythmias. With regard to complete pump failure, have you any reason to suspect that this is related to any drug regime?

Dr Lown. By complete pump failure we mean that there is a loss of blood pressure, the patient looks as if he is dying or dead but the electrocardiogram still shows an unchanged pattern for the first few seconds of this occurrence although thereafter and within a minute or so the electrocardiogram deteriorates and shows asystole. This we have observed in six patients; two of these patients had cardiac rupture. We examined whether the use of anti-arrhythmic drugs was implicated. In three of the patients they had not received any anti-arrhythmic drugs. One of the two patients who had cardiac rupture had received ouabain 30 minutes earlier, and this may have been a causal relationship. So we now think it is failure of pump action which in the first instance is the provocative event. The electrical activity is essentially normal and ultimately deteriorates because of no blood flow.

Your second question concerns the miscellaneous mechanisms. Two were patients who had complete heart block and were effectively paced. One had systemic lupus erythematosus and after seven days we withdrew the pacing catheter, because normal sinus rhythm had been established. The patient was febrile and critically ill and the private physician did not want to reinstitute any drastic measures; she redeveloped complete heart block and succumbed. The second patient had terminal renal failure and as the azotaemia got worse we found it more and more difficult to pace. This was carried out for two or three days and eventually even with the use of steroids and isoprenaline we were unable to pace. A third patient, a diabetic, in the miscellaneous category may have died from hypoglycaemia since a large amount of insulin was administered by mistake. I do not recollect the fourth.

Dr Sloman. I wonder if you could tell us any previous experience where you saw ventricular standstill, and into which category you would put it. Do you believe that there is any place for drug treatment in an attempt to prevent ventricular standstill?

Dr Lown. Ventricular standstill has not been a common mechanism. It is most unusual if the bradycardia is properly treated so we have not observed it. In the first 130 patients we had one patient who was approaching asystole, with a rate of 12, and then with 1·2 mg. of atropine the rate accelerated. Ventricular asystole is a common mechanism in the secondary pattern of electrical derangements of heart beat. In patients with profound

19

shock the majority of deaths are due to asystole. For asystole to be a primary mechanism seems most unusual. The major mechanism of arrhythmic death is ventricular fibrillation.

Dr Oliver. Could you tell us some figure, maybe a four-hour or six-hour figure, about numbers admitted. Obviously your low incidence of primary ventricular fibrillation may be directly dependent upon the delay in arrival of your patients. One would like to know a little about how many of these are occurring, for example, in the admission area or as they enter your unit. This will also relate to the speed of admission.

Dr Lown. Dr Oliver has been asking me this question for a year or so.

Dr Oliver. I hope you have prepared your answer.

Dr Lown. I have not! Firstly, I believe it is very difficult and I am impressed with the figures that I have given about arrival times in relation to onset of symptoms. Primarily one depends on history, and history is frequently extremely vague. One makes an assessment on other ancilliary factors. If you look at the patient what is of interest is the following. About 50 per cent. of our patients are not diagnosed as having acute myocardial infarction—this would reflect on their coming early because this is an extremely low figure; there is a 90 per cent. incidence of arrhythmias; and also the incidence of ventricular tachycardia, which is certainly a very early arrhythmia, is 28 per cent. In studying creatine phosphokinase we find that 80 per cent. of the patients have a normal level at the time of arrival, and then it subsequently rises. Without assessment of the history it would seem to us that the arrival is early but it could not be considered very early in a big city or in any big metropolitan community with traffic and endless other problems. I would say probably that our figures simulate those which Dr Sloman presented.

Dr Nixon. I would like to ask Dr Lown if in the group of patients he regards as having pump failure, he distinguishes in any way between parts of the pump, such as atrial failure or whether it is regarded as the whole pump?

Dr Lown. In the first 100 patients, all of whom had central venous catheters, right ventricular failure was rare in patients who had the first episode of acute myocardial infarction without cardiomegaly, and without preceding overt coronary artery disease. It is our view, then, that this is probably left ventricular failure from which atrial failure may very well drive. It may well be that some of these arrhythmias of pump failure are due to atrial infarction in which case the extent of the infarct would be large and they would form the same category prognostically.

Dr Killip. Dr Lown, did you have autopsies on all six patients who had so-called primary pump failure? We certainly have seen this syndrome also but I believe with only one exception, when autopsies have been done, all of the patients have had ruptured ventricles.

Dr Lown. We had autopsies in four of the six. Two had ruptures and two did not.

ROYAL POSTGRADUATE MEDICAL SCHOOL, HAMMERSMITH, LONDON

JOHN SHILLINGFORD

SOME six or seven years ago we became increasingly concerned at the high death rate following myocardial infarction. We were concerned not only at the mortality itself but by our lack of knowledge of the circulatory and other changes taking place during the acute phase, and which often lead to the death of the patient. In order to increase our knowledge and attempt to reduce the appalling mortality we decided to make a detailed study of the haemodynamic and other changes taking place in such patients. Little work had previously been done in this direction as it had been considered that the patients had been too ill to move to a laboratory for haemodynamic studies. Moreover, at that time the cause of death was not always clear, but we thought that it might be classified for practical purposes under the following headings: (1) a disturbance of rhythm; (2) cardiac weakness and failure; (3) peripheral vasodilatation and hypotension; (4) biochemical changes; (5) embolism; (6) respiratory disturbances from secondary effects in the lungs; (7) the misuse of drugs. I want to say that our emphasis was on intensive research as well as exploring the possibility of the value of continuous supervision of the patient. For this reason in our unit we have only cared for one patient at a time to enable us to study the haemodynamic and other changes, in depth. The patients are unselected and only those with a frank infarct are admitted to the unit. One hundred and sixty patients have so far been studied with an overall mortality of 19 per cent. In view of the specialised nature of the unit, further breakdown is probably of little value and I will describe briefly the research carried out during this period.

21

We have, and are studying (1) the natural history of the cardiac output and blood pressure changes during the acute phase following a myocardial infarction; (2) the incidence of arrhythmias and their effect on the circulation; (3) the haemodynamic effects of morphia, oxygen and pressor agents; (4) studies on the vasovagal syndrome and its management; (5) the pulmonary arterial pressure and its relation to pulmonary oedema and left ventricular failure; (6) changes in respiratory function; (7) changes in renal function; (8) studies on aneurysm formation in the ventricle; (9) the value of the right atrial electrode in assisting in the interpretation of the difficult arrhythmias; (10) the haemodynamic effects of lignocaine; (11) the effects of posture; (12) catecholamine excretion and its relation to cardiac failure.

A side-ward attached to the main male medical ward has been set aside entirely as a care and study room for patients with acute myocardial infarction. The recording apparatus installed includes a multi-channel direct-writing recorder with two pressure, two electrocardiographic, one phonocardiographic and one respiration channel. The outputs are recorded on a direct writer and displayed on a four-channel oscilloscope. A dye dilution curve recorder is used for measuring the cardiac output. Electrical signals from this ward may be transmitted via a cable and stored on eight-channel magnetic tape recorder in a nearby laboratory. This instrument has five D.C. channels, two A.C. channels, and one channel for speech, and will run continuously for 24 hours.

The following observations are made: the clinical state, electrocardiogram, arterial pressure, venous pressure, cardiac output, phonocardiography, cardiac pulsations, serum electrolytes and serum enzymes, blood gases, catecholamines.

In the near future we expect to extend our facilities by building a new three-bed ward for intensive care and research.

DISCUSSION

Dr Sloman. May I ask Professor Shillingford if he has any idea of the mortality of acute myocardial infarction in patients in general wards in his hospital? He quoted the mortality in his unit as 19 per cent.

Professor Shillingford. Yes, it's the same in nearly all hospitals, approximately 30 per cent. But, I suspect it is probably improving with the introduction of anti-arrhythmic therapy and also increasing knowledge of how to handle these complications.

Dr Marquis. With this experience of catheterisation in myocardial infarction, have you evidence of any particular risk such as the onset of arrhythmias following introduction of the catheter?

Professor Shillingford. With the insertion of the catheter into the right atrium as far as I know there has been no problem at all. With insertion further into the pulmonary artery, as one goes through the right ventricle, extrasystoles are sometimes produced. We have had no instance of a serious arrhythmia. These catheters are all PE 50's or 60's of very fine soft tubing which are floated through on the stream. It is not as though one is using a hard catheter. However, like all these manoeuvres, I think they must be in expert hands especially on the arterial side, and one must use a certain amount of circumspection.

NEW YORK HOSPITAL-CORNELL MEDICAL CENTER, NEW YORK

Thomas Killip

There are many parallels between my presentation and that of Dr Sloman. Our approach to the analysis of data is rather similar, although we do differ on some details.

In any evaluation of the results of coronary care there are at least five factors which should be considered when weighing the data from one unit in contrast to that of another (Table I).

Table I. *Factors influencing mortality in acute myocardial infarction*

1. Criteria for diagnosis.
2. Interval from onset to admission.
3. Selective or random admission.
4. Competence of nurses.
5. Aggressive management.

Each of the factors listed above may have a bearing on clinical results, yet it is disappointing how few reports available to date provide sufficient information to enable the disinterested observer to evaluate the report. As yet in this conference no one has mentioned their criteria utilised for diagnosis of myocardial infarction. If obscure complaints and minor electrocardiographic changes are diagnosed as myocardial infarction, mortality may be low. On the other hand if only patients with transmural infarction are treated, mortality will be high. It is now abundantly clear that the

23

interval from onset of illness to admission is critical in evaluating mortality.

The incidence of primary ventricular fibrillation is highest in the first few hours after infarction. The longer the delay in admission to hospital the fewer survivors.

The criteria which we utilise for diagnosis of acute myocardial infarction at the New York Hospital-Cornell Medical Center are as follows:

(a) *Transmural myocardial infarction.* Pain, Q-waves, changing electrocardiogram, characteristic enzyme pattern abnormality in blood.

(b) *Myocardial infarction (not transmural).* Pain, ST-T abnormalities on the electrocardiogram which progress towards normal, confirmed by a characteristic blood enzyme pattern abnormality.

(c) *Possible infarction.* Pain which appears to be of cardiac ischaemic origin, abnormal electrocardiogram with ST segment and T-wave changes, which may not fluctuate on repeated tracings, and a non-specific blood enzyme pattern abnormality.

(d) *No myocardial infarction.* No objective evidence on electrocardiogram or blood enzyme analysis of cardiac abnormality.

When the data from three years' operations of our coronary care unit are analysed according to the diagnostic criteria listed above, we find the following distribution of diagnoses: 62 per cent. of patients had definite myocardial infarction, 15 per cent. had possible myocardial infarction, 23 per cent. did not have myocardial infarction although they were admitted to the unit on the basis of the initial impression of an experienced physician that they might be having acute infarction. Of this last group, approximately one-third had angina, one-third had primary arrhythmia, and one-third had a wide variety of other diagnoses.

The 70 patients with possible infarction had a mortality of 3 per cent. Only two of these patients died, and both died several weeks after transfer to regular care. This observation has important implications. If a patient is admitted to a coronary care unit with ischaemic cardiac pain, and if the pain subsides in the first 24 hours after admission, and if the tentative diagnosis of acute myocardial infarction cannot be confirmed by objective tests including serial electrocardiograms and blood enzyme assay, the patient has an excellent immediate prognosis and may be transferred to regular care for further evaluation without significant hazard. Perhaps some of these patients have the impending coronary syndrome, perhaps some have prolonged angina, and perhaps some have had microscopic losses of functioning myocardium. When the group

24

is taken as a whole, however, it has different clinical characteristics, different prognosis, and therefore may be managed differently from those patients with established infarction.

It is reasonable to postulate that the functional severity of the infarction influences both morbidity and prognosis. The patient is therefore classified into one of four groups:

1. *No heart failure*—no signs of pulmonary or venous congestion.

2. *Moderate heart failure*—râles at lung bases, development or intensification of a gallop, tachypnoea or dyspnoea, or signs of right heart failure including venous and hepatic distension.

3. *Severe heart failure*—pulmonary oedema diagnosed by standard clinical signs.

4. *Shock*—systolic pressure less than 90 mm.Hg and evidence of peripheral constriction including cold extremities, diaphoresis, peripheral cyanosis, mental confusion, decreased urine output.

The incidence of arrhythmia varies with the functional severity ranging from 83 per cent. in patients without failure to 100 per cent. in patients with cardiogenic shock. The distribution of patients admitted to the coronary care unit according to their functional severity is as follows: no heart failure, 30 per cent.; moderate heart failure, 42 per cent.; severe heart failure, 11 per cent.; cardiogenic shock, 17 per cent. Thus, approximately one-third of our patients comprise the highest risk group, those with pulmonary oedema or shock.

It is now known that the incidence of arrhythmias is much higher than had been recognised in the premonitoring era. Some arrhythmias are trivial but others are life-threatening, the recognition of which should impel an immediate therapeutic decision.

The life-threatening arrhythmias include:

1. Sinus bradycardia or sinus arrest with or without escape rhythm.

2. Second or third degree atrioventricular block.

3. Frequent ventricular premature complexes or ventricular tachycardia.

4. Ventricular fibrillation.

5. Ventricular asystole.

The incidence of life-threatening arrhythmias (Table II) can be related to the functional severity of the infarction.

The incidence of sinus arrest or sinus bradycardia was similar whether or not shock was present. However, heart block was three times more common in the presence of shock. Ventricular arrhythmias were slightly more common in the presence of shock. Most striking, however, is the effect of shock on the incidence of ventricular asystole. Asystole is uncommon in the absence of shock, occurring in only 2 per cent. of instances. In the presence of shock, however, 30 per cent. of the patients developed ventricular asystole.

Table II. *Incidence of life-threatening arrhythmia*

LTA	Shock absent per cent.	Shock present per cent.
Sinus arrest, bradycardia . . .	8	11
A-V block, 2nd or 3rd degree . . .	11	30
VPCs, ventric. tachycardia . . .	29	36
Ventric. fibrillation	2	9
Ventric. asystole	2	30

The different varieties of supraventricular dysrhythmias appeared to be equally common whether or not shock was present. We agree with Dr Lown that most of these arrhythmias are self-limited and heroic measures of treatment are generally not indicated, except in the rare instance when the sudden onset of a supraventricular tachycardia is associated with cardiovascular collapse or cardiac arrest.

Table III. *Incidence of bradyarrhythmia*

	No shock (per cent.)	Shock (per cent.)
Bradyarrhythmia-total	26	81
Sinus arrest, bradycardia . . .	13	17
A-V block, 2nd degree	7	4
A-V block, 3rd degree	5	60
{ Nodal, ventric. escape	73*	50*
{ Ventric. asystole	27*	50*

* Per cent. of those with 3rd degree A-V block.

As shown in Table III, slow ventricular rates are much more common in patients with cardiogenic shock than in those who do not develop shock. The difference is largely due to the high risk that patients in shock have of developing complete heart block. Of interest also is the fact that half of the patients who developed complete heart block as a complication of cardiogenic shock failed to have adequate escape of lower pacemakers and thus had cardiac arrest due to ventricular asystole with onset of block. In contrast, ventricular asystole occurred in only approximately one-quarter of the patients who developed complete heart block in the absence of shock.

We believe that the high incidence of bradycardia and ventricular asystole in patients with cardiogenic shock supports the view that it is reasonable to insert a pacemaker electrode on a standby, prophylactic basis because of the high risk of subsequent serious dysrhythmia.

Coronary care units are designed to improve mortality from myocardial infarction. Yet when we analysed the results of treatment of the first 100 patients with definite myocardial infarction who were admitted consecutively to the coronary care unit, and compared these data with that from 100 patients admitted consecutively to regular care facilities during the same period of time, we were disappointed. Mortality on regular care was 29 per cent. Mortality in the coronary care unit was 32 per cent. These figures refer to mortality during the total period of hospitalisation, and not just during their sojourn in the coronary care unit.

During our initial experience in the coronary care unit we did not have strong central control of treatment, and considerable authority was delegated to the house officers. Experience and interest varied among the junior staff and we found that a variety of treatment programmes had been utilised for entirely similar conditions with disparate results. Close analysis of the data suggested that perhaps the mortality could have been reduced by one-third if each patient had been treated with maximum efficiency. We subsequently instituted a programme of strong central control by the senior cardiac staff, set down a series of guidelines for treatment of cardiac conditions and undertook a rather intensive educational programme with each new house staff member who came into the unit.

Following these changes in the management of the coronary care unit, there has been sustained improvement in our clinical performance. Analysis of our results since the changes reveals the following mortality rates: no heart failure, 0 per cent.; moderate heart failure, 4 per cent. (ventricular rupture); severe heart failure, 13 per cent.; cardiogenic shock, 82 per cent. Overall mortality in the coronary care unit is now 21 per cent. whereas the mortality on regular care continues to be approximately 30 per cent.

It is of course difficult to evaluate the influence of change in therapeutic programmes, the growth of clinical experience, and the

27

change in the administrative orientation of our coronary care unit with regard to the steady improvement in the clinical record. It would appear that most coronary care unit teams go through a period of progressive improvement in clinical care. My associate, Dr John T. Kimball, Jr., and I are convinced that the major change responsible for the improvement in medical care in our unit was the development of a strong management policy for the coronary care unit itself. In our institution with a tradition of private practice and delegation of large responsibilities to the house staff in training, we were able to improve the care of the patient with myocardial infarction when the prerogatives of the attending and house staff physicians were deliberately proscribed by a senior cardiology staff. We believe that these observations have important implications for the delivery of coronary care in hospitals throughout the world. As important as the management of the patient is the management of the coronary care unit.

DISCUSSION

Dr Lown. In changing responsibility, did you initiate any new therapeutic manoeuvres such as anti-arrhythmic drugs?

Dr Killip. No I do not think that we did. We have had a choice of therapeutic manoeuvres from the start in the coronary care unit. We have been using lidocaine, for example, for almost four years. What we did was to take away the choice and this is a point of philosophy in medical care about which we feel rather strongly. As you know, in the States, many of our teaching hospitals give a great deal of responsibility and authority to junior House Officers and all of us went through this stage of being the primary physician and making all the decisions. My own view is that, at least in the field of cardiology and, I suspect, in a number of other medical fields also the clinical judgment and the choice of therapeutic interventions is so demanding of experience that this policy of delegating a great deal of responsibility to junior House Physicians can no longer be defended in a teaching hospital such as ours. It is easy to say that, but hard to change. The only place where we have changed this attitude is in the Coronary Care Unit where the policy for care is essentially that prescribed by the senior cardiologist there.

THE LONDON HOSPITAL

LAWSON MCDONALD

THE Coronary Unit at The London Hospital, and the findings on the first 150 patients with cardiac infarction, who were treated in it have been described by Restieaux *et al.* (1967), with details of age, sex, and type of infarction. The Unit consists of five beds. The London Hospital is a large undergraduate university hospital which acts partly as a community hospital.

Between November 1965 and December 1966 150 patients with recent cardiac infarction were admitted to the Unit. Current policy may be viewed in the light of experience with these patients; it remains similar except for minor modifications which are made for specific research programmes.

The criteria for diagnosis of cardiac infarction were those of Wood (1961). All except 22 patients were admitted to hospital within 24 hours of the onset of severe pain; the times of their admission are shown in Table I.

Table I. *Times of admission after the onset of pain*

Hours	No.
0–4	24
5–6	19
7–12	52
13–24	33
25–48	10
> 48	12
Total	150

Management

The patients were unselected and were admitted to the Unit for at least 48 hours; they remained longer if complications developed. Subsequently they were transferred to a general medical ward. Whilst in the Unit heart rate and heart rhythm were monitored continuously by equipment which consisted of a rate-meter, an oscilloscope, an audible alarm system, an electrocardiogram (ECG) sampling device, and a memory tape loop.

Treatment of patients while in the unit was uniform. Humidified nasal oxygen was given for 48 hours at a flow-rate of 4 litres per minute. Pain was relieved by morphine or diamorphine (heroin).

29

An intramuscular injection of 15 mg. morphine sulphate B.P. and 25 mg. promethazine hydrochloride B.P. was used, but if pain was very severe a small dose of intravenous morphine sulphate was used.

Patients were treated with anticoagulants unless there were contraindications, such as a history of active peptic ulcer or the presence of a pericardial friction rub; 88 per cent. of the patients received anticoagulant therapy. An initial intravenous dose of 10,000 units of heparin was followed by an intravenous heparin infusion for 48 hours. This contained 40,000 units of heparin in 1 litre of 5 per cent. dextrose per 24 hours, a concentration which kept the whole-blood-clotting time at approximately twice normal. Oral phenindione tablets B.P. were given on admission and the dose was adjusted to give a prothrombin ratio of 2–2·3: 1 (patient: control).

Left ventricular failure, as indicated by dyspnoea, gallop rhythm and pulmonary venous congestion, was treated with digitalis and diuretic therapy. The development of complete heart block was treated by the immediate insertion into the right ventricle of a bipolar endocardial pacemaker catheter via an antecubital vein (Portal et al., 1962; Samet et al., 1963; Paulk & Hurst, 1966). Pacing was continued until sinus rhythm returned and the catheter was left in position for a further five days. Ventricular fibrillation was treated by immediate external cardiac massage and positive pressure ventilation followed by direct current shock (Lown et al., 1962).

The Unit was staffed day and night by a cardiac registrar who was immediately available. All cardiac arrests were treated by the emergency resuscitation team for the hospital.

Mortality

The mortality-rate for the period of admission to hospital was 14 per cent. and the mortality-rate for the first 48 hours in the Unit was 4·7 per cent. Patients remained in the Unit for from 48 hours to three weeks with an average stay of 72 hours. Five patients were readmitted to the Unit from the medical wards on one or more occasions.

The time of death and the terminal dysrhythmias were recorded in the 21 patients who died (Fig. 1). In the first 48 hours seven patients in pulmonary oedema died from asystole. Necropsy showed extensive cardiac infarction. Death from ventricular fibrillation was recorded in eight patients and was sudden and without any preceding clinical deterioration in five. It was particularly common from the fourth to the fifteenth day.

Dysrhythmias

Serious dysrhythmias were recorded in 28 of the 150 patients (19 per cent.), all of whom had transmural cardiac infarction (Fig. 2). One or more episodes of ventricular fibrillation were

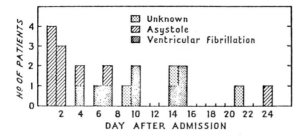

FIG. 1. Mortality and the terminal dysrhythmias after cardiac infarction.

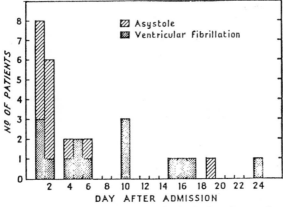

FIG. 2. The incidence of serious dysrhythmias after cardiac infarction.

recorded in 15 patients (10 per cent.) and this dysrhythmia occurred throughout the first four weeks. The incidence of ventricular fibrillation has fallen with the prophylactic use of lignocaine and procaine amide. Asystole developed in 13 patients (9 per cent.) and was more common in the first 48 hours. This was due to the number of patients in pulmonary oedema and cardiogenic ' shock ' who developed asystole as the terminal dysrhythmia. A high percentage of the patients with dysrhythmias had other serious

31

complications after their infarction, and a number had conditions such as diabetes mellitus or hypertension which are known to affect mortality adversely.

Resuscitation

Resuscitation was attempted in 25 patients and was initially successful in 14. However, four subsequently died in hospital from severe heart failure. Ten patients left hospital and were alive one to twelve months later, giving a success-rate of 40 per cent. Of these 10 patients, six had had ventricular fibrillation and four had had ventricular asystole.

Comment

The possible need for readmission to the Coronary Unit for at least three weeks after infarction is apparent from these results, and therefore the desirability for patients to be nursed in wards adjacent to the Unit, after their discharge from it. The medical staffing of coronary units, even in a university hospital, presents considerable demands on medical manpower. Both these aspects of coronary care merit discussion, as does the management of patients from the onset of cardiac infarction to the time of their admission to a coronary unit (Pantridge & Geddes, 1966).

REFERENCES

Lown, B., Amarasingham, R. & Neuman, J. (1962). New methods for terminating cardiac arrhythmias. *J. Am. med. Ass.* **182**, 548.

Pantridge, J. F. & Geddes, J. S. (1966). Cardiac arrest after myocardial infarction. *Lancet*, **1**, 807.

Paulk, E. A. & Hurst, J. W. (1966). Complete heart block in acute myocardial infarction. *Am. J. Cardiol.* **17**, 695.

Portal, R. W., Davies, J. G., Leatham, A. & Siddons, A. H. M. (1962). Artificial pacing for heart block. *Lancet*, **2**, 1369.

Restieaux, N., Bray, C., Bullard, H., Murray, M., Robinson, J., Brigden, W. & McDonald, L. (1967). 150 patients with cardiac infarction treated in a Coronary Unit. *Lancet*, **1**, 1285.

Samet, P., Jacobs, W. & Bernstein, W. H. (1963). Electrode catheter pacemaker in the treatment of complete heart block in the presence of acute myocardial infarction. *Am. J. Cardiol.* **11**, 379.

Wood, P. (1961). *Diseases of the Heart and Circulation.* London: Eyre & Spottiswoode.

Discussion

Professor Shillingford. Your incidence of ventricular fibrillation is perhaps the same as found in a number of centres before the more rigorous use of anti-arrhythmic drugs. Have you been treating the development of extrasystoles as put forward by Dr Lown and others?

If you are able to control them by lignocaine and other drugs, the incidence should be somewhat smaller.

Dr McDonald. During the particular period of the analysis, this approach was being developed. We are now adopting it, and I think it is going to result in a falling incidence of ventricular fibrillation. We have not suppressed all dysrhythmias, however, even with adequate doses of lignocaine.

Dr Killip. The group of patients that you mentioned with late complications after transfer is very important. In our initial experience, something like 30 per cent. of our deaths occurred after transfer from the coronary care unit, and when we looked at these more closely we found that every single one of these patients had had one of these dysrhythmias before. With this in mind we became a lot more conservative and, although our initial plan was to keep the patient in the coronary care unit from three to five days, we now keep them in 48 hours after all evidence of complications, particularly a ventricular arrhythmia has been handled. Now the average stay in the coronary care unit is seven days and the late death problem has dropped dramatically and represents 10 per cent. or less of our total death rate. I don't know whether this is the right answer or not, but I would be interested in whether you were able to pick up in retrospect any clues about these deaths.

Dr McDonald. If you are going to pick out these dysrhythmias you have either got to have a monitor which is very sophisticated, or else you have got to have somebody looking at a film strip 24 hours a day. Even then you may miss them, I think myself the kind of patient who is going to die may be picked up in the first 24–48 hours by high enzyme levels. In other words, it seems to me the higher the enzymes the bigger the infarct and the worse the outlook.

Dr Lown. I would like to make a comment as regards the question of late deaths. Of the deaths we had a third were late, and initially some of them were sudden but if one carries on and maintains the therapeutic programme in the very patients that Dr Killip mentioned—those that had serious life-threatening dysrhythmias— there is a significant reduction of these, so that in the last year we had few late sudden deaths. We maintain therapy now in these patients for three months beyond the hospital stay.

Dr McDonald. Not with lignocaine?

Dr Lown. No, it was impossible to do so with lignocaine. We give them procaine amide and make sure that they do not have arrhythmias at discharge. We maintain them on 2 or 3 g. of procaine amide daily.

Dr McDonald. We are very attracted to this currently as being even preferable to lignocaine because I think when you transfer these patients to the general ward it is very often difficult to get the physician to keep up intravenous therapy.

Dr Lown. While they are receiving lignocaine they remain in the unit, but in those who continue to show a dangerous arrhythmia when lignocaine has been discontinued, procaine amide is instituted and procaine amide given orally is less likely to be hypotensive. Without wishing to put this point too strongly, three of these late serious dysrhythmias had no warning though they have been very carefully watched.

ROYAL INFIRMARY, EDINBURGH

Desmond Julian

The Royal Infirmary is the major community hospital of this City, as well as its principal teaching hospital. Its Coronary Care Unit has, therefore, had the dual purpose of making the maximum impact upon the mortality of acute myocardial infarction in the area, and of conducting research.

The Unit has had the active support of all the physicians of the hospital, who set up an Executive Committee of three to administer it. Seven physicians in rotation take clinical charge of the Unit for periods of one week at a time. There are three junior medical staff specifically attached to the Unit, and there is a rota of 30 members of the junior medical staff to undertake night duties. There is at all times a doctor in the Unit, together with a minimum of two nurses, one of whom is fully trained.

The Unit has six beds provided with Sanborn monitors, a central monitoring station, battery-powered standby pacemakers, two defibrillators and a portable image intensifier. The therapeutic policy in recent months has largely followed that of Lown *et al.* (1967) except that endocardial pacing electrodes have been inserted in all patients with greater than 1st degree heart block and recently, in all patients with bundle branch block.

We have attempted to accommodate as many patients as possible who would be likely to benefit from the facilities of a Coronary Care Unit, and our admission policy for patients with acute myocardial infarction has therefore been as follows:

1. Patients under 70 years of age suspected of having sustained a myocardial infarction within the preceding 48 hours ('routine' admission).

34

2. Patients of any age with serious arrhythmias developing either elsewhere in the hospital or outside the hospital, irrespective of age of infarct (' transfer ' admission).

During the 16-month period from the opening of the Unit in April 1966 to mid-August 1967, 800 patients were admitted. The final diagnosis in the 800 patients is as shown in Table I.

Table I. *Royal Infirmary, Edinburgh, Coronary Care Unit*

Admissions April 1966–August 1967

Definite Myocardial Infarction . . . . . $\begin{cases} \text{Routine 500} \\ \text{Transfer } 52 \end{cases}$	552
Possible Myocardial Infarction	144
Arrhythmias not due to Infarction	63
Non-cardiac conditions	41
Total admissions	800

In patients with myocardial infarction, the principles determining transfer to the general medical wards are as follows:

1. Uncomplicated cases are transferred either at 9 a.m. or 6 p.m. after a minimum period of 48 hours in the Unit.

2. Those who have experienced serious arrhythmias are not discharged until a complication-free period of at least 24 hours has elapsed. If they have experienced ventricular tachycardia, ventricular fibrillation or advanced heart block, a period of at least three days free from arrhythmia is demanded before transfer.

Approximately 75 per cent. of patients were discharged in under 72 hours, and the average length of stay in the Unit was just over three days.

The overall hospital mortality in 552 patients with acute myocardial infarction was 19.2 per cent. That in the ' transfer group ' was very high at 46 per cent., as would be expected in a group in whom there had been many cases of cardiac arrest before admission.

The 500 routinely admitted patients are of some interest as they may be regarded as reasonably representative of patients under 70, seen soon after the onset of acute myocardial infarction. The average age was 58 years.

Fifty-five per cent. of these patients were admitted within four hours of the onset of their symptoms, 72 per cent. within six hours and 87 per cent. within 12 hours.

Of the 500 'routine' admissions 39 developed ventricular fibrillation, if we exclude those in whom this arrhythmia was precipitated by pacing or drugs, or was agonal. Fifteen of these patients were free of shock or failure at the time of their ventricular fibrillation and 14 of these survived to leave hospital. In 24 patients, shock or failure preceded the onset of ventricular fibrillation, and of these six survived.

Of the 500 routinely admitted patients 66 died in the Coronary Care Unit, and 16 more after transfer to medical wards, making a total mortality in the 'routine' admissions of 16.4 per cent.

Further details of the Unit have already been published (Lawrie *et al.*, 1967).

REFERENCES

Lawrie, D. M., Greenwood, T. W., Goddard, M., Harvey, A. C., Donald, K. W., Julian, D. G. & Oliver, M. F. (1967). A coronary care unit in the routine management of acute myocardial infarcation. *Lancet*, **2**, 109.
Lown, B., Fakhro, A. M., Hood, W. B. & Thorn, G. W. (1967). The coronary care unit, new perspectives and directions. *J. Am. med. Ass.* **199**, 188.

Discussion

Professor Shillingford. The incidence of ventricular fibrillation is approximately 2 per cent. Where is the other improvement of mortality coming from?

Dr Julian. I think it is quite possible that we are in fact preventing cases of ventricular fibrillation. We are treating patients with heart block who would otherwise die, and the management of arrhythmias complicating failure and shock is a factor of importance. I believe most of the effect is in treating arrhythmias, but I don't think at this time we can say, in fact, what effect we have had on mortality.

CORONARY HEART DISEASES SECTION, U.S. PUBLIC HEALTH SERVICES, WASHINGTON
A CO-OPERATIVE STUDY

EDWARD B. CROSS

EARLY in the history of the Coronary Care Units, the Heart Disease Control Program, U.S. Public Health Service, accepted the responsibility for evaluating this new concept. The primary objective of such an evaluation was the determination of the effectiveness of Coronary Care Units in reducing morbidity and mortality in hospitalised acute myocardial infarction patients. Secondary objectives were concerned with determining factors or problems which would adversely affect the successful establishment and operation of such Units. In essence, the Coronary Care Unit concept logically appeared as an ideal way to care for acute myocardial infarction patients. Our concern was to find ways of making such Units more effective.

The design of the evaluation study not only consisted of a retrospective and a prospective aspect, but also involved two basically different types of institutional set-ups. Several more or less standardised demonstration study Coronary Care Units were established and operated with significant financial support from the Heart Disease Control Program. The staffing, physical design, equipment, length of stay in the Unit and laboratory studies were standardised in these study Units. On the other hand, in an attempt to accumulate rapidly a signficant number of cases in a relatively short time, a number of existing Units were selected for data collection only. The later type of Units were rather heterogeneous in most respects and data on both Coronary Care Units and regular care patients were mostly of a retrospective nature. On the Coronary Care Unit patients in the demonstration study units, the data collected was of a prospective type and rather detailed.

In measuring the overall effectiveness of the Unit in reducing morbidity and mortality, data were collected on three groups of patients; namely acute myocardial infarction patients treated in the hospital prior to the opening of the Unit, concurrently treated regular care patients and Coronary Care Unit patients. We also collected data on patients admitted to the hospital for one to two years immediately prior to opening the Coronary Care Unit. By such a plan we could compare the Coronary Care Unit with both the prior and concurrent regular care experience in treating acute M.I. patients. Further, one could also compare the overall hospital experience before and following establishment of the Unit.

Age and severity considerations
In a first attempt to correct for bias due to patient selection for admission to the Unit, we utilised a modification of the severity index of Freis, and more recently used by Dr Sloman in Australia as follows:

Class I . . No hypotension or congestive failure
Class II . . Hypotension and/or congestive failure
Class III . . Cardiogenic shock
(Cardiac arrest cases on admission were added to Class III.)

It must be apparent to all that there are inherent defects in such a severity classification system, particularly in the Class II category. In this group there is found the full range of congestive failure, i.e., from basilar râles to the frank acute pulmonary oedema syndrome. In addition, in this category hypotension may exist alone or in combination with various degrees of congestive failure. Such a classification system does not take into account some of the commonly accepted bad prognostic signs such as major arrhythmias, conduction defects and previous history of myocardial infarction. Similarly the patient's classification may be affected by the time preceding the examination or the effects of any earlier treatment.

In an additional attempt to overcome patient selection bias, age comparisons of patients were also made.

Coronary care unit results
1. *Hospital Fatality Experience (Crude Age and Severity Rates).* In examining fatality experience data of this type, it is quite important not only to look at crude rates but to examine specific severity and specific age rates. This, in essence, is an attempt to compare results on more homogeneous or similar patients, thereby reducing the effect of patient selection in the study. In looking at the crude mortality rate in a series of 2,617 Coronary Care Unit treated patients, representing 11 heterogenous hospitals, i.e., university affiliated hospitals, and community hospitals with and without full time house-staff, the following individual results were noted.

Fatality rates for the individual hospitals ranged from a low 20·9 per cent. to a high of 32·8 per cent. (Table I).

Table I. *M.I. fatality rates 2,617 CCU treated patients in participating hospitals*

Hospital	Number of Patients Treated	Fatality Rates (per cent.)
A	425	20·9
B	153	23·5
C	250	24·8
D	367	25·3
E	115	26·1
F	203	26·6
G	321	26·8
H	302	26·8
I	163	27·6
J	196	28·1
K	122	32·8

When one reviewed the specific severity rates according to the previously described severity index for the 2,617 CCU treated patients in these same hospitals, the following ranges in each of the three severity classes were noted:

Class	Range	Median (per cent.)
I.	9·9–22·8	(15·3)
II	24·7–55·6	(38·6)
III	50·0–84·6	(72·5)

(*See* Table II)

Table II. *M.I. fatality rates 2,617 CCU treated patients in participating hospitals. Severity Groups*

Array of Rates	ADMISSION SEVERITY I	II	III
	(per cent.)		
	9·8	24·7	50·0
	10·6	25·9	60·0
	11·5	26·9	63·3
	14·1	33·3	65·0
Lowest	15·1	33·9	70·0
to	15·3*	38·6*	72·5*
Highest	17·4	38·9	76·3
	18·2	40·9	80·0
	18·6	41·9	81·3
	18·6	50·0	81·8
	22·8	55·6	84·6

* Median

Reviewing age specific fatality rates on these same patients, the following results were noted:

39

Age	Range (per cent.)	Median (per cent.)
Under 55 years	6·5–25·0	(14·7)
55–64 years .	17·2–31·0	(22·8)
65 and over .	29·5–46·9	(27·3)

From this type of approach one can see readily that although the severity index used is somewhat crude, severity classification on hospital admission is a very important prognostic sign in regard to mortality rates. Age is also noted to be a prognostic indicator, but not as significant as that of congestive failure or shock on admission.

2. *Previous history of coronary heart disease and myocardial infarction.* In a series of 2,647 hospitalised patients (Unit and Non-Unit), without and with a past history of coronary heart disease (angina pectoris only or myocardial infarction), the following fatality rates were noted in the three categories:

History	Rate (per cent.)
Negative history for CHD .	21·8
Angina pectoris only . .	26·9
Previous M.I.. . . .	37·3

(*See* Table III)

Table III. *M.I. fatality rates with and without prior CHD 2,647 patients*

Age Groups

History	All Ages (per cent.)	Fatality Rates Under 55 (per cent.)	55–64 (per cent.)	65 and over (per cent.)
No CHD	21·8	8·8	19·8	37·4
A.P. only	26·9	19·2	22·2	35·2
Prior M.I.	37·3	27·7	31·3	47·7

Age specific rates on this same group of patients show the following:

History	AGE 55 and Under (per cent.)	55–65 (per cent.)	65 and Over (per cent.)
No CHD . . .	8·8	19·8	37·4
Angina pectoris . .	19·2	22·2	35·2
Prior M.I.. . .	27·7	31·3	47·7

It is noted, for all ages, the patients with a history of angina pectoris have a slightly greater risk of death in hospital over the non-CHD patient; however, the history of a previous M.I. carries a much greater risk, i.e., almost a two-fold risk over the patient without a history of CHD. When one examines the effects within age groups, it is noted that the patients under 55 had a two-fold risk with a history of angina pectoris only and a three-fold risk in the presence of a history of prior M.I. For the two older age groups the differences were in the same direction, however not as striking.
3. *Cardiac arrest.* A review of the records of 2,174 CCU treated patients revealed the following:

Arrhythmia	Incidence (*per cent.*)	Fatality (*per cent.*)	Survival (*per cent.*)
Ventricular fibrillation .	10·3	58	42
Ventricular standstill .	7·4	94	6
All cardiac arrests . .	17·7	73	27
No cardiac arrest . .	82·3	17	83
All Patients . . .	100·0	26	74

It is readily apparent that ventricular fibrillation is a much less ominous complication than ventricular standstill. In situations where these types of cardiac arrest are seen, the fatality from unsuccessful cardio-pulmonary resuscitation in association with cardiac arrest, the results in ventricular fibrillation have always been greater than that noted in ventricular standstill. Further, as would be expected the mortality rate increases with severity on admission indexing, i.e., Class II and III patients experiencing cardiac arrest show a marked increased mortality rate over Class I patients.
4. *Heart block (atrioventricular).* An analysis of data on a series of 930 CCU treated patients revealed that heart block (A.V.) is significantly related to fatality rate. The incidence of heart block among this group of patients was noted as follows:

Type of A-V Block	Incidence (*per cent.*)
All Types . . .	21·4
1st Degree . .	8·6
2nd Degree . .	4·6
3rd Degree . .	8·2

The fatality rate in this series of patients revealed:

Type of A-V Block	Fatality Rates (per cent.)
All patients (930) . .	23·3
None	19·0
1st Degree . . .	21·3
2nd Degree . . .	48·3
3rd Degree . . .	51·3

It is noted that the fatality rate in 1st Degree A-V Block patients is not significantly greater than that in those without heart block. However the rate is markedly increased in association with 2nd and 3rd Degree A-V Block.

Coronary Care Unit—regular care comparison

In an analysis of 4,509 cases treated in Coronary Care Units, regular care prior to the CCU, and concurrent regular care, it was noted that in most hospitals there was a decrease in adjusted mortality rates among CCU treated patients versus prior regular care. The overall mortality reduction was 14 per cent. There was no difference between current and prior regular care.

Impact of CCU on hospitals fatality

The analysis of 4,500 hospitalised M.I. cases (including 1,600 treated before the start of the unit and 2,900 since), consisting of

Table IV. *Impact of Coronary Care Unit in two selected hospitals*

| | ADJUSTED RATES | |
| | Hospital A | Hospital J |
Current	(per cent.)	(per cent.)
Regular Care	27·8	37·5
CCU	18·9	29·2
% Change	−32·0	−22·0
Hospital		
Prior	29·4	29·5
Since	20·8	32·4
% Change	−29·0	+10·0

eight reporting hospitals, revealed a wide range of changes. The individual hospitals ranged from a decrease in mortality of 29 per cent. to an increase in mortality of 10 per cent. since the CCU.

42

The combined hospital experience shows an overall decrease of 10 per cent. in mortality in the hospitals since establishment of the units. Closer scrutiny reveals that this change in hospital mortality was attributable to the units' results. For example, a comparison noted in two of these hospitals (A and J) revealed that hospital A had reduction in mortality in the CCU as well as in concurrent regular care, which resulted in an overall favourable effect. On the other hand, hospital J had a decreased mortality in the CCU and an increased concurrent regular care mortality, thereby resulting in an increased death rate for the hospital.

SUMMARY

Proper and valid assessment of the effectiveness of Coronary Care Units requires a common system of categorising patients, as well as usage of commonly accepted definitions. These requisites are essential not only for intra-institutional evaluation of results but for proper evaluation of published reports and studies as well.

Ideally any evaluation of CCU's should include a comparison between the Unit and prior regular care, the Unit and current regular care, and the hospital before and after establishment of the Unit. Problems posed by such a plan of evaluation are: (1) lack of comparable data on regular care hospital records; (2) more thorough examination and diagnostic work-up in CCU patients and, (3) usually a higher calibre and a more adequate number of trained personnel in the CCU than in the general medical wards.

It has been amply demonstrated that Coronary Care Units can reduce the morbidity and mortality in hospitalised acute myocardial infarction patients. However, the effect is maximal if the following desirable features are present.

1. An adequate number of properly trained and highly motivated medical and nursing personnel in the Unit and the entire hospital as well.

2. A Unit of sufficient size to admit all acute myocardial infarction patients.

3. A Unit which practises aggressive treatment policies as appropriate.

4. A Unit which functions as an integral part of the hospital.

5. A Unit which is designed and equipped in a manner to be favourable for patient comfort and welfare, and also allow for maximum efficiency of operation.

It is not enough for a Coronary Care Unit to merely reduce morbidity and mortality in the Unit; it must play a major role in reduction of overall hospital mortality from acute myocardial infarction. This is the only way we can consciously justify the establishment and operation of Coronary Care Units.

Finally, it is realised that Coronary Care Units have not yet reached their maximal potential. We must look for better monitoring techniques, better methods for treating cardiogenic shock and better training and utilisation of health personnel to attain this goal.

CORONARY CARE UNITS:

ADMINISTRATION

Chairman: Professor K. W. DONALD

TRAINING OF NURSES AND PHYSICIANS FOR CORONARY CARE

THOMAS KILLIP

Cornell University Medical College, New York, New York

IN discussing the training requirements for nurses and physicians in positions of responsibility in the management of patients with myocardial infarction, we are literally deep into the heart of one of the great difficulties facing medicine in the Western world. How to provide meaningful postgraduate education on a continuing basis for doctors and nurses remains an important unsolved problem as we search for quality medical care for all the people. We must remember that in most of the countries of the world there are serious medical personnel shortages. We do not utilise our medical personnel efficiently. Moreover, medical educators have not been able to create a successful programme for continued postgraduate education.

The shortage of medical personnel in the United States is a national calamity. We have an inadequate number of physicians. They are overworked and are generally expending their talents inefficiently. We could utilise an increase of 30 to 50 per cent. There are approximately 800,000 registered nurses in the United States and it has been estimated that a minimum of 400,000 more are needed.

With each new innovation in the practice of medicine and the organisation of medical care we eat up more manpower. Open heart surgery and valve replacement require close supervision of the patient by competent medical and nursing teams for many days following operation. The development of chronic dialysis and renal transplant procedures has led to the creation of renal medical and nursing teams which require more manpower and many hours of specialised training. The development of the intensive care unit and its logical outgrowth, the coronary care unit, has put new responsibilities upon the nurse and physician and created a new manpower demand.

The postgraduate training of the physician remains an unsolved problem. As you all know the immediate graduate training of the newly fledged physician is rather well organised in most of our countries. Following graduation from medical school the physician spends several years as a house officer before moving into the

47

practice of medicine or an academic role. In my medical school, Cornell Medical College, the average medical graduate is 26 years old and faces an average of four years of postgraduate training as a house officer before he becomes a medical specialist. Many take five, six or even seven years of training. Very few of our graduates become general practitioners. In addition, unfortunately, in the United States the physician almost invariably must serve two years in the armed forces.

The postgraduate training of the house officer, which may be termed a preceptorship with progressive responsibility, has produced physicians and surgeons of the highest quality trained to perform modern medicine. Unfortunately, once this preceptorship period is completed, the problems begin. I am not aware of any successful programme of continuing education designed for the physician who has completed his postgraduate training. Once the doctor goes into practice in his early or mid-thirties, be he academic or community orientated, he is on his own. There is little or no supervision of quality and there is no formal organised programme of postgraduate refresher education.

A number of studies have shown that as a general rule the physician practises the quality of medicine created by his environment. The physician in the large academic centre with multiple checks and balances controlling patient care and with a plethora of educational and research conferences, generally practices medicine of high quality. The physician in an environment in which there is little supervision of day to day practice and in which postgraduate educational opportunities are few indeed must invest a great effort to keep abreast of the trends of modern medicine. It becomes increasingly difficult for him to practise quality medicine. There are conspicuous exceptions to these general statements, but such are the facts.

The development of the intensive care unit, the increased use of the emergency room, at least in the United States, as an acute care centre, and the creation of specialised care units such as the coronary care unit, the pulmonary care unit or the renal care unit suggest to me that we are going to see the creation of a new group of physician specialists. These men will be specialists in the acute care of the severely ill. In a hospital of 300 to 500 beds or more, the activities of an intensive care or coronary care unit may support one or more full-time physicians whose major interest and responsibilities are in the care of the acutely ill patient. Our own experience at the New York Hospital has convinced us that the well-trained team of nurses, physicians and medical technicians does a far better job of caring for the acutely ill patient than does the 'pick-up' group which is created anew for each special problem.

How should the physician taking responsibility for patients in the coronary care unit be trained? To answer this question successfully I believe that we must create a programme of continuing education for the physician. The physician responsible in a coronary care unit must be a trained cardiologist. I suggest that to become a clinical cardiologist one must have a minimum of three years' experience in general medicine and two years' experience in clinical cardiology. I would also insist that at least one additional year and preferably two years be spent in a laboratory discipline in which active clinical or physiological investigation is being carried out.

In some ways the modern cardiologist is a frustrated surgeon. He must be able to perform cut-downs, to insert pacemaker catheters, to cannulate arteries and to perform endotracheal intubation or resuscitation. Perhaps in the near future as cardiopulmonary assisting devices become available the cardiologist may be required to attach such a device to an acutely ill patient within minutes. Many of these techniques are utilised by cardiologists who perform angiography or cardiac catheterisation and such training is an essential part of the programme to create a modern cardiologist.

Once the cardiologist has been created, it is our responsibility to see that his education continues. I believe the heart associations or cardiac societies in various countries throughout the world have a distinct responsibility in this area. As we are all aware, there are many conventions, seminars, postgraduate courses and the like, but I am far from convinced that such devices truly provide a useful postgraduate experience for the physician who is practising in the closed medical environment of the community hospital.

Those of us in academic centres must develop and take prime responsibility for an active ongoing postgraduate experience which directly involves the physician in the learning experience. Perhaps you in the audience are better learners than I am. I know, however, that when faced with a new field of medicine I learn rather poorly from the illustrated lecture given by the renowned authority. I learn far more rapidly on rounds when seeing the patient, discussing the problem with my peers and following up this active experience by reading the literature. This type of experience must be available to all physicians. It is not available in the typical postgraduate course or seminar. As the educators, or perhaps the word is

49

educationalists, have pointed out, there are very serious obstacles to translating the course-learned material to application in a bedside situation. I believe that we have a unique opportunity to develop a new kind of postgraduate educational experience utilising the coronary care unit, its facilities and its personnel.

The challenge that coronary care presents to medicine should be clearly stated. Medicine, in contrast to surgery or obstetrics, has traditionally had few areas in which quality control could be seriously applied. The surgeon utilises the tissue review committee with its careful scrutiny of pathological material removed at operation as a check on the quality and accuracy of surgical diagnosis and care. At the present time the obstetrician is perhaps the only specialist who is able to invoke quality control in his field for the obstetrician operates under the premise that no woman should die in childbrith. In the United States and I suspect in many other areas also, most communities have a maternal mortality committee. Should a woman die during childbirth, the circumstances of the situation are carefully reviewed by a committee of experts and a judgment is rendered. Those of you who read the *New England Journal of Medicine* must be astounded, as am I, by the frank discussion and strong authoritative opinion that is rendered, in print, regarding the lapses in medical care which may have been responsible for a maternal mortality. Recently, the obstetricians and pediatricians have been developing the premise that no infant should die following birth and have utilised a similar approach in neonatal death.

In contrast to surgery and obstetrics, medicine has not had a technique for quality control until the development of the coronary care unit. This conference is adequate witness to the fact that we are beginning to develop standards of diagnosis and standards of care for patients with acute myocardial infarction. In the coronary care unit we can evaluate medical care literally on a day to day basis. The physician in charge of the unit can ask himself each day: What is the mortality? How many patients had cardiac arrest? Were arrhythmias successfully controlled? As the computer engulfs medicine with its almost infinite permanent memory, we shall shortly be able to compare the success in management of myocardial infarction in hospital X with that in hospital Y. We may even be able to contrast therapeutic success or failure of Doctor A with Doctor B.

Thus the coronary care unit will lead, in my opinion, to the development of firm medical standards for certain conditions. The community will not hesitate to hold these before us and demand

50

that we meet them. For the first time in the history of medicine in my country the consumer is beginning to play an active role and we, the producers, must be prepared to meet their demands.

Postgraduate education of the nurse is equally as important as for the physician. In the United States at the present time we have three types of nursing education. (1) The baccalaureate programme is college oriented and generally requires five years to produce a registered nurse who has a Bachelor of Science degree. The baccalaureate graduate is generally a superior individual. (2) For many years hospitals had three-year schools of nursing. These institutions accepted girls who had finished high school and gave them a diploma in nursing, hence the name diploma school. Unfortunately, in many instances the students were being exploited and the hospital nursing school was little more than attempt to create manpower for the hospital. The diploma schools are gradually being phased out in our country and are being replaced. (3) Community college schools are training young women in nursing and after two years provide an associate degree and a registered nurse. The replacement of the three-year hospital programme by the two-year community college programme is an attempt to upgrade the educational experience of the student nurse. Following graduation from the two-year programme the nurse will probably take several months of specialised training before becoming a fully trained bedside nurse.

The growth of specialised care techniques administered by nurses, perhaps first begun by the surgeons in the operating room and the recovery room, has created the need for specialised training programmes for nurses. The demands of the coronary care unit are no exception. We find that young, aggressive and rather restless nurses who wish to continue working at the bedside are attracted to coronary care. They enjoy their new authority and are eager to increase their direct responsibility for patient welfare. In our Coronary Care Unit, as in common with many others, nurses diagnose arrhythmias, resuscitate patients, perform electrical defibrillation and, under specially defined circumstances, administer emergency intravenous medication. They do not hesitate to suggest to the doctor a needed therapy. As will no doubt be developed in subsequent discussion in this conference, our group and many others believe that the nurse is the key individual in the successful coronary care unit. The nurse is the one professional person who is at the patient's bedside at all times. To provide quality care she must have the training and authority to perform many tasks which previously had been reserved for the physician.

51

At the New York Hospital-Cornell Medical Center, the development of our nurse training programme has been the result of a close co-operation between the Division of Cardiology in the Department of Medicine and Cornell University School of Nursing. We began with a training programme for our own staff nurses. It entailed some 40 hours of course work given by the doctors. A year and a half ago, we developed a programme to train the nurses from community hospitals to become coronary care specialists. The course is six weeks long and includes a review of anatomy and physiology, pharmacology and therapeutics, some 30 hours of instruction in electrocardiography, practical experience with supervised nursing in the coronary care unit, and experience in the dog laboratory in the technique of defibrillation and cardiac pacing. We enrol 20 to 30 students per course and emphasise individual instruction and seminar-type learning.

Recently, a number of our graduates from the first-year training programmes were visited in their own hospitals. Most of them have achieved positions of responsibility in their community hospitals and have maintained a strong bedside orientation. Most of them are heavily involved in postgraduate teaching programmes in their local community. We find that the one area which should be emphasised more extensively is that of pharmacology and the management of patients.

DISCUSSION

Dr Fox. The need for competent personnel has been emphasised. In the United States we still hold to the principle that you need two people to man a resuscitation team even though there is evidence that, if you cannot convert the person's arrhythmia with a de-polarizing current application, the need for closed chest cardiac resuscitation is probably diminished because of the lack of fruitful results. I think that from a policy standpoint nobody is willing to accept this at the moment and therefore we work with the concept that you need two competent people. That does not mean that you have to have two highly skilled nurses, not to speak of the physicians one would like to have there as well. In looking at our problem in the United States we find that one-quarter of all deaths in the United States are due to coronary heart disease and that one-third of all male deaths from age 35 to 64 are due to coronary heart disease. The socio-economic implication obviously is such that it commands the most serious attention. Lacking a preventive approach, how can we set up a system of care when the following statistics apply in the United States?

There are approximately 3,700 hospitals which have less than 100 beds, some 2,300 hospitals with bed capacities of 100 to 199, and 1,200 hospitals with over 200 beds—in other words, 7,200 hospitals. Half of our population then depends on small hospitals for their care, including acute coronaries, and these are hospitals which at the moment are having great difficulty seeing a way of cost-accounting the support of a coronary care type of facility.

The following figures show the demands that we think are not unrealistic for personnel to man these units on a round the clock, round the week, round the year basis. It would be necessary to have a supervisory person in the nursing paramedical area as well as four individuals on a weekly round the clock basis for the hospitals with units less than 100 beds. That represents some 14,000 to 15,000 individuals for a nation of just under 200 million individuals. For hospitals of intermediate size (100–199 beds) we have calculated 12,000 and for the larger hospitals some 20,000. This is 47,000 individuals to man a system of in-hospital care and this does not take account of the replacement or turnover. It does not take account of any of the extended services in the community nor does it take into account progressive care extending beyond the acute care in the unit.

Our Congress, very fortunately, saw the need and provided one million dollars to be applied to setting up specific units for the training of personnel—almost exclusively at this time graduate nurses. Dr Killip's unit in New York had already been started. There have been 12 more started in the very recent past and an attempt has been made to get a balanced geographic distribution so that the travel expenses involved were not too great. We are only going to be able to turn out 1,100 individuals per year even though some of these courses, as contrasted to Dr Killip's six-week course, are as short as three weeks. We are going to try to evaluate the difference in approach in these units to see if we can improve upon the way in which we can turn out more people with reasonably adequate training in lesser time and particularly with lesser investment of time, effort and resources in their training. Dr Killip mentioned the necessary needs to get paramedical personnel. It seems perfectly obvious that we will not have enough young nurses for these units in the United States and we are assured this is true elsewhere. I suggest that possibly what we need to generate is a cadre of individuals whom I would like to see considered as clinical physiologists rather than technicians or rather than physicians' assistants. This group should in time have the senior professional status such as we accord to nurses now. That doesn't mean that they do not work under the general supervision of the medical profession. I think this is absolutely necessary, but, we cannot have them indefinitely playing second fiddle to another profession, and enlist enough of them from the brighter groups into a baccalaureate type of training programme. Practical experience could be of an internship sort and then they could go back to graduate work, be it towards a higher degree or not. Dr Wilson of the English Ministry of Health raised a very important question over discussions on this. What is the eventual goal for a man who in his twenties may have aspired to a medical career but doesn't find himself sufficiently convinced, able to assemble the resources or academically able to meet the requirements of the medical curriculum but who would like to do something of this sort in clinical physiology in the early years of this life? What do we provide for him as a later in life opportunity?

There is a great need in the United States for senior administrators of hospitals and medical services and I think this need will be greatly extended in the future. I suggest that these medically interested people could graduate into that type of role and achieve the resources in their personal living whereby they could support their children through higher education and the like. As such, I think that we have a particular need to look at the paramedical side and want to emphasise that.

Professor Donald. There is certainly quite a group of people, some of which Dr Fox has mentioned, people who haven't quite made the grade as medical students or have not had the money or haven't settled down early enough in life, people who get tired of industrial electronics, who want to do something more related to human activities and so on. These people have not yet been used enough by the community, but they certainly will have to be given a proper career. Are there any views particularly about whether one should press with the nursing developments or whether one should also think of other paramedical activities or both?

Dr Nixon. I do not know whether this system of recruiting paramedical people will come into being or not, but we have a real problem and that is the shortage of nurses. If you are going to form a coronary care unit you have got to have a group of nurses who are capable of being trained to do certain things. They have to monitor distress, cyanosis, changes in the peripheral circulation, respiration, central venous pressure by a saline manometer and also the electrocardiogram, although I think this is the least valuable of the monitoring methods. They must know how to give intravenous medication and must know how to produce deep sedation. They need to know how to treat cerebral oedema in the unconscious patient. They need to know about the various techniques of artificial ventilation, cardiac arrest and resuscitation, and they must have familiarity with different sorts of catheters. These nurses and the physicians who train them are key people in that they can do a lot in the small general hospital that could not be done before and make a lot of difference to mortality. They have got to teach the junior doctor and they cannot be dominated by the therapeutic whims of changing house staff and registrars. But there aren't enough of these nurses anywhere and hospitals cannot undertake the setting up of a whole lot of different specialised units. I think coronary units are a phase and would like to see a movement towards solving the nursing problems of hospitals by setting up intensive care units and providing room or accommodation in such a unit to provide architecturally the coronary patient with the peace and quiet he needs.

Professor Shillingford. I think that everybody here has pioneered the conception of better medicine for acute illnessess. I think that we shall find very shortly that the respirologists, the renal experts and the neurologists will hold similar meetings. Each will ask for and assemble their own special units, and this will create chaos among the nurses. I have a strong suspicion that within 15 or 20 years, we will have to divide our hospitals into three areas, the high care, the medium care and the convalescent area where no nursing is needed. We have got to be extremely careful over setting up one little section in a high-powered fashion without considering the services as a whole.

Dr McDonald. I would like to congratulate Drs Fox and Killip for putting this problem into a very good perspective. I am not quite sure about these "professional defibrillators". Should they be in sole charge of the patient or work with the doctor? I personally find that the electrocardiogram is the most important thing that you can monitor in these patients. An alternative approach to training a very specialised group is what we are doing in the London hospital. Every student nurse early on is told the basic principles. We aim that everybody near coronary patients should be able to treat them. That might be a better answer than selecting a few people, because I think the care of these patients is going to get simpler and simpler.

Dr Meltzer. The nurses in our institutions have probably had as pleasant an experience as a nurse could have. They have been

55

paid a good deal more than other nurses, and they have been on a continuous educational programme which lasted three to four months preparing them. Recently we reviewed the experience of 38 nurses whom we trained in the past four years and to my dismay the nursing life-expectancy is 8·6 months. This is incredible. After spending three months teaching these women, this is how long they have lasted. We have been looking into the problem of why they quit. Many of the girls got married and now have children. That is a position one has to anticipate. But another one which I had not considered is a certain boredom with the job. We have let the nurses assess their own experiences each month as to how they were doing. A rather peculiar thing appeared— the curve of confidence and security kept going up but interest kept coming down. At first the nurse likes the responsibility but it wears off, and after eight or nine months the nurse resigns.

Those numbers mentioned by Dr Fox of 47,000 nurses would mean 47,000 original nurses. If my figures are correct and they last about nine months, you can see how this problem would be exaggerated and become impossible. I do not think the answer will be with paramedical personnel, and I think it probably has to be within the nursing profession itself. Nursing simply has to be changed. It just cannot exist in its current form. Nurses are trained in foolish trips, such as bedpan rounds and passing out diet trays and that sort of thing. There just has to be an entire reorganisation in nursing. I suspect that physicians rather than nurses are going to have to accomplish this in order to get nursing to do what medicine needs of it now. Nursing education should teach to an undergraduate level in regard to coronary care so that every nurse in the hospital would be trained rather than the 47,000 specialised nurses. If this transition is as high as it seems to be in our experience you would have a constant flow and make nursing more attractive to more people than it is currently, so I think the answers could be within nursing itself rather than trying to create a new group of people.

Professor Donald. I feel that the medical profession must also reorganise itself. There are far too many of us who live comfortably on the plains of manoeuvre rather than in the front lines. You see very highly qualified teams going around ponderously discussing cases of pernicious anaemia or of mild thyrotoxicosis or a patient with diarrhoea and passing blood, and, after great rumination, they all come to the diagnosis of ulcerative colitis. This is a low level activity and the profession has got to get back into the front line.

THE DESIGN OF THE CORONARY CARE UNIT AND ITS INSTRUMENTATION

Peter L. Frommer,

Myocardial Infarction Branch, Artificial Heart—Myocardial Infarction Program, National Heart Institute, Bethesda, Md.

Modern concepts of care for the patient with acute myocardial infarction include three key resources which the coronary care unit (CCU) must provide: skilled, specially trained personnel who are in immediate attendance, special apparatus for patient monitoring and therapeutic manoeuvres, and a comfortable environment conducive to recuperation. The design of a unit must permit the fulfilment of these three needs, taking into account the characteristics and requirements of the hospital in which it is to be situated.

Coronary care units generally have four to eight beds, although a few have been built to accommodate 16 or more patients. One CCU bed for about every 40 or 50 regular beds is typical of the needs of those community hospitals in the U.S.A. which keep patients five to seven days.

In planning its unit, each institution must examine its own experience—how many patients are admitted annually with myocardial infarction? How many will leave the unit prematurely because this diagnosis is quickly excluded? Or because of death? How frequently will the unit be used for patients with rhythm problems? In addition consideration must be given to the erratic rather than predictably regular admission of patients. Each unit must plan its policies: How long will patients be kept in the CCU? Will certain groups of patients with myocardial infarction be excluded? Will the establishment of a CCU predictably modify the pattern of patient referral? How will the unit be related and integrated—physically and administratively—with relevant organisations in the hospital?

Turning now to the architectural design, provision must be made for the surveillance of each patient by the staff, both from a monitoring station and during the course of their routine activities. In most units this has been accomplished by the strategic positioning of windows and doors. In a few CCU closed circuit television systems have been utilised to avoid extensive architectural renovation.

Of equal importance to the adequacy of surveillance is the need for providing privacy, i.e., single rooms, curtains for observation

57

windows, doors, etc. This is essential for ensuring rest and quiet and also for avoiding exposure of patients to emergency situations which will inevitably arise.

An environment favourable to recuperation should also include provisions for patient comforts such as sound-proofing, temperature and humidity control (in many parts of the world), attractive furnishings, television, and the maintenence of normal cycles of day and night. All monitoring equipment should be out of ear-shot and out of the line of vision of every patient.

The size of the patient rooms must be sufficient for ready access to the bed from the end and both sides, and for bringing relatively bulky equipment to the bedside. Rooms of at least 12 square meters are recommended. Similarly, doors and corridors must be of sufficient dimensions for the ready movement of beds, portable X-ray apparatus, emergency carts, etc.

Parenthetically, consideration has been given by some groups to the use of beds which are non-opaque to X-ray and will permit the fluoroscopy of the patient in his regular bed.

Each room should be supplied with adequate utilities. These should include six or eight electrical power outlets with a common ground for safety (but not all on a single fuse or circuit breaker), power for portable X-ray apparatus, and standby emergency electrical power. Bedside outlets for oxygen and suction are important. High intensity lighting should be available for emergency procedures. Apparatus should be off the floor and out of the way whenever possible; wall-mounted monitoring equipment and provision for hanging bottles of intravenous fluids from the ceiling are advantageous.

In addition to these patient needs, facilities must be provided for the staff so that they can remain on or near the unit at all times.

The CCU is generally considered a totally self-sufficient and independent unit. Yet, economic considerations impose a certain minimum number of beds for a totally self-sufficient group, perhaps four beds if a staff of two is considered essential at all times. Thus if a smaller hospital is to provide its patients with the benefits of a CCU, the unit can probably not be made totally self-sufficient. Careful design can nevertheless fulfil the above criteria for patient comforts and for the availability of staff on or in the immediate proximity of the unit at all times.

Monitoring equipment of many types, from the simplest instruments to rather elaborate systems, is being utilised in CCU. The most important function of any system is the constant automatic monitoring of the cardiac rhythm throughout the patient's stay in the unit. Small electrodes, in which a salt paste forms the only electrical contact between the conductive surface and the patient, can provide long-term tracings with minimum artifacts, especially if they are carefully applied with double surface adhesive tape after appropriate skin preparation. Positioning electrodes on the thorax minimises artifacts in the signal and reduces the encumbrance upon the patient. Some have advocated the use of a radio-telemetry link between the patient and a bedside receiver. This permits free activity by the patient not only in bed, but also in the vicinity of his room. Perhaps this technique may be most effective in the later stages of hospitalisation as part of the ' progressive care ' concept.

The display of the electrocardiogram should be both at the bedside where it is most useful for patient care, and at a central station where it is of greatest value for surveillance. The display at the central monitoring station may be on a multi-trace oscilloscope, but the use of individual scopes has the advantage of avoiding inactivation of the entire system by the failure of a single element. Either system is useful, but most importantly, the electrocardiogram of each patient must be on display at all times at the central station.

Provision for the direct write-out of any of the monitored electrocardiograms is necessary at least at the central station and it is extremely valuable at each bedside. A readily portable direct writing device should be available for connection into the monitor at the bedside if a recorder is not dedicated to each bed.

An automatic alarm system for each electrocardiogram is an essential element of every monitoring system. Some alarm systems are triggered only by transgression of high or low rate limits after a number of beats, but most are triggered by a single abnormal RR interval. It is important to recognise that automatic alarm systems do not generally respond to changes in the configuration of the electrocardiogram unless rate limits are transgressed. Accordingly, the appearance of a nodal or ventricular pacemaker, firing within the rate limits set, will generally go undetected. While the automatic detection of QRS duration by relatively simple analogue computational techniques has been accomplished and has been used for alarm purposes, it is not widely utilised.

The reliability of an alarm system is dependent not only upon the intrinsic characteristics of the instrument, but also upon the care with which alarm limits are set for each particular patient at each point in time.

Some alarm systems have incorporated pacing apparatus to be automatically activated in the event of bradycardia. Many contend that this mode of therapy is needed with sufficient infrequency that such apparatus can be brought to the bedside when necessary. Perhaps more importantly, in the patient with a prophylactically inserted intracardiac pacing catheter, the use of a battery-operated standby pacemaker is of less hazard.

Arrhythmia alarms are activated only after an arrhythmia has developed. To aid in the interpretation of the genesis of arrhythmias, a knowledge of prior events may be of great value. A magnetic tape loop system to provide a brief memory, which is continuously updated on one end while it is being erased at the other end, is in fairly wide use. When the arrhythmia alarm is triggered, a direct writing apparatus can be automatically started and the tape loop stopped; this arrangement is necessary if both the arrhythmia and its initiating events are to be recorded. For patient care, relatively brief loops (one-half to two minutes) seem the most satisfactory, since they permit a relatively rapid recall of prior events. Longer recordings, though of interest, require longer playback time and are generally less useful for clinical purposes. Tape loop switching should permit playback without erasure as an optional feature to permit repeated scrutiny of the record.

Automatic inscription of the electrocardiogram should be initiated not only by the arrhythmia alarm. In many circumstances, brief recordings at predetermined time intervals may be of value in detecting and following morphological changes in the electro-cardiogram, as well as in providing brief records of the rhythm.

Monitoring systems have been built to include a variety of automatic display and recording systems for parameters other than the electrocardiogram, particularly the heart rate, respiratory rate, temperature, and the blood pressure. These may be of some convenience in the routine care of patients with myocardial infarction, and perhaps they offer an efficient means of charting extensive data in the larger unit. However, before incorporating such measurements into a monitoring system, their cost effectiveness must be judged individually for the coronary care unit in question.

In research settings, quite extensive measurements of cardiovascular, pulmonary, renal and other organ system performance have been conducted on patients with acute myocardial infarction. It has been demonstrated that such measurements can be performed safely by skilled hands when appropriate facilities are available. These studies have not only improved our understanding of myocardial infarction and its treatment, but they have suggested the value of certain additional measurements in specific circumstances. Accordingly, some groups are almost routinely measuring central venous or other right sided pressures from indwelling catheters. These signals can be readily connected to simple, self-contained display and alarm devices and recording instruments. With the use of a catheter which incorporates an electrode at its tip, the same catheter will yield the intracardiac electrocardiogram which will permit the better interpretation of arrhythmias and generate more reliable alarms; the intracardiac electrode may also serve for pacing in the treatment of bradycardia.

In patients with complications, some groups have found considerable value in the continuous direct measurement of arterial pressure from an indwelling catheter; on-line cardiac output determinations with the use of special purpose on-line computers have aided others in the more rational treatment of patients with shock or congestive failure. Monitoring of the depth of respiration, of mixed venous or arterial blood gases and pH, and of indices of cardiac dynamics have been undertaken on a limited scale.

The design for these more complex instrumentation and monitoring systems must keep in mind specific needs, interests and expected utilisation. Certain characteristics which are likely to be of value in such a system may be summarised, e.g., the system must be reliable and it must be compact, integrated and sufficiently easy to use that it will be of value to the personnel on the unit; the system should be controllable from the bedside; a direct write-out of all data should always be provided, at least in summary form; for continuously recording magnetic tape systems, rapid playback and special display systems must be available and time and event encoding and recognition are important. For some of the most complex systems, digital computers have been designed for on-line data reduction, computation and for rapid data retrieval.

It must be remembered that none of these additional measurements discussed above are yet of proven value for routine coronary care. In the patient with complications, some may be of importance as well as of interest, and they can probably be obtained without these very elaborate instrumentation systems.

At the present time, the monitoring needs of the coronary care unit which can be fulfilled by commercially available equipment and which seem reasonable for routine use are simply highly reliable rhythm monitoring and arrhythmia detection. With future developments additional parameters will undoubtedly be found useful and important. Systems for their sensing, recording and display will be developed.

The safety of instruments connected to patients, particularly those with intracardiac catheters, is a topic of great importance

61

and the hazards of faulty grounding and minute leakage currents have been emphasised. These are real and important considerations. However, it must be remembered that the safety of patients in the CCU, in terms of their survival, will depend in part upon the reliability and performance of the monitoring system, which includes such factors as the assurance of arrhythmia detection, the avoidance of erroneous or confusing data and a minimum of down time for repairs. All of these points must be considered in the design and utilisation of monitoring equipment.

The challenge in the design of the CCU and its monitoring system is in making available the resources of these units as defined above on a practical and economic basis to the great mass of patients with acute myocardial infarction.

DISCUSSION

Dr Sandøe (Copenhagen). I would like to focus on some principles in monitoring which are of great practical importance and which have caused a lot of headaches in many coronary care units and in the Coronary Care Unit at the Medical Department B in the University Clinic of Copenhagen, with which I am associated.

Firstly, what is necessary to ensure the safety of the patient during his stay in the coronary care unit?

Secondly, how can electrical signals be obtained without too much interference from electrical noise?

Thirdly, how can we create a pool of medical engineers whom we can consult concerning the design and development of good monitoring equipment. We have been discussing the problem of staffing these units, but with good electronic advice we should be able to reduce the staff and monitor more patients with fewer nurses.

First, the safety of the patient. This is at risk because some patients have a low conductor pathway linking the surface of the skin directly to the heart; the conductor may be a catheter filled with electrolyte solution or it may be a pacemaker cable. Furthermore, his safety is hazarded by pieces of electrical apparatus which very often have a certain voltage on their surface due to some fault. These two things together make it possible for a current to pass directly through the heart and thus provoke ventricular fibrillation, I think it is essential to realise that many instances of ventricular fibrillation provoked by the set-up in coronary care units are unidentified errors. There are very often periodic failures in the apparatus. The conductor between the patient and the failing apparatus may be a nurse who is standing with one hand on the catheter and with the other hand on the apparatus, or it may be, as it was once in our unit, different flooring in the monitoring room and the flooring may have a different effect with different electrical machinery. Thus when a machine is started, for example an X-ray machine, the voltage of one of the floorings may change and this will create a voltage on the ground which will go to this machine and give a source for electricity to run along the electrical points and thence to the heart. The precautions against these accidents should be approached from two different aspects. First, there should be precautions in respect of the construction of electrical medical apparatus and, secondly, there should be precautions as regards the installation of this apparatus. I shall not go into detail as regards the construction of the apparatus because I do not know anything about it, but I would suggest that there are certain countries, Britain among them, where there is a very good safety code for electrical medical apparatus. On the other hand, there are countries, among them my own, with a very poor safety code —one which is only aimed at protection of housewives from electric shock when they are using a flat iron or a vacuum cleaner. This safety code is not good enough to protect the patients who are so unlucky as to arrive in our coronary care unit.

This I think should be a challenge for most Health Authorities in any country—to put up compulsory safety codes both for the electrical medical apparatus and for their installation. I think it must be made compulsory because at present in many care units there are still two-point plugs and varying grounding in each room.

The second problem will be partly solved by proper grounding, but only partly. The real solution is in the design of the electrical installation in the unit. To change this installation is a very expensive affair but, if you are going to build a hospital, it would be very little more expensive to fit it correctly than in a bad way. We have counted on that as we are going to have a new hospital unit in the University of Copenhagen and it will increase the instalment expenses by only 10 per cent.

This brings me to the last point—how do we get over these problems? The only way is to create a pool of medical engineers who can be used as consultants. It has been proved that no doctor can learn engineering and no engineer whose building ways are different from day to day can be a good medical engineer. You have to have premedical grounding. I would like to hear about experiences of the paramedical Faculties which have been set up in several Institutes of Technology in the United States.

Dr Fox. I would just like to mention a recent article in the *Journal of the American Medical Association* of 28th August entitled ' Delirium in a Coronary Care Unit '. This indicates the concern of these authors about the sensory deprivation that perhaps accompanies the more scientific approach to the measurement of the physiological parameters. It accentuates the need to maintain a degree of connection with real life so that we do not have this added complication, which occurred in 11 individuals in a total experience of 500.

Dr Oliver. I would like to take up one or two rather important points that I believe Dr Frommer has covered. None of us here has both total and immediate surveillance of arrhythmias in any unit. I doubt if this exists and if we accept that this is so, then we have got to devise a system to produce just that—total and immediate surveillance. In parenthesis, earlier Dr Lown commented on our low incidence of ventricular tachycardia and he is quite right. The reason is that we did not at that time appreciate the importance of slow ventricular tachycardia at 70 or 80 per minute which was not triggering any R-R interval alarm system. We have all I am sure seen this frequently and as we have become aware of it, so has our recorded incidence of ventricular tachycardia increased. Therefore we cannot rely completely on R-R interval alarm systems. We cannot rely on breadth counting systems, because these are at present inadequate. I would suggest in relationship to some of the remarks made earlier that perhaps investment of the order that you are trying to achieve—one million dollars producing 1,100 individuals and you have shown very clearly how inadequate that is going to be in terms of your demands—should not be in this area at all. It should be devoted to an international co-operative effort to produce a small and cheap on-line computer for all of us and I cannot see there is any short cut to this.

Dr McDonald. We felt some time ago that it was very important in evaluating drugs which might suppress various dysrhythmias to have a system which we could have 12 hours on, 12 hours off and know exactly what was happening. A recording method has, therefore, been developed by my colleague Mr John Norman who is at the National Heart Hospital and Institute of Cardiology which does these things for 16 hours: there are recorded alarms and there is an event marker and the usual immediate display of these parameters. This is the kind of research I like because you can come in next morning and start the play back and if there is not too much on it, it will play back 16 hours experience in 8 minutes and it tells us exactly what has been happening with high-speed search.

Dr Sloman. Along the lines that Dr McDonald has just mentioned we have developed with our medical electronics department a piece of equipment which has the benefits of being very cheap. We have a standard Tanberg, two-channel stereo-tape recorder. This is a commercial piece of equipment designed by a biomedical engineer. This small machine has a modulated device which will record ECG, pressure and pulse waves or trace continuously or intermittently. It will run for four hours or eight hours depending on the selected speed and play back the records on an oscilloscope. This equipment is cheap and available and we think that it will give us the type of surveillance that will enable us to predict more from our various physiological parameters.

RADIOLOGY IN THE CORONARY CARE UNIT

ERIC SAMUEL

Department of Diagnostic Radiology, University of Edinburgh

RADIOLOGICAL assistance has to cope with two separate demands in the coronary care unit, namely the production of chest radiographs and the control of fluoroscopy for the insertion of cardiac pacemakers.

These two distinct requirements are difficult to reconcile as the former demands a portable unit capable of high outputs, whilst the latter requires a light and flexible mobile unit. Compromise is always unsatisfactory and in our prototype unit, we have stressed fluoroscopic aspects although the unit is capable of producing extremely satisfactory chest films.

A shorter focal film distance than the normal 6 feet for chest radiography must be accepted under conditions of coronary care and in all patients with rapid respiration a drop of 40 in. or even 30 in. must be accepted. The consequent distortion can be allowed for in interpretation of the film.

For the fluoroscopic control the following medical conditions were suggested:

1. The unit should be sufficiently light and mobile to be manipulated and controlled by a single operator.

2. The controls of the unit should be arranged so that they can be used by a single operator.

3. The fluoroscopic viewing should be on a T.V. intensifier, 625 line chain.

4. The viewing monitor and controls should be on a separate console.

5. The tube and intensifier should have independent movement.

The commercially available units (Philips BV 20, Siremobil, CGR, etc.) are all constructed on the arc principle whereby the tube and intensifier are mounted at each end of a half circle and are free to move through a half circle. In its turn the pivot of the arc can be raised and lowered. These units are connected to a T.V. intensifier system.

These units have the serious disadvantage, in regard to their use in coronary care, namely they are heavy and bulky in view of their mechanics and they do not provide sufficient coverage of a patient in a coronary care bed (Fig. 1). It was found in our

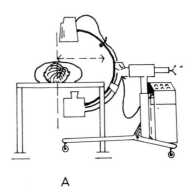

A

Fig. 1A. This figure shows diagrammatically the coverage of a patient in a hospital bed by the conventional commercially available television fluoroscopic mobile unit. The width of the hospital bed prevents full coverage of the chest as the unit is primarily designed for an operating table with a central support.

experience of such a unit that it was not possible to screen across the chest without displacing the patient to one side of the bed, a feature of considerable disadvantage when it is considered that the operator is working from the opposite side of the bed. The following unit was therefore devised which allows a 28 in. coverage across the bed. The average breadth is 36 in. and allows full coverage of the whole of the chest.

The tube movement is independent of the intensifier in an upward

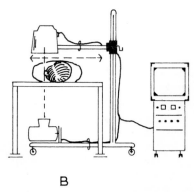

B

FIG. 1B. Illustrates the Cardiovision with full coverage of the patient's chest in a hospital bed.

and downward direction but is arranged so that it cannot move from side to side. No danger from radiation from a primary beam thus arises but full use can be made of the inverse square law to keep the radiation at minimum when particularly thick patients are being examined.

The diaphragm control on the stand allows the field size to be kept to a maximum. The intensifier is a 6 in. Mullard unit coupled to a 625 line system and a 14 in. T.V. monitor allows good vision of the cardiac outline (Fig. 2).

The separation of the controls to a separate console (which can be clamped to the unit for moving) has allowed the development of an extremely light weight stand.

The supporting column is of such length that the intensifier can be elevated sufficiently to allow the tube to be raised and isolated to allow a chest film to be taken. The radiographic maximum output of the unit is 90KV at 15 mA and for fluoroscopy the factors used have been 80KV at 1 to 1·5 mA.

Other uses for such a unit will soon become apparent in a medical ward. Thus, the follow up of a pneumothorax or the rapid screening of a suspected pulmonary collapse or embolus may have advantages over a chest film.

Certainly in those units, e.g., assorted respiratory units and thoracic surgical units where daily chest X-rays are needed, the use of such a unit may limit the number of chest films needed and thus effect a considerable saving in expense and labour.

We are also investigating the possibilities of connecting the unit to videotape and obtaining a record of the fluoroscopic procedures.

67

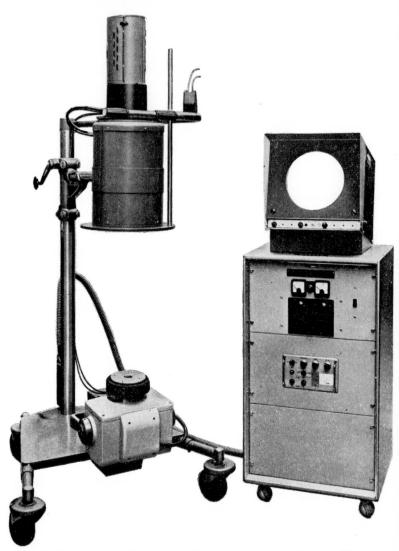

FIG. 2. Represents a photograph of the completed unit. The television and X-ray controls are mounted on a separate console but the exposure button and diaphragm controls are mounted on the unit.

Its use in contrast studies for pulmonary emboli without removing the patient from his bed will have to be considered.

To date we have used a foam rubber mattress on a hard-board bed base.

The unit has been produced by Messrs. Watson & Sons.

ACKNOWLEDGEMENTS

I am grateful to Drs Oliver, Julian, Lassers and Godman for their assistance and to Messrs. Watson & Sons for their co-operation in the development of this unit.

ARRHYTHMIAS

Chairman: Dr. M. F. OLIVER

THE MANAGEMENT OF ATRIAL ARRHYTHMIAS

PATRICK MOUNSEY

Royal Postgraduate Medical School, Hammersmith London

Classification of atrial arrhythmias

In an attempt to simplify the subject of arrhythmias after acute cardiac infarction, we proposed a broad classification based on the over-all cardiac response to the dominant arrhythmia. In this classification, the atrial arrhythmias were divided into three main groups:

1. Supraventricular tachycardia, comprising atrial tachycardia, flutter, and fibrillation, often interchanging with one another.

2. Supraventricular bradycardia, that is sinus bradycardia, vasovagal attacks and partial heart-block.

3. Atrial transport dysfunction, consisting of various forms of nodal rhythm or atrio-ventricular dissociation.

We have found this simple grouping useful in that a patient's detailed arrhythmias usually vary within the same group, as when short bursts of atrial tachycardia, flutter or fibrillation follow one another in quick succession. It also has the advantage of emphasising some of the main circulatory disturbances resulting from the arrhythmias either in heart rate or loss of atrial transport function.

Incidence

The incidence of the various groups of atrial arrhythmias is shown in Table I (Fluck *et al.*, 1967); the commonest was supraventricular

Table I. *Classification of arrhythmias after acute cardiac infarction*

(103 consecutive episodes continuously monitored)

	No. Episodes
1. Supraventricular Tachycardia Group (A.T.—A. Flutter—A. Fib.)	16
2. Supraventricular Bradycardia Group (Sinus B. and Vasovagal)	20
3. Atrial Transport Dysfunction Group (A–V Dissociation and A–V Rhythm)	5
4. Ventricular Tachycardia Group	5
5. Ventricular Bradycardia Group (Complete Heart Block) . .	12
6. Extrasystoles only (Atrial, A–V, Ventricular)	25
7. Unheralded Cardiac Arrest (V.F.) (24 hrs.)	3
8. No Arrhythmias	17
	103

bradycardia. The supraventricular tachycardia group was almost as common and the rarest was the atrial transport dysfunction group. Altogether, there were 41 instances of atrial arrhythmias in 103 episodes of cardiac infarction, making atrial arrhythmias twice as common as ventricular, of which only 20 episodes occurred. In arriving at these figures, cases with extrasystoles alone were excluded.

Natural history

In our series, the atrial arrhythmias were usually transient, self-limiting and relatively benign. The natural history of the arrhythmias differed in the three groups. In Figure 1, representative examples of one patient from each group are shown. Although no clear-cut relationship between the site of the cardiac infarct and the nature of the arrhythmia was found, none the less, an anterior cardiac infarct was commoner in the supraventricular tachycardia group, while a posterior cardiac infarct was usually found in the supraventricular bradycardia group. Evidence of left ventricular failure on admission was the rule in patients in the supraventricular tachycardia group, but with supraventricular bradycardia, this was seldom present. In patients with atrial transport dysfunction, those with larger cardiac infarcts had evidence of left ventricular failure. There was a difference also in the time of occurrence of supraventricular tachycardias and of vasovagal attacks with supraventricular bradycardia. Whereas the former occurred any time within the first week and usually ceased spontaneously by the end of the first week, the latter occurred only within the first 24–48 hours, usually at a time when patients were in considerable pain and requiring frequent analgesics. Atrial transport dysfunction was seen at varying times during the first week after infarction and sometimes lasted up to two or three weeks after the date of the infarct.

Management

We believe that treatment should be primarily directed to improving the general state of the patient and correcting any haemodynamic deterioration resulting from the arrhythmia. Oxygen and diuretics are helpful in combating heart failure; transient hypotension can often be corrected by postural means alone, nursing the patient flat and if necessary, raising his legs. These manoeuvres

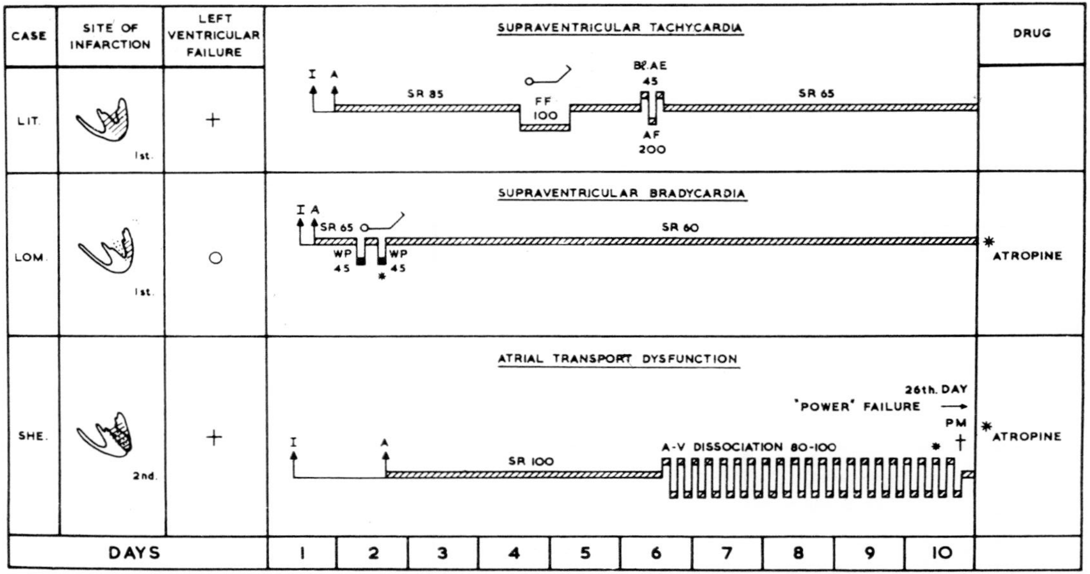

FIG. 1. The natural history of atrial arrhythmias after acute cardiac infarction. A representative example of each group is shown. The first arrow, marked I, indicates the time of the infarct; and the second arrow, marked A, the time of admission to hospital. The horizontal hatched line indicates sinus rhythm. Interruption of this line indicates the development of an arrhythmia: If upwards, the blood pressure is maintained; if downwards, the blood pressure falls. SR = sinus rhythm; FF = flutter fibrillation; BlAE = blocked atrialect opics; AF = atrial fibrillation; WP = wandering pacemaker; the horizontal mannikin with legs in the air indicates postural treatment for hypotension. Cross-hatching indicates an anterior cardiac infarct, and stippling a posterior infarct. For interpretation, see text.

No CASES	ARRHYTHMIA		NO ANTI-ARR. TREATMENT	DRUG ANTI-ARR. TREATMENT	ELEC. ANTI-ARR. TREATMENT	SURVIVORS
16	SUPRAVENTRICULAR TACHYCARDIA		7	DIGITALIS 9	CARDIOVERSION 1	14
20	SUPRAVENTRICULAR BRADYCARDIA	11	11			10
	WITH VASOVAGAL A.	7	2	ATROPINE 5		6
	WITH PARTIAL H.B	2		ATROPINE 2		2
5	ATRIAL TRANSPORT DYSFUNCTION		2	ATROPINE 2		4

FIG. 2. Management of the atrial arrhythmias.
(With vasovagal a. = with vasovagal attack.)

are usually sufficient to maintain the blood pressure at an adequate level and patients can usually lie flat without discomfort even with early left ventricular failure.

Turning to specific forms of anti-arrhythmic treatment, this was not considered necessary in about half our patients (Fig. 2). Where, however, the arrhythmia was more prolonged and was associated with profound disturbances of the circulation, specific therapy was undertaken. In the supraventricular tachycardia group, cardiac glycosides are the method of choice and are a well-tried form of therapy whose possible complications are recognised. Frequent coupled atrial extrasystoles are sometimes prodromal to atrial tachycardia or fibrillation; in such cases the prophylactic use of intravenous lignocaine may suppress the extrasystoles and help prevent the onset of a more serious atrial arrythmia.

In the supraventricular bradycardia group, no treatment is required for simple sinus bradycardia. On the other hand, our experience suggested that these patients were at special risk of developing vasovagal episodes during the first 24–48 hours and therefore constant 24-hour observation throughout that period was of the utmost importance. When a vasovagal episode occurred, the pulse rate fell precipitously to between 30–50 a minute with a simultaneous fall in blood pressure, which sometimes became temporarily unrecordable, and pallor, sweating, nausea and sometimes mental confusion. The attacks quickly respond to postural treatment and to intravenous atropine (0·4–0·6 mg. intravenously). Since many of these patients are complaining of severe cardiac pain, special care should be exercised in the use of analgesics because of the tendency of morphine and pethidine to lower the blood pressure. Frequent small doses of these are probably preferable to a single large dose.

The patients in the atrial transport dysfunction group often require no treatment where the general circulation remains good and the blood pressure well maintained. In the presence of a large cardiac infarct however, loss of atrial transport function may produce serious circulatory disability with a considerable fall in systemic blood pressure. In these patients, intravenous atropine will restore sinus rhythm for a period of 15 to 30 minutes, and this may sometimes be a useful form of treatment, pending spontaneous reversion to sinus rhythm.

Although electrical shock therapy is usually effective in converting atrial arrhythmias after cardiac infarction to sinus rhythm, we have seldom found it necessary to use it, bearing in mind that so many of these rhythms take the form of short paroxysms in a

heart whose rhythmicity is temporarily disturbed following the acute
ischaemic episode.

Prognosis

Although 5 out of the 41 patients with atrial arrhythmias in our
series died, only one of these appeared to die an arrhythmic death,
the other four being already severely ill from other complications
such as renal failure, ruptured ventricular septum or the development
of a large cardiac aneurysm. The atrial arrhythmias *per se*, therefore,
appeared to carry a relatively good prognosis, although they were
also frequently associated with seriously damaged hearts. This
association is clearly shown in Table II, where certain major factors

Table II. *Relationship of certain general factors to death
and survival in patients with atrial arrhythmias*

	Died	Survived
Number of Patients	5 {3 Men / 2 Women}	36 {32 Men / 4 Women}
Average age	60 years	57 years
Hypertension	2	12
Left ventricular failure . . .	5	9
Average duration of ischaemic heart disease	41 months	27 months
L.B.B.B.	3	1
L.D.H. enzymes	919 i.u. Heat Stable 63%	394 i.u. Heat Stable 64%

are listed, likely to influence the overall prognosis after cardiac
infarction. It will be seen that the average age of the five patients
who died was slightly higher than of those who survived. Hypertension was almost equally common in the two groups. Left
ventricular failure was present in all those who died, but in only
a quarter of those who survived. Similarly, the average length of
the history of ischaemic heart disease was longer in the patients
who died. Left bundle branch block was also found to carry a
very poor prognosis. Finally, the average level of the lactic dehydrogenase enzymes was about 2½ times higher in those who
died, suggesting that these patients probably had larger cardiac
infarcts.

CONCLUSIONS

In general, atrial arrhythmias after acute cardiac infarction, are frequent, occurring in nearly 50 per cent. of patients. They are usually relatively benign, short-lived and self-terminating. Treatment should be primarily directed to improving the general state of the circulation and to combating heart failure. Specific drug treatment for arrhythmias is only required in about half of the patients, special emphasis being laid on cardiac glycosides and atropine. Intravenous lignocaine may sometimes be beneficial in suppressing frequent atrial extrasystoles, often prodromal to atrial fibrillation. The place of quinidine or procaine amide in treating supraventricular tachycardias after acute cardiac infarction is debatable. Similar caution should be used in the prophylactic employment of beta-blocking agents because of their myocardial depressant action. The indications for electrical cardioversion in this group of arrhythmias are probably limited, due to their short paroxysmal nature and the temporary arrhythmic instability of the heart. None the less, where an atrial arrhythmia is prolonged, rapid and resistant to other forms of treatment, cardioversion may sometimes be valuable, effective and life-saving.

REFERENCE

FLUCK, D. C., OLSEN, E., PENTECOST, B. L., THOMAS, M., FILLMORE, S. J., SHILLINGFORD, J. P. & MOUNSEY, J. P. D. (1967). The natural history and clinical significance of arrhythmias after acute cardiac infarction. *Br. Heart J.* **29**, 170.

DISCUSSION

Dr. Dalle. I consider that arrhythmias are bad either because they warn of death-producing arrhythmias which occur later on or because they affect haemodynamics adversely. They do so for four reasons: 1. They can be too rapid. 2. They can be irregular. 3. They can cause the loss of the atrial contribution to ventricular filling. 4. Aberrant intraventricular conduction may cause decreased efficiency of ventricular contraction.

Whether or not atrial arrhythmias are a sign of atrial infarction or a sign of left ventricular failure with left atrial dilatation, is important because therapy has to be very different. If ventricular failure is present we have to be aggressive and I would like first to ask Dr Meltzer what he would do with a patient in good condition, without overt signs of congestive failure, who develops rapid atrial fibrillation in the course of otherwise uncomplicated infarction.

Dr Meltzer. I would defibrillate the patient immediately and I would *not* digitalise him. I would stop atrial fibrillation as soon as I found it and would not tolerate it for one minute. It is a decompensating mechanism.

Dr Dalle. You believe that atrial fibrillation is bad because it is sometimes rapid, always irregular and it always takes away the atrial contribution to ventricular filling? Dr Lown believes that it is generally, if not always, caused by left ventricular failure so we will leave him to answer Dr Meltzer.

Dr Lown. The majority of atrial arrhythmias evolve out of some power failure. This has been our view and the effiicacy of digitalis supports this. It is striking how short lived atrial arrhythmias are. It is also striking how often they are recurrent and at times long-lasting, and therefore the objective is not to engage in a technical legerdemain of cardioversion which I wish I could support and sponsor, but rather to go to the fundamental basis of the arrhythmia and digitalise these patients, Dr Mounsey indicated that anterior infarcts are more frequent in this group and that severe ischaemic heart disease was more frequently present: in effect these are serious infarcts. At present, our capacity to diagnose incipient left ventricular failure is weak, and until better techniques come along, we regard these arrhythmias as good markers of the unrecognised presence of left ventricular failure. If this is so, digitalisation certainly is an appropraite therapeutic procedure. We have had an incidence of atrial flutter of 5·3 per cent. and of atrial fibrillation of 13 per cent. The prognostic implication of these arrhythmias is that in atrial flutter we have had a mortality of 44 per cent. and in those with atrial fibrillation of 33 per cent. These figures indicate the magnitude of the infarction and the coincidence of heart failure. These are the factors—not the arrhythmia itself. The arrhythmia is merely a barometer indicating the functional state of the heart and therefore cardioversion is not an appropraite first approach.

Dr Dalle. Would you agree with the statement that it is hard to predict which arrhythmia will recur after termination and which will not recur?

Dr Lown. This is so. Our therapy therefore goes further and those people who have exhibited such atrial arrhythmias we maintain on quinidine.

Dr Dalle. In other words, therefore, it is not only a barometer, it also participates in the eventual further deterioration of the patient. It would probably be good to start with drugs. Either you terminate it with drugs or you do not. If you do not, it would not probably harm anyone to cardiovert the patient and then to look for a good maintenance therapy—for instance, quinidine or digitalis.

Dr Lown. I agree entirely, Cardioversion is not a major heresy.

Professor Shillingford. What evidence do you have, Dr Lown, that it is fibrillation that follows power failure rather than power failure that follows fibrillation?

Dr Lown. We are not able to say dogmatically that this is so, but we are able to suggest it.

Professor Shillingford. How often do you hear a third heart sound before the onset of fibrillation? How often do you have a fall in blood pressure before the onset of fibrillation? In my experience, fibrillation occurs absolutely out of the blue.

Dr Dalle. I think this comes back to the two aetiologies of atrial fibrillation, one being the possibility of atrial injury and the other that a dilated left atrium is prone to develop atrial fibrillation. Probably both occur. We are unable to detect left ventricular end-diastolic pressure elevation early enough. We are only measuring pulmonary artery pressures or listening to sounds or trying to find a gallop. Left ventricular failure may, in fact, have developed much earlier.

Dr Meltzer. If 33 per cent. of the people with atrial fibrillation die, I suggest you try my approach. We don't have anywhere near a 33 per cent. mortality. Professor Shillingford is quite right. Since we have been monitoring the cardiovascular system as a functional mechanism we have noticed people go into failure after the arrhythmia rather than the other way round as you suggest, and the major therapy should be to terminate this arrhythmia promptly by cardioversion and digitalise the patient thereafter.

Dr Wallace. Just one comment with regard to the incidence of atrial infarction. James has described the histology of the atrium in, I believe, 10 or 12 patients with myocardial infarction and atrial arrhythmias, and found that all of them had infarction involving the sinus node. We have had six patients whom we have studied this way, and so far all have had infarction involving the atrium. Whether they were in failure or not I think is a debatable issue, but the current evidence does support the contention that they do have atrial infarction even though we cannot diagnose it clinically.

Dr Mounsey. In our group we had autopsies in both of the two patients with supraventricular tachycardia who died. In neither was there evidence of atrial infarction and in neither were either of the arteries to the node blocked. Although atrial infarction and damage to the node is obviously a real entity in some patients, it would be an unlikely explanation for the arrhythmias in our patients, as these were transient and they soon went back into sinus rhythm. One of them died six weeks later after being in sinus rhythm for a month.

Dr Dalle. I think there is a striking difference between atrial fibrillation and atrial flutter. I think almost everyone will agree that digitalis is rather unreliable and certainly unpredictable with atrial flutter and that cardioversion is advised as the first measure. There may be a case for initial administration of a small dose of digitalis but certainly not full digitalisation.

Dr Killip. I do not think there is much doubt that supraventricular arrhythmias tend to recur and immediate electrical treatment will not prevent that. Our own view is that what is really important is the ventricular rate and I think we can be led astray by being primarily concerned with a supraventricular arrhythmia, rather than primarily concerned with the patient's heart.

Professor Shillingford. These rhythms change frequently and our policy is to watch the patient, not his rhythm, to see what the circulation is doing, especially the cerebral circulation. If there is any evidence of deterioration in the circulation then he will treat the arrhythmia but if you wait half the cases will come out of the arrhythmia spontaneously. I think if you shock the heart you will get a little further damage perhaps.

Dr Semple (Glasgow). May I at this stage mention briefly a new method of treating such arrhythmias? I think it has some significance in the present discussion. I would like to describe a single patient. A man of 75, known to have had two myocardial infarcts, came into hospital with supraventricular tachycardia and we digitalised him. He was not in failure on admission but by next morning he had developed failure and we decided to convert his arrhythmia. Possibly Dr Lown would criticise us for giving as big a shock as 100 watt seconds. He developed ventricular fibrillation and we shocked him out of that into sinus bradycardia. Then he developed A.V. dissociation and later V.F.; he was shocked into asystole. Again he developed A.V. dissociation and then V.F.; after further D.C. shock supraventricular tachycardia returned. I do not know why but once more we shocked him and again produced V.F. Eventually after this exciting procedure he came out of his anaesthetic and said, ' Did it go quite well doctor? ' He was well after that, but had ventricular extrasystoles. We put him on a lignocaine drip and two days later he was back into supraventricular tachycardia with right bundle branch block. I just could not face another cardioversion in this man, but we did something just as good and restored sinus rhythm. After this we kept him on the lignocaine drip as he still continued to have extrasystoles. The next day he again developed supraventricular tachycardia this time with left bundle branch block. Once more the procedure led to a few extrasystoles, and then sinus rhythm with ventricular ectopics. He did very well after this. Indeed he left hospital apparently well but was readmitted 10 days later again with supraventricular tachycardia. The same procedure again put him back into sinus rhythm. Since then he has been on procaine amide and had no further arrhythmias. The procedure we used was a sharp blow over the apex of the heart. I am not saying this is a safe procedure and that you can get rid of all your cardioverters, but you will agree that in this case it was safer than cardioversion. On each occasion this man was on the monitor and an intravenous drip was ready for anti-arrhythmic drugs. We took all possible precautions in case he went into V.F. This is an unsynchronised shock and in each case it produced ectopic beat. There is no doubt that that ectopic beat could fall on a T-wave and I would not suggest anyone trying this without full precautions.

Dr Sloman. In our experience of atrial fibrillation there has been an overall mortality of 40 per cent. and we have found that the prognosis has been related to the clinical state at the time of their first admission to the unit, and was not made any worse by the occurrence of atrial fibrillation alone. However, arrhythmias in addition to atrial fibrillation have made the prognosis worse. We feel that it is not quite right to call atrial fibrillation a benign arrhythmia but it is not as malignant an arrhythmia as has been reported in the literature, where mortalities of up to 50 and 60 per cent. have been recorded. We have had no patients with embolism, whereas in the literature there are records of high proportions of patients with embolism associated with atrial fibrillation. Dr Julian's paper mentioned this and his incidence of embolism associated with atrial fibrillation is also very low. I should mention, though, that we have felt obliged to revert two of these patients who had atrial fibrillation when this was associated with quite obvious haemodynamic deterioration.

Dr Nixon. I have difficulty with the definition of left ventricular failure. There are distinct stages in its development—where the atrium is overacting, where the patient is breathing a little more quickly because his lungs are stiffening up, and the terminal stage of pulmonary oedema. Dr Mounsey seems to treat it like a pregnancy

—it's either there or not. Will you please say what your definitions were?

Dr Mounsey. I think you have made a good point and it's not possible without careful monitoring of the pressures to define with certainty exactly what you are dealing with. Most of us are unable to measure directly left atrial pressure. Our estimate in these patients of the presence of left ventricular failure was based on the overall picture, and most of them were not in frank pulmonary oedema. They had daily chest X-rays, which were looked at critically by the radiologist, and we recognised early signs of congestion there. They had a raised respiratory rate, but were often not breathless and could lie flat even when the evidence of failure on chest X-rays was quite obvious. In many of the patients we had a catheter in the pulmonary artery and, although this is only an indirect measurement of what is going on in the left side of the heart, in all of these patients the pulmonary artery pressure was raised. Crepitations at the bases are also an important sign but are to be interpreted with reservation.

ELECTRICAL INSTABILITY OF THE HEART

BERNARD LOWN

From the Medical Clinics of the Peter Bent Brigham Hospital and the Cardio-vascular Research Laboratories, Department of Nutrition, Harvard School of Public Health, Boston, Massachusetts.

THE lessons learned from coronary care will probably find most important application to the high risk ambulatory patients with coronary artery disease. Actually, the major problem exists outside the hospital. The findings of Kuller and his colleagues (1966) indicate that in Baltimore City 20·6 per cent. of all coronary deaths between ages 40 and 64 occurred outside the hospital and 46·2 per cent. were dead on arrival. Thus 67 per cent. were dead before hospitalisation.

This larger problem will remain until a number of questions are answered and dealt with. Is sudden death in ambulatory patients due to ventricular arrhythmias? Are there premonitory rhythm disorders as are observed in the patient in the coronary care unit? If this is indeed true, what is the interval between the innocuous disorder and the electrical catastrophe? Is the time sufficient to permit effective medical intervention? What clinical factors distinguish the group susceptible to sudden death? Did these patients have electrical instability of the heart beat? Is this instability determinable? If so, how? These are but some of the many questions. The content of the answers will determine the direction of medical endeavour. One possibility is the monitoring of selected high risk coronary patients. However, the large scope of such effort required to yield any significant results would preclude this as an undertaking except with investigative intent. A prerequisite to such effort is the evolvement of tests which will predict the individual susceptible to sudden death, namely, the patient with electrical instability of the heart beat. By this is meant the susceptibility of the heart to repetitive ventricular response.

EXPERIMENTAL STUDIES

Ventricular vulnerability

I would like to review certain animal experiments which suggest a possible approach to this problem. In dogs, following a two-stage occlusion of the left anterior descending coronary artery there is no alteration in the position of the vulnerable period with relation to the Q-T interval. The only change is an increase in duration of the ventricular vulnerable period by about 21 per cent. Following myocardial infarction, there is no change in threshold energy for ventricular fibrillation. The threshold to transthoracic shock remains at 1 Joule (J) and for internal stimulation the figure is about 40,000 microjoules. Following coronary occlusion, however, ventricular tachycardia can be elicited from the vulnerable period for the first time. This arrhythmia has been designated as $VT_{(vp)}$. A typical example is illustrated in Figure 1. This arrhythmia follows whether the discharges was delivered transthoracically or directly to the myocardium by unipolar electrodes. It was never observed in the non-ligated animal. Low energy shocks administered in any other parts of the cardiac cycle did not result in $VT_{(vp)}$.

The vulnerable periods for $VT_{(vp)}$ and for ventricular fibrillation (VF) were of identical duration. The median threshold energy of shock for producing $VT_{(vp)}$ was 29 per cent. that required to produce VF. The lowest discharge energy which produced $VT_{(vp)}$ was 0·01 J or watt seconds (Fig. 2).

An analysis of 253 episodes of $VT_{(vp)}$ showed a number of distinctive features. The ventricular rate was extremely rapid; the mean rate was 359 ± 114. As one might expect there was a significant compromise of systemic pressure with this arrhythmia.

85

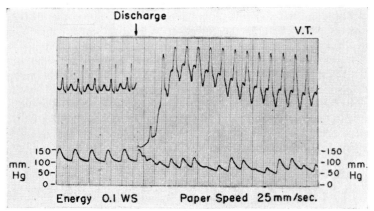

FIG. 1. Ventricular tachycardia of the vulnerable period—VT$_{(vp)}$—is produced by a 0·1 Joule (or w.s.) shock delivered in the ventricular vulnerable period. The animal had ligation of the left anterior coronary artery 72 hours earlier.

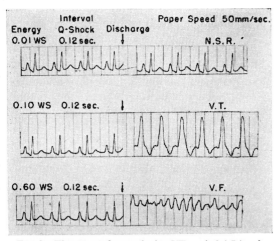

FIG. 2. The energy for producing VT$_{(vp)}$ is 0·1 J (w.s.) while for ventricular fibrillation (VF) it is 0·6 J (w.s.). The synchronisation from the Q wave is the same, or 0·12 seconds. The shock falls at the apex of the T wave and coincides with the ventricular vulnerable period.

However, in some animals there was a restoration of pressure toward normal though the heart rate remained unaltered. This occurred because of sequential changes in cycle length simulating coupled pacing of the heart (Fig. 3). The arrhythmia was always unifocal. The energy for restoring sinus mechanism was of the same order as that required to initiate the arrhythmia. In 39 episodes the minimal energy for reversion was 0.65 ± 0.23 J. This contrasts strikingly with the energy required to revert VF by

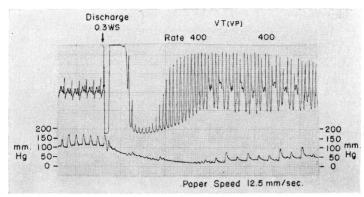

FIG. 3. $VT_{(vp)}$ at a rate of 400 with a marked compromise in systemic pressure which is improved as soon as irregularity in ventricular rhythm is spontaneously established.

electrical discharge. While in 65 per cent. of normal dogs VF can be restored to normal sinus rhythm at an energy of 70 J or less, after myocardial infarction the energy for transthoracic shock increases to 190 J. When VF was produced in the same animal during the same experiment, the energy needed to revert VF was 200 to 400 times greater than that needed to abolish $VT_{(vp)}$.

When $VT_{(vp)}$ was not controlled, in 75 per cent. it resulted in VF. Thus it is a prefibrillatory disorder. It can be produced within an hour after the coronary artery ligation and for about five to seven days thereafter. In the second week 90 per cent. of animals are immune to further development of $VT_{(vp)}$. In a small percentage, however, this susceptibility lasted indefinitely. This can be predicted by persistence of an aneurysmal type of current of injury in the electrocardiogram. If catecholamines are administered when this response is waning, it redevelops and then the animal behaves as though acute myocardial infarction had been induced more recently.

A similar phenomenon has been observed in patients with acute myocardial infarction. $VT_{(vp)}$, as shown in Figure 4, occurred in this patient within the first 72 hours. An extrasystole falling early in the cycle will trigger bursts of ventricular tachycardia. In order to do so, there has to be an interruption of the T wave. Generally this can be expressed as a function of the Q-T interval. When the QR'/QT ranges from 0·60 to 0·85, $VT_{(vp)}$ will occur.

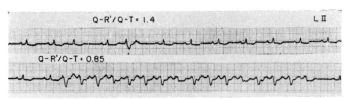

FIG. 4. Patient within 24 hours after onset of acute myocardial infarction. When Q-R'/Q-T is 1·4, ventricular ectopic beats are single. However, when this ratio is abbreviated to 0·85, $VT_{(vp)}$ results.

SOME THEORETIC CONSIDERATIONS

The myocardium is not an absolutely homogeneous tissue as regards propagation of excitation. Recovery from the refractory period is a slower process and is even more dispersed. When an impulse is delivered to the heart during the vulnerable period, it encounters an irregularly excitable field and is forced to propagate at a subnormal velocity and over a tortuous pathway. This favours re-entry of the depolarisation wave and self-sustained activity. Each successive re-entry augments the initial non-uniformity. Fibres responding early will exhibit a shorter refractory period than those responding later. This further contributes to the inhomogeneity and results in increased dispersion of both duration of refractoriness and velocity of conduction. The work of Moe and his colleagues (Han *et al.*, 1966; Han & Moe, 1967; Moe *et al.*, 1967) has provided much evidence indicating that those agencies which increase temporal dispersion of recovery from the refractory state predispose to fibrillation. Since $VT_{(vp)}$ can be provoked in the animal with acute myocardial infarction by delivering an electrical pulse during the vulnerable period, a mechanism of re-entry is also the probable basis for this arrhythmia.

Perpetuation of a re-entrant wave form arrhythmia requires four conditions: an obstacle around which the wave may propagate, a tissue mass of sufficient size, a mean refractory period sufficiently brief and a slow conduction velocity. These conditions are met at the perimeter of an infarct. It is of interest that studies in our laboratory with multiple bipolar leads in the animal with myocardial infarction have shown that $VT_{(vp)}$ cannot be evoked except from the area of infarction itself or from its very closest proximity. It may be that a low energy shock activates a single pathway around the perimeter of the infarction which becomes self-sustaining. Higher energy shocks would then activate multiple sites which would lead to fractionation of the pathway of propagation and thereby favour VF.

The elicitation of repetitive ventricular response (RVR) from the vulnerable period therefore suggests the existence of electrical instability, a possible precondition for ventricular fibrillation and sudden death.

Digitalis drugs

Electrical instability can also be demonstrated to exist in the diastolic period outside the ventricular vulnerable period. In the non-digitalised animal, when a single electrical discharge was delivered directly to the myocardium, a single propagated response resulted. In order to produce RVR from a single stimulus delivered outside the ventricular vulnerable period, energies of several Joules were required. In a large number of animals the mean energy for ventricular tachycardia was 5·9 J. These are massive energies. There was, however, a remarkable change in threshold in the digitalised animal. After recovery from ouabain-induced ventricular tachycardia, the energy for RVR was reduced by six orders of magnitude. The results were the same whether stimulation was from the right ventricular cavity, the surfaces of the right or left ventricles or from the left ventricular myocardium. The phenomenon of RVR was not dependent on the type of wave form employed. Of greatest interest is that the point of initial as well as maximum sensitivity was well beyond the outer boundary of the vulnerable period and usually coincided with the very terminal portion of the T wave. This phenomenon lasted for more than four times the usual duration of overt drug toxicity.

During progressive digitalisation with acetyl strophanthidin, electrical sensitivity was first detected when 400 to 600 micrograms of drug was administered. This represented about 40 to 70 per cent. of the toxic dose. The initial response was a dual coupled beat. As more drug was infused, the response to a single stimulus became increasingly repetitive with emergence of paroxysms of long lasting ventricular tachycardia. At the onset of electrical sensitivity the zone of multiple response was of 20 msec. duration. With increasing doses of glycoside it rapidly extended into diastole and also into the relative and absolute refractory periods. Before the onset of a digitalis toxic response the sensitive zone embraced over 60 per cent. of the cardiac cycle. What relevance does this have to the problem of myocardial infarction? Our recent investigations indicate a number of changes in the digitalised animal with acute myocardial infarction. The threshold for RVR is remarkably reduced during the ventricular vulnerable period. The phenomenon of RVR is much longer lasting and it takes less digitalis to evoke this response in the ischaemic heart.

These two approaches present but preliminary studies of the problem of determining whether susceptibility to ventricular fibrillation and tachycardia can be detected. The area of electrical instability must be carefully investigated, for the challenge is indeed great.

Supported by grants HE-07776-04, 5 TI-HE-5242, PO 1-HE-11306-01 from the National Institutes of Health; the John A. Hartford Foundation; the Fund for Research and Teaching, Department of Nutrition, Harvard School of Public Health.

REFERENCES

HAN, J. & MOE, G. K. (1967). Non-uniform recovery of excitability in ventricular muscle. *Circulation Res.* **14**, 44.
HAN, J., JALON, G. P. D. DE & MOE, G. K. (1966). Fibrillation threshold of premature ventricular responses. *Circulation Res.* **18**, 18.
KULLER, L., LILIENFELD, A. & FISHER, R. (1966). Epidemiology study of sudden and unexpected deaths due to arterio-sclerotic heart disease. *Circulation*, **34**, 1056.
MOE, G. K., ALBIDSKOV, J. A. & HAN, J. (1967). Factors responsible for the initiation and maintenance of ventricular fibrillation. In *Sudden Cardiac Death*, p. 56, ed. SURAWICZ, B. & PELLEGRINE, E. D. New York: Grune & Stratton.

DISCUSSION

Dr Leatham (London). I think there should be a general discussion of factors increasing the vulnerability of the heart to ventricular fibrillation. The threshold for ventricular fibrillation is clearly lowered, as has been shown by Dr Lown, following cardiac infarction and digitalis. What other factors make the heart clinically (that is in the bedside care of patients) more vulnerable to electrical instability or more electrically unstable? One is pericarditis and I think that Dr Sowton has reported previously six patients, four of whom died, with ventricular fibrillation. These deaths occurred in patients who were in the post-operative period following the insertion of epicardial pacing electrodes. Admittedly, the power of the pacemakers that we were using at that time was much higher than we use at present and this may have been a factor; following this report we always use low-power pacemaking. But one wonders whether the post-operative period and perhaps pericarditis were not factors. Perhaps this is one of the reasons for using endocardial pacing systems. I would like to ask Dr Sowton whether he thinks pericarditis is a factor or whether he thinks there were other factors in the cases that he reported.

Dr Sowton. I think pericarditis is a factor but there were also other factors in those patients. They had surgical trauma at the site where the impulse had been applied, which may have led to irritability in that region. Some of them were having drugs at the same time. The pace-makers were producing rather long impulses and there was a big area of contact between the electrodes and the heart. Under those particular circumstances, there were many other factors not present after myocardial infarction.

Dr Rossi (Rome). In addition to digitalis, susceptibility to ventricular tachycardia can be due to other causes—some known and others improperly understood—for example inhibited membrane exchange and electrolytic disturbances, hypoxia or different degrees of myocardial oxygenation in different parts of the heart.

Dr Oliver. You have approached this largely from the point of view of digitalis, Dr Lown, but your opening remarks were concerned with increased excitability due to infarction. It would be interesting in view of what Dr Rossi has said to examine what might be operating in the absence of drugs; in other words, to what extent hypoxia and altered membrane exchange may contribute.

Dr Lown. Digitalis is but one special case. The objective of describing experiments is not so much to show that you can reduce cardioversion energy in the presence of digitalis but to indicate that possibly we now have a method of assessing the degree of digitalisation. By electrically pulsing the heart and finding repetitive responses—in the dog at least—we can now assess the degree of digitalisation, a problem that has been with us since Withering in 1785 launched the drug. But digitalis is one of many factors that will be conducive to instability. It is of importance that unless there is inhomogeneity ventricular fibrillation is not favoured. For example, it has been long known that asphyxiated animals die from asystole and not from ventricular fibrillation. In this circumstance the effect is global and there is less likelihood of ventricular fibrillation. Inhomogeneity of adjacent fibres is, therefore, a very important factor. Again, stimulation of the vagus predisposes to atrial fibrillation. The reason, perhaps, for this is that vagal stimulation shortens the refractory period only of those fibres that are innervated and the adjacent fibres that are not innervated therefore have a different refractory period, permitting the development of multiple wavelets of depolarisation. Inhomogeneity is one very important factor and drugs which produce it will favour ventricular fibrillation. Changes in potassium may also be important and certainly digitalis does induce profound changes in the exchange flux of potassium from myocardial as well as other tissues —red cells, skeletal muscle, etc. Whether change in membrane stability is a factor I do not know.

Dr Wallace. I think there are a variety of influences that can lead to inhomogeneity which generally tend to reduce the fibrillation threshold. One awkward experiment that has been performed demonstrated that quinidine enhances inhomogeneity but presumably it does not enhance vulnerability; at least in the work we have done it seems either to do nothing or to raise fibrillation threshold. I would be interested to know whether you have ever studied quinidine to see whether it makes the heart more or less vulnerable.

Dr Lown. It makes the heart less vulnerable to electrical instability. Both quinidine and potassium make it less vulnerable.

Dr Wallace. I think one of the more practical aspects of the problem of inhomogeneity relates to the recovery of the heart following premature excitation. We have found that with premature ventricular beats and premature atrial beats, the vulnerability of the heart is markedly increased following one premature beat, even more so after three or four in a run. From experiments in dogs we have been able to show a 30 to 40 per cent. drop in fibrillation threshold after four premature ventricular beats and we have become very concerned about the potential lethality of a pacemaker operating in a patient who is having bouts of ventricular tachycardia. The fibrillation threshold with a square wave pulse of 2 milliseconds duration can be as low as 0.5 ma. after three or four premature beats whereas it is 25 or 30 ma. after a normal beat. This is true whether the premature beat is atrial or ventricular in origin. Another area for consideration is the problem of temperature gradients. We became interested in the phenomena of fibrillation during recovery from cardiac surgery, where measurements have shown that there are significant temperature gradients of as much as 4 or 5 degrees Centigrade between the endocardium and the epicardium. This degree of inhomogeneity resulting from temperature differences will certainly favour the development of ventricular fibrillation. So I think that lack of homogeneity in response is a very real factor that can be induced by physical phenomena, such as premature beats or temperature gradients and can be accentuated by drugs that we use commonly.

Dr Dalle. Quinidine has been shown to enhance the possibility of repetitive firing in dogs being paced during its administration. The experiments were simple—the dogs were paced asynchronously so that the vulnerable period of the T wave was hit repetitively and then relatively high therapeutic dosages were administered—this induced repetitive firing in these animals. Another thing which may be important is that quinidine and procaine amide are known to be deleterious in ectopic rhythms when there is also a prolonged QT interval—for instance, with complete heart block or myocardial infarction, hypokalaemia or administration of other drugs. On the one hand, therefore, we have an increase in the fibrillation threshold and on the other, we have inhomogeneity facilitating the induction of fibrillation.

Dr Lown. The classification of arrhythmias suggested earlier this morning is an attempt to get away from the arbitrary anatomical classification and proceed to a physiological one. For example with ventricular ectopic beats, there is a good deal of physiological evidence to show that small currents passed along Purkinje fibres lower the threshold of automaticity. If an electrical beat falls on a vulnerable period the interesting question is ' How does it activate ventricular fibrillation? ' If you have a pacemaker beating asynchronously it will fall in the vulnerable period hundreds of times or more in the course of a day without activating a vulnerable period. What happens in myocardial infarction in addition to generation of ectopic beats is that an ectopic beat has the capacity somehow to lower the threshold for ventricular fibrillation and repetitive beats lower it more so.

Dr McDonald. It seems to me there is a difference between ectopic rhythms in cardiac infarction and cardiomyopathy. The latter may show any of these ectopic rhythms but they do not have the same likelihood of going on to ventricular fibrillation.

Dr Lown. I think that the peri-infarction area differs in several ways. One is that potassium gradients may exist and small gradients may produce an impulse and activate fibres. There may be differences in the gradients of catecholamines and of oxygen concentration. Many years ago the current of oxygen differential was considered responsible for arrhythmias. We know that if we stimulate the heart of a healthy animal we cannot get repetitive responses; if we stimulate the intact part of the heart in an animal with infarction, we cannot get any repetitive responses either. The closer we come to the infarcted area the more likely they are to occur. Therefore the area of instability is around the infarct. The brady-arrhythmias are of great interest because it has been shown that the tendency to ectopic beats increases as the heart slows. It does not matter what the factor is provoking ectopic beats—be it hypothermia, be it coronary ligation, be it pressure-overload of the heart—in all these circumstances the onset of ectopic beats is inversely related to cycle length. Furthermore in bradycardia there is a great dispersion of the duration of refractory periods, therefore the threshold to ventricular fibrillation is lowered and bradycardias are potentially true arrhythmias. Inhomogeneity is, thus, something that will have to receive a lot more attention. As regards treatment the warning signal to us is whenever the QT is prolonged, it is possible that some inhomogeneity of the heart and the tendency to ventricular fibrillation exists.

VENTRICULAR TACHYCARDIA

YVES BOUVRAIN

Hôpital Lariboisière, Paris

DURING a period of six years we have noticed bouts of ventricular tachycardia (V.T.) in 51 patients during the early stage of the myocardial infarction in the intensive Cardiac Care Unit of the Hôpital Lariboisière.

We did not take into account either short sequences of ventricular extrasystoles happening against a background of sinus rhythm or slow ventricular rhythms as described by Puech (of which we had some examples) but exclusively those episodes which were sufficiently long and at such a fast rate as to need emergency treatment. Neither did we take into account the bouts of V.T. occurring during the course of an A.V. block in myocardial infarction. These 51 patients have been selected among a total of 556 with acute myocardial infarction; but on account of the selection of the cases sent into our Unit, this has no statistical value. Moreover these observations are about a third of the whole of our ventricular tachycardias.

Occurrence

Our patients included 40 men and 11 women, ranging in age from 39 to 83.

The localisation of the infarct was posterior in 30; and anterior and/or septal in 21.

The time of onset was:

1st day . . .	12
From 2nd to 7th day .	17
From 8th to 20th day .	12
From 21st to 28th day .	6
After the end of bedrest	4

This shows a prevalence of the bouts of V.T. during the first week (58 per cent.) but this is less distinct than for other disturbances of the rhythm, chiefly A.V. blocks (96 per cent. in our statistics). This distribution is noteworthy since 20 per cent. of the V.T. took place after the third week.

Electrocardiogram

The ECG findings are the same as those of V.T. of other aetiologies and the oesophageal leads are always very useful for differentiating it from supraventricular tachycardias with bundle branch block, V.T. with retrograde conduction and multifocal V.T.

We had some cases of retrograde conduction with Wenckebach periods, the RP interval increasing progressively until a P wave falls out. With retrograde conduction 1/1 the diagnosis might be impossible, but pressure on eyeballs is sometimes helpful.

Clinical aspects

In spite of contrary opinions episodes of V.T. happening in the early stages of the infarction can often be well tolerated, at least during the first hours; such was the case with 17 of our patients, but the tolerance was poor in 10 and very bad in 24, in whom acute circulatory failure developed.

It is important to note that syncope occurred with the onset of the bout in eight patients, for then it is difficult to distinguish between V.T. and fibrillation, especially when we do not have three synchronous leads (and is often the case in emergencies). Indeed these very high speed, syncopal V.Ts., sometimes described as ventricular flutter, imply a prognosis very different from that of actual fibrillation. This fact perhaps explains some discrepancies between statistical results of resuscitation in myocardial infarction.

Treatment

In seven patients the episode of V.T. ceased spontaneously or after an injection of hydroxizin-morphine administered as premedication before the electric shock.

In 31 patients the shock was applied. We had 23 successes, generally after one or two shocks. The conversion failed in eight patients, with two deaths in two patients already dying when admitted into the Care Unit. In three cases the shock started a V. F. and with a second shock sinus rhythm was at once obtained.

In 13 patients 50 mg. of Ajmalin were injected intravenously with 10 successes and 3 failures. This drug was responsible for two episodes of asystole, both quickly ended after cardiac massage. This risk is well known and is possible with all depressive drugs, but Ajmalin has the advantage of being promptly catabolised, so the critical period is short.

In four patients who had long runs of V.T. separated by some sinus beats the disappearance of the ectopic activity was obtained with a perfusion of procaine amide.

It would seem, therefore, from the data presented that there is no significant difference between effect of shock and Ajmalin; the former can be used everywhere, but on account of its depressive effect, the latter is to be preferred only in the hospital.

RESULTS

After immediate treatment 44 patients recovered sinus rhythm, two died, and in five the V.T. continued, but in all these five cases sinus rhythm was re-established within one or two days either by another shock or by Ajmalin. We can also emphasise the fact that in one patient, it was impossible to stop the V.T. and the condition deteriorated. We then inserted a catheter electrode into the right ventricle and it was possible, using coupled stimulation, to decrease the frequency by half. Improvement was obtained and after some hours conversion became possible.

LATER RESULTS

Nine patients had one or more recurrent bouts of V.T., the maximum being 11 recurrences. But after a few days, Ajmalin or procaine amide being administered first intravenously, then orally, the ventricular hyperexcitability ended in most cases.

Finally, 13 patients died within a few days or weeks of admission, two owing to uncontrollable V.T., five sudden deaths (and among them 3 fibrillations) and six acute myocardial failures with sinus rhythm.

CONCLUSION

The data of 51 patients having had one or more bouts of V.T. during the early phase of myocardial infarction are presented.

Thirty-six patients were discharged alive in apparently good condition. Three of them only had very late recurrence. Fifteen died, two immediately after admission, the others during the course of the first month. The mortality rate, therefore, was 30 per cent. This is approximately the same as in all our patients with infarction.

VENTRICULAR FIBRILLATION

DUNCAN LAWRIE
Royal Infirmary, Edinburgh

As reports of ventricular fibrillation (V.F.) occurring in coronary care units accumulated over the past years, it soon became apparent that it arises in a variety of clinical situations. The concept of primary and secondary V.F. (Meltzer & Kitchell, 1966)—primary in the absence of shock or marked circulatory failure—emphasised the totally different prognosis in the two groups. However, after some experience of our own we felt that a wider spectrum existed and the following classifications was proposed (Oliver *et al.*, 1967):

1. Primary   In the patient without signs of cardiac failure and/or hypotension (systolic blood pressure < 100 mm. Hg.).

2. Complicating   Complicating pre-existing cardiac failure and/or hypotension.

3. Agonal   In patients who before the development of V.F. have already lost a vital function such as blood pressure or respiration.

4. Pacemaker induced.

5. Drug induced.

The importance of this classification is to differentiate complicating V.F. from agonal V.F. as well as pointing out that, on occasion,

V.F. may be produced by therapy. The essence of an agonal rhythm is that it appears after some vital function has disappeared— it represents continuing electrical activity despite mechanical death. Table I shows our total experience of V.F. over a 16-month period.

Table I. *Patients with ventricular fibrillation*

Type	Routine	Non-Routine	Total
Primary	15	2	17
Complicating	23	10	33
Agonal	4	0	4
Pacemaker	5	2	7
Drug	3	1	4

Our patients are from two sources (1) routine admissions to the Coronary Care Unit, and (2) emergency or non-routine patients who are first admitted to the general wards and subsequently transferred to the CCU because of the development of dangerous arrhythmias. I wish to deal briefly with the last three groups and more fully with the primary and complicating patients.

Agonal V.F., in our experience, is an uncommon rhythm and appears confined to those patients who have been given sympathomimetic drugs (Lown *et al.*, 1967).

Pacemaker induced V.F. is now well recognised and I do not need to mention it further (Paulk & Hurst, 1966).

It may be extremely difficult if not impossible to decide when V.F. has occurred as the result of drug therapy. We have only placed patients in this category when there has been a very clear temporal relationship between the giving of a drug and the onset of V.F. Three of our cases were due to digoxin, the remaining one to isoprenaline.

Some of the earliest literature on V.F. suggested that it was more common in males and particularly in the younger patient (Julian *et al.*, 1964). Table II deals only with 'routine' patients as the 'non-routine' group is obviously a highly selected one and cannot be included when analysing results. You will note that we did not find an undue number of males. However, in the primary group, the average age was considerably less than that for all patients and 47 per cent. were under 50 years of age, whereas of all routine cases only 19 per cent. were in this age range. You will see from Table II also that the incidence of V.F.—only primary

Table II. *' Routine' patients with ventricular fibrillation*

Type	Male	Female	Average Age	No. <50 yrs of age	
Primary . . .	11	4	53·0	7	(47%)
Complicating . .	17	6	60·0	4	(17%)

and complicating cases—was almost 8 per cent. This is as encountered by many other units (Julian *et al*, 1964; Conference Report, 1966; Goble *et al.*, 1966). It is when one comes to consider the timing of the arrest that I think one finds the chief characteristic of V.F. It is a complication which occurs early in the course of myocardial infarction. This is especially so in the primary group (Table III) for, as you will see, more than half the

Table III. *(' Routine' and ' non-routine' patients.)   Timing of ventricular fibrillation*

Primary V.F.—17 patients
   10 (60 per cent.) within 4 hours of onset of symptoms
   14 (82 per cent.) within 12 hours of onset of symptoms
   13 (76 per cent.) within 2 hours of admission

Complicating V.F.—33 patients
   13 (40 per cent.) within 4 hours of onset of symptoms
   21 (64 per cent.) within 12 hours of onset of symptoms ·
   18 (55 per cent.) within 4 hours of admission

patients had their first arrest within four hours of onset of symptoms. Of the 17 with primary V.F., 14 had an arrest within 12 hours of the onset of symptoms and 13 had their first arrest within two hours of admission. The timing in the complicating group is less striking but still over 60 per cent. had their arrest within 12 hours of onset of symptoms and more than half within four hours of admission. Recently, Pantridge & Geddes (1967) have emphasised this point. They found that the risk of developing V.F. in the first four hours was 15 times as great as the risk of developing it in the period 4–12 hours and 25 times as great when compared with the period 12–24 hours.

   Prevention of V.F. is obviously crucial and therefore much effort has been expended in attempting to identify vulnerable patients. Several points are worthy of mention. Firstly, on two occasions, we have observed a normal ECG just prior to an arrest. Secondly, once the infarct pattern has appeared on the ECG, we have not found any particular site of infarction to have an unduly high incidence of V.F. All our patients developed pathological Q waves on the ECG although in two cases these were confined to chest leads V_6–V_9. We have not been impressed with signs of clinical deterioration in patients just prior to the arrest, a finding in agreement with others (Restieaux *et al.*, 1967).

The only prodromata of ventricular fibrillation are arrhythmias. The classical sequence which we have seen on many occasions is initiated by multiple ventricular ectopic beats, some of which are of the R on T variety. One of these triggers off a paroxysm of ventricular tachycardia and this merges into V.F. as the RR interval diminishes. Because of this sequence, it has been suggested that V.F. should not occur often in an efficient unit as there are specific arrhythmic warnings allowing time for the institution of therapy. We would agree that where we have had an ECG immediately preceding the arrest, arrhythmias have always been present but we have been impressed with the rapidity with which V.F. can develop—sometimes within 30 seconds of the first arrhythmia first appearing. Table IV shows the arrhythmias noted

Table IV. *Arrhythmias noted prior to arrest*

Primary

No monitoring	5 patients
No arrhythmias noted	9 patients
Arrhythmia noted but no therapy possible	2 patients
Arrhythmia noted and therapy given .	1 patient

Complicating

No monitoring	17 patients
No arrhythmia noted	5 patients
Arrhythmia noted and therapy given .	11 patients

prior to the arrest in primary and complicating cases. A proportion of patients arrested so soon after admission that no monitoring information was available. Similarly, those who arrested in general medical wards were not being monitored at the time. Nevertheless, disregarding these groups, there were a surprising number of ' primary ' patients in whom no arrhythmias were noted despite monitoring. It can be argued that this is due to a deficiency in the monitoring system and that arrhythmias were overlooked. It would only be possible to prove this point by constant ECG recording and unfortunately we do not have the facilities for this. Our personal belief that V.F. frequently develops abruptly with little warning has been strengthened by observation of two patients in the primary group. While watching the ECG on the oscilloscope of these patients, V.F. developed with 20–30 seconds of ectopic beats first appearing, and in neither case was it possible to give suppressive therapy.

Again, in the complicating group, there is a proportion in whom no arrhythmias were noted but there is a larger group in whom arrhythmias were noted and suppressive therapy given. This illustrates a further point, that in our experience there are certain patients in whom drug therapy, and often multiple drug therapy, does not prevent ventricular fibrillation. These are patients who usually develop V.F. at a late stage comparatively; they frequently have multiple episodes of V.F. and their chances of survival are considerably less (5 of 15) than the patient who develops V.F. abruptly at an early stage in the infarction. By and large, this 'early' group more often have single episodes of V.F.; suppressive therapy controls the tendency to V.F. easily and the prognosis is relatively good (21 of 35 left hospital).

The therapy of V.F. is in many respects the simplest aspect. We are convinced that D.C. defibrillation should be done as speedily as possible and all other therapeutic considerations are of secondary importance. Normally, defibrillation is done in the Unit within 30–40 seconds of the arrest and with this time interval we have not found acidosis a problem. In the early days of the Unit there were occasions when bicarbonate was given over-liberally and now we recommend that 100 mEq. be given initially and the blood gas figures which we have suggest that this is adequate. External cardiac massage and intubation are seldom required following defibrillation.

As a result of our resuscitative measures, we have now 26 patients who survived V.F. and were eventually discharged home.

Like others (e.g., Goble et al., 1966) we have found that the chances of long-term survival depend very much upon the clinical state of the patient at the time of arrest. Thus, our 'primary' patients have done extremely well and only 1 of 17 did not survive. The relationship to clinical state is well shown if one divides the complicating group into mild, moderate and severe according to the clinical signs of cardiac failure. Six of ten mild cases left hospital, whereas in the severe group there were no long-term survivors, although nine were successfully resuscitated. The overall mortality of those admitted directly to the Unit has been reduced by 4 per cent. as a consequence of successful resuscitation from V.F. This 4 per cent. represents a 20 per cent. reduction in mortality rate and is all the more important as there is now evidence that these persons who survive V.F. and leave hospital have as good a prognosis as other patients in a similar clinical state who did not suffer a cardiac arrest (Geddes et al., 1967).

REFERENCES

Conference Report (1966). Training Technics for the Coronary Care Unit. *Am. J. Cardiol.* **17**, 736.

GEDDES, J. S., ADGEY, A. A. J. & PANTRIDGE, J. F. (1967). Prognosis after recovery from ventricular fibrillation complicating ischaemic heart disease. *Lancet*, **2**, 273.

GOBLE, A. J., SLOMAN, G. & ROBINSON, J. S. (1965). Mortality reduction in a coronary care unit. *Br. med. J.* **2**, 1,005.

JULIAN, D. G., VALENTINE, P. A. & MILLER, G. G. (1964). Disturbances of rate rhythm and conduction in acute myocardial infarction. *Am. J. Med.* **37**, 915.

LOWN, B., FAKHRO, A. M., HOOD, W. B. & THORN, G. W. (1967). The coronary care unit, new perspectives and directions. *J. Am. med. Ass.* **199**, 188.

MELTZER, L. E. & KITCHELL, J. R. (1966). The incidence of arrhythmias associated with acute myocardial infarction. *Progr. cardiovasc. Dis.* **9**, 50.

OLIVER, M. F., JULIAN, D. G. & DONALD, K. W. (1967). Problems in evaluating coronary care units. Their responsibilities and their relation to the community. *Am. J. Cardiol.* **20**, 465.

PANTRIDGE, J. F. & GEDDES, J. S. (1967). A mobile intensive-care unit in the management of myocardial infarction. *Lancet*, **2**, 271.

PAULK, E. A. & HURST, J. W. (1966). Complete heart block in acute myocardial infarction. *Am. J. Cardiol.* **17**, 695.

RESTIEAUX, N., BRAY, C., BULLARD, H., MURRAY, M., ROBINSON, J., BRIGDEN, W. & McDONALD, L. (1967). 150 Patients with cardiac infarction treated in a coronary unit. *Lancet*, **1**, 1285.

DISCUSSION

Dr Sloman. I would like to present briefly some of our results in ventricular fibrillation and then link these with those of the previous speakers. In our series of 300 patients with proven myocardial infarction there were 72 clinical deaths with nine successful long-term survivors. There have been many short-term survivors but the point I would like to emphasise is that in our experience which extends from 1963 until now, we have only had nine long-term survivors and all of these have come from the ventricular fibrillation group. Now that was in our Coronary Care Unit. We also had the responsibility of looking after people who had cardiac arrests elsewhere in our hospital. Of 116 cardiac arrests in a 12-month period prior to July of this year, there were 52 patients with myocardial infarction, 11 with pulmonary embolism and 53 miscellaneous cases occurring in operating theatres and various other places around the hospital. Of 51 patients with ventricular fibrillation there were nine survivors. Of 37 with ventricular standstill—of course, this is the arrhythmia that is

102

identified at the time the resuscitation team gets there—there was one survivor. I would agree with Dr Lawrie that it is correct in Coronary Care Units to defibrillate the patient immediately ventricular fibrillation occurs, although, as has been suggested by a number of speakers, this arrhythmia should not occur in such units. A Coronary Care Unit is a place where one can prevent these arrhythmias easily and, in fact, we have only had one primary ventricular fibrillation in the last 12 months. However, if it does occur defibrillation should be carried out straight away and if the doctor is not present our nurses are instructed to do this. We will then proceed to correct the acidosis and give other drugs. In other parts of the hospital, it is the usual practice to apply external cardiac massage, assisted ventilation and correction of acidosis prior to the resuscitation team arriving and ventricular fibrillation is later treated with D.C. counter-shock. So there are two different methods in most hospitals for dealing with ventricular fibrillation.

The comments of the two previous speakers raise two problems. First, that a number of patients develop ventricular fibrillation out of the blue without any predictors that these patients may develop ventricular fibrillation. Should we deduce from this that all patients, irrespective of their clinical state on admission to the Coronary Care Unit, or previously, should be given an anti-arrhythmic drug either intravenously or intramuscularly? It seems to me, from what Dr Lawrie has said, that this is quite a reasonable deduction. Secondly, Professor Bouvrain emphasised that ventricular tachycardia occurs outside Coronary Care Units in the second and third week after myocardial infarction. The deduction here surely must be that we must prolong the period of anti-arrhythmic treatment after the patient leaves the Coronary Care Unit—perhaps for three or four weeks. Therefore, we have two suggestions to consider: the prophylactic use of anti-arrhythmic drugs in the home, and the continuation of anti-arrhythmic treatment for much longer than most of us have been doing up to now.

I would like to ask Professor Bouvrain a question regarding his five patients who remained in ventricular tachycardia and his two deaths. Could he tell us what type of defibrillator he was using? Our experience has been that we have always been able to defibrillate people with ventricular tachycardia. Often there has not been a successful outcome but we are always able to put them into sinus rhythm or ventricular standstill. Was he using an A.C. defibrillator? This may explain the difference.

Dr Oliver. I believe Dr Lawrie said that practically all the primary V.F. occurred in the first 12 hours. How many patients did you have that had primary V.F. after the first 24 hours?

Dr Lawrie. There was only one after 24 hours with primary V.F., and all the other late instances of V.F. occurred in very ill patients.

Dr Killip. It seems to me reasonable to ask if we can always be sure of ventricular tachycardia. It is often very difficult to separate a supraventricular arrhythmia with aberration from a truly lower than nodal focus. Retrograde conduction and the shape of the complex do not really help and I suspect myself that a significant number of the patients we see with the slower ventricular tachycardias, who tolerate them well, actually may not have their focus site below the AV node. This may well have an important therapeutic significance. It certainly has important functional significance. I agree with a number of the previous speakers about the demand for instant response to both ventricular tachycardia and ventricular fibrillation and it is worth pointing out, in relation to the earlier discussion of the genesis of sustained tachycardias, that everything we said about dispersion of recovery period and the importance of vulnerability and ectopic activity can be applied to the atria. All these factors are important in the genesis of supraventricular tachycardia and a sustained tachycardia for reasons that are mysterious may accelerate and this in turn can lead to further deterioration. This, I think, is why it is so important to define the nature of the arrhythmia.

Dr McDonald. There is an important point to clarify. I agree with Dr Lawrie that both in primary and secondary V.F. there is a significant number of patients in whom, in spite of good monitoring, there do not appear to be any premonitory dysrhythmias at all. What I would like to do is to try and equate this with Dr Lown's experience. I think that the incidence of ventricular fibrillation is falling in every unit but he is claiming a fantastically low rate. Therefore, if we accept this, we must conclude that for some reason or other his patients show premonitory dysrhythmias and ours do not.

Dr Lown. If you compare experience in coronary care units where there has been no aggressive therapy of arrhythmias, there is a mortality not dissimilar to that which existed prior to the introduction of intensive coronary care. Dr Killip's study is one of the best of its type because he ran intensive coronary care simultaneously with regular care. If I remember his mortality correctly, 32 per cent. died in coronary care and 30 per cent. in regular care. But the moment aggressive management was introduced, the mortality went down substantially to about 20 per cent. In effect by the doctrine of early therapy the reduction in death approaches the very figures that Dr Cross presented for the United States. With anti-arrhythmic therapy we are not improving circulation, haemodynamics, coronary flow, but what are we doing?. One thing alone—the cutting out of arrhythmias—that is why our figures are different. I cannot give any experience about primary V.F. because we do not see it. Even the three patients we presented had congestive heart failure. These exclude agonal cases. Dr. Lawrie pointed out that when arrhythmias were noted, therapy was given in about 11 patients and they nonetheless had ventricular fibrillation. One important thing we have learned goes back again to this classification of arrhythmias. There are certainly arrhythmias that are brady-cardiac and, in these people, anti-arrhythmic drugs may provoke arrhythmics. The bradycardias cannot be defined in terms of a rate because some patients have bradycardias at the rate of 150! In a patient with a rate of 150 and ventricular tachycardia, we pre-cipitated V.F. consistently with lignocaine and with procaine amide or with whatever anti-arrhythmic drug we used. The only thing we could do was to over-ride at a rate of 190. This patient survived. We have had four such patients in whom we had to over-ride the heart at 120, 130, 140 and higher rates. The moment we see patients who develop ectopic arrhythmias after anti-arrhythmic drugs we place them in the category of bradycardia and then try to utilise measures to accelerate the heart rate. I would like to make one more point about what Dr Killip said. Physiologically it is hard to concede that slow rate ventricular tachycardias are supraventricular or junctional with this degree of aberration. It is difficult, as Dr Killip quite properly said, to make a diagnosis electrocardio-graphically even if one probes the atrium with atrial leads and oesophageal leads to be certain about ventricular tachycardia because aberrant conduction may be a function of rapid rate. If you have aberration or even if you have fusion, there is no certainty that you are not dealing with a supraventricular arrhythmia. And so my interpretation would be the very converse of Dr Killip's: the rapid arrhythmias may be supraventricular with bundle branch block but the slow arrhythmias are probably ventricular.

Dr Oliver. Thank you very much. I do not think we should become too involved in this question of whether one can treat a condition that does not occur. In fact we are probably not so far apart as might appear. As I recall your figures, a minority—perhaps 40 per cent.—are admitted to the Brigham within 12 hours of the onset of their symptoms. Dr Lawrie has shown that our experience is that 35 out of 50 V.F.s were admitted within 12 hours. We see a different and more vulnerable population. What we want to know, is this: is early primary V.F., of which we see more than you, just as responsive to anti-arrhythmic drugs or is it not? May be it is not. I do not think we know that.

Dr Julian. In view of his success with V.F., I want to know why Dr Lown is so unsuccessful in preventing ventricular tachycardia—more unsuccessful than anybody else with a 27 per cent. incidence.

Dr Lown. The success or lack of success depends I think on the way we classify V.T. We have only a 3 per cent. incidence of rapid V.T.s—that is those with a rapid rate of over 100—and are probably suppressing this arrhythmia because the incidence of rapid V.T. should be more.

THE USE OF LIDOCAINE IN THE TREATMENT OF ARRHYTHMIA

THOMAS KILLIP

Cornell University Medical College
New York, New York

AT the present time there are five drugs which are commonly utilised in the United States to suppress arrhythmia. These drugs include (1) digitalis, (2) quinidine, (3) procaine amide, (4) diphenyl-hydantoin, and (5) lidocaine. The beta-blocking drug propranolol is not included in this list since in my opinion it is an experimental drug whose usefulness remains to be evaluated in the treatment of myocardial infarction.

Digitalis, as is well known, is effective in certain supraventricular and ventricular arrhythmias. We have utilised this drug extensively in the management of patients with myocardial infarction both for heart failure and the treatment of arrhythmia. Since, however, digitalis will be discussed extensively at a later point in this Symposium, it will not be further considered in this presentation.

Quinidine, procaine amide and lidocaine have many actions in common. They are all, of course, local anaesthetics and their effect on the myocardial action potential appears to be essentially similar. Not quite as much is known about diphenylhydantoin which has recently been advanced as a useful agent by a number of workers. There is some evidence that diphenylhydantoin may have a different locus of action from other agents namely on the sodium pump.

Quinidine, of course, is the prototype of all anti-arrhythmic drugs. Techniques of administration have been developed through trial and error. Quinidine depresses atrial and ventricular automaticity by decreasing the rate of spontaneous depolarisation of the diastolic prepotential. Quinidine slows conduction and prolongs recovery time. Due to a so-called vagolytic effect the drug enhances atrioventricular conduction. This effect is particularly evident in the presence of rapid atrial rates and A-V block such as atrial fibrillation or flutter. Quinidine also is a peripheral vasodilator and depresses myocardial contractility. It would appear that all of the anti-arrhythmics mentioned above share to a greater or lesser extent the therapeutic as well as the adverse reactions of quinidine. Thus, the anti-arrhythmia agents in common use may in appropriate dosage and clinical circumstance, enhance A-V conduction, depress myocardial contractility and cause peripheral vasodilatation.

Utilising an ingenious experimental preparation, Regan has recently shown that in experimental myocardial infarction, potassium efflux from the infarcted area can be correlated with the onset of ventricular arrhythmia and fatal ventricular fibrillation in the dog. Administration of procaine amide in adequate dosage will suppress the ventricular arrhythmia and coincidentally inhibit the potassium efflux. It is possible, but by no means proven, that anti-arrhythmic agents are effective by virtue of their ability at the plasma membrane to control ion movement. Since however the cause of arrhythmia in acute myocardial infarction as well as other conditions is unknown, the mechanism of drug action must remain speculative.

Our approach to ventricular arrhythmia complicating acute myocardial infarction is as follows. Generally, ventricular arrhythmia is actively treated at its first recognition. When there are more than three ventricular premature complexes per minute, or two or more consecutively, intravenous lidocaine is the therapy of choice. Lidocaine is given as a bolus injection in an immediate initial dose of 1 to 2 mg. per kg. If this treatment is not effective within three to five minutes, a second dose of 0·5 to 1 mg. per kg. is administered. Successive doses are administered until a total of 3 to 4 mg. per kg. have been injected. In certain urgent situations the total dose may be even higher. If effective, drug action is usually recognised within 30 to 90 seconds. Once the arrhythmia has been suppressed a constant intravenous drip of lidocaine is initiated. The rate of infusion varies from 1 to 5 mg. per minute. At the faster rates of administration the patient may receive 6 to 8 g. of lidocaine in a 24-hour period. In urgent clinical situations considerably higher doses have been administered.

When the constant infusion rate is adjusted and the arrhythmia is suppressed, the infusion is continued for 24 to 36 hours. Usually the rate of infusion is gradually decreased and, if no arrhythmia appears, is terminated at the end of this time. Should arrhythmia recur, it is treated first with a bolus injection of lidocaine of approximately 1 mg. per kg. and then the infusion rate of the constant drip is increased. It has not been useful in our experience to treat recurrent arrhythmia by increasing the infusion rate without administering a bolus first, since the time required to achieve a higher drug concentration may be rather prolonged.

Lidocaine may also be useful in the treatment of supraventricular arrhythmia, particularly atrial premature contractions. Relatively few patients have been treated in our Unit with this technique. More commonly digitalis is utilised.

In common with the other anti-arrhythmic drugs mentioned, lidocaine enhances atrioventricular conduction. The drug should therefore be utilised with care in patients with rapid atrial rates and A-V block. Figure 1 shows the effect of lidocaine in a

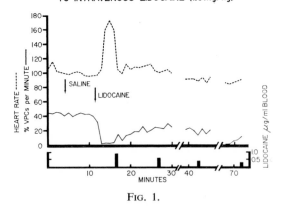

RESPONSE OF VENTRICULAR PREMATURE COMPLEXES
AND HEART RATE IN ATRIAL FIBRILLATION
TO INTRAVENOUS LIDOCAINE (1.0 mg/kg)

Fig. 1.

patient with atrial fibrillation and ventricular arrhythmia. The drug suppressed the ventricular ectopic beats and enhanced A-V conduction. Thus, the ventricular rate became very rapid.

The effectiveness of lidocaine in a typical ventricular arrhythmia is shown in the Figure 2A. In this patient multifocal ventricular premature complexes with short coupling intervals repeatedly led to ventricular fibrillation and cardiac arrest. This patient had a complex arrhythmia which we interpret as atrial fibrillation with A-V block and nodal escape complicated by multifocal ventricular premature complexes. This arrhythmia is almost certainly an excessive digitalis-low potassium toxicity problem. Following the injection of lidocaine as shown in Figure 2B, the ventricular

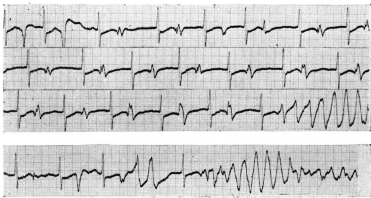

Fig. 2A. Atrial fibrillation with A-V block and nodal escape complicated by multifocal ventricular premature complexes.

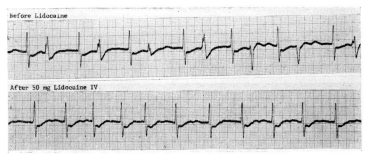

Fig. 2B. The effect of lidocaine in obliterating multifocal ventricular complexes but with increase in ventricular rate.

rate is increased, probably reflecting the enhancement of A-V conduction due to the drug, and the multifocal ventricular premature complexes have been obliterated. This latter effect is probably a combined one reflecting both the increased ventricular rate and the suppressive effects of the drug.

In our experience, both procaine amide and lidocaine are useful in the management of cardiac arrest. In some patients defibrillation is followed immediately by reappearance of the ventricular arrhythmia. It is important to evaluate carefully the cause of failure of defibrillation. For this reason we insist that an electrocardiogram be running continuously throughout the procedure. Defibrillation was attempted several times in one patient with cardiac arrest due to ventricular fibrillation. The defibrillation was successful in each instance but was immediately followed by multifocal ventricular premature complexes and relapse to fibrillation. After three consecutive defibrillations, 200 mg. of procaine amide was administered intravenously and three minutes later a fourth defibrillation was successful and was followed by sustained sinus rhythm. This experience occurred several years ago and at the present time we would almost certainly utilise 100–150 mg. lidocaine in the same therapeutic situation.

To obtain objective information on the effectiveness of lidocaine in the treatment of ventricular arrhythmias we administered the drug intravenously under carefully controlled conditions to 24 patients with frequent (20 to 50 per cent. of ventricular rate) ventricular premature complexes. The electrocardiogram was monitored continuously. Blood pressure was measured at frequent intervals and blood samples were taken for analysis of the plasma drug concentration.

Half the group spontaneously complained of discomfort due to transient lightheadedness or sleepiness. Specific questioning revealed however that all had experienced the symptoms. Convulsions were not observed. In our experience convulsions have been observed only in the situation of high dosages of lidocaine combined with evidence of cerebral anoxia. Thus, the patient who is suffering from cardiac arrest, severe heart failure or cardiogenic shock and who is given large doses of lidocaine intravenously may have a seizure syndrome. In several desperate clinical situations, despite the initiation of seizures by the drug, we have continued giving high dosage of lidocaine and controlled the seizure with anti-epileptic medication. We believe that this programme has been life-saving in a small number of patients.

In no patient have we observed a fall in blood pressure, a significant effect of the drug on the sinus discharge rate or any detectable effect of the drug on QRS duration. Interventricular block or bundle branch block has never been observed. In 19 comparable studies the effect of lidocaine on ventricular premature complexes was: complete ablation in ten, marked decrease in six, slight decrease in two, and no discernible effect in one. Thus, the drug had a therapeutic effect in 95 per cent. of the patients studied. The duration of the drug effect was quite variable. It appeared that the patients could be separated into two groups by virtue of the therapeutic response (Figure 3). In eight subjects, Group A,

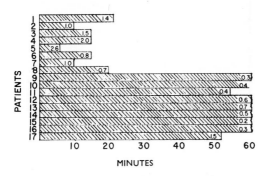

FIG. 3. Duration of effect in relation to blood level of lidocaine in micrograms per ml.

the therapeutic effect persisted for an average of 15 minutes (range 6–25 minutes). In 9 subjects, Group B, the therapeutic effect persisted 50 minutes or longer. In some patients it persisted for several hours.

The wide variation in duration of therapeutic effect for an effective cardiac agent is not surprising. In some patients the improvement in cardiac function secondary to ablation of the arrhythmia may so influence those factors which precipitated the original arrhythmia, that further ectopic beats do not occur. It is well known that if drugs are withdrawn from a patient previously in heart failure it may take many weeks, considerably longer than the duration of the drug effect, for heart failure to return. On the other hand, in some patients it is apparent that those factors which produce the arrhythmia are so overpowering, that high concentrations of drug are needed for therapeutic effect and as soon as blood or tissue levels fall below a threshold value, arrhythmia returns (Fig. 4).

Lidocaine blood levels were performed through the kind co-operation of the Astra Drug Company. The blood level 15 minutes after injection of 1·0 mg. per kg. averaged 1·0 micrograms per ml. for Group A. Despite the longer duration of therapeutic effect in

111

RESPONSE OF VENTRICULAR PREMATURE COMPLEXES
TO INTRAVENOUS LIDOCAINE (1.5 mg/kg)

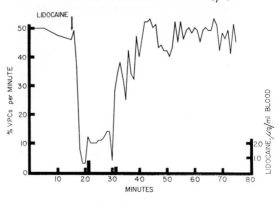

FIG. 4.

Group B the blood level one hour after injection averaged 0·5 micrograms per ml. The blood level of lidocaine 4 minutes after the anti-arrhythmic effect following 1·0 mg. per kg. averaged 1·2 micrograms per ml. with a range of 0·8 to 1·8 micrograms per ml.; the t½ of lidocaine in blood approximated 20 minutes. The peak blood level did not correlate with the duration of anti-arrhythmic effect, and this lack of correlation presumably reflects the secondary effects on heart function of the ablation of the arrhythmia mentioned above.

In a series of experiments in unanaesthetised trained dogs with complete heart block, it was observed that lidocaine did not affect the atrial rate, but slowed the ventricular rate. Moreover, the drug prolonged the asystole following abrupt cessation of ventricular driving. In this experiment the dog's heart was driven for three minutes at a rate of 90 per minute. Under controlled conditions asystole following cessation of ventricular driving averaged six seconds. With lidocaine in a dose of 2 mg. per kg. the duration of asystole was doubled. Dose response experiments in the dogs revealed a minimal effect with 0·5 mg. per kg. and systemic toxicity at levels of 4 mg. per kg. The blood level decay curve appeared to be multi-exponential. It is our impression that man can tolerate higher doses of lidocaine than can the dog.

Our current views on the use of lidocaine in the management of ventricular arrhythmia in the presence of acute myocardial infarction may be summarised as follows. The ability to administer

112

the drug rapidly, intravenously, is a distinct therapeutic advantage. Its short duration of action, from a few minutes to perhaps a hour or more, is not necessarily disadvantageous. Following initial administration one can evaluate the therapeutic response and decide whether procaine amide, quinidine, lidocaine or some other drug should be administered on a continuous basis. The drug is effective in a high percentage of cases and cardiac toxicity is essentially nil. Most patients will have minor central nervous system symptoms and in the presence of cerebral anoxia or in-adequate cerebral blood flow, convulsions may occur.

In my opinion, lidocaine is the drug of choice in the immediate treatment of ventricular premature complexes.

DISCUSSION

Dr Oliver. Most of us who have used lignocaine to any extent would support the contention that Dr Killip has put forward that this drug is a very effective agent for suppressing ventricular ectopic beats and ventricular tachycardia, and for preventing ventricular fibrillation. It might be reasonable to take that as read and then examine whether we all feel, as Dr Killip has suggested, that it has no cardiotoxic effects. I am not sure that we would agree. We have been six patients out of the first 200 or so who received lignocaine, in whom there was depression of the pacemaker or increasing A.V. block and, in one case, complete heart block, and in another complete pump failure occurring in the presence of normal sinus rhythm. This is a very difficult subject to discuss because these complications occur anyway as part of the history of acute myocardial infarction. All that we could say on this point is that we know for sure that two patients have received an overdose of lignocaine. Once, in error, a patient was given a bolus of 500 mg. instead of 50 mg. This was one of these things that happen in the best-regulated circles and this patient developed convulsions and died in normal sinus rhythm although mechanical failure had occurred. The other patient had had an infusion over 12 to 14 hours of up to 1 g. of lignocaine and then suddenly got a bolus of about 200–300 mg. when the flow rate through his drip altered as he moved around in bed. He had convulsions immediately although he had been perfectly well beforehand. We have also seen suppression of atrial pacing occurring in people who had lignocaine but again this could perhaps be related to the natural history of the condition. We have found that these complications have occurred after a considerable amount of lignocaine and they have not occurred at the beginning of an infusion. It might be interesting to see if anybody else has had adverse experiences. I should say hastily that we do not feel that these few experiences indicate that this is not the drug of choice. All I am saying is that we are being a little cautious.

Dr Lown. I agree entirely with Dr Killip's thesis that at the present time this is the drug of choice for ventricular ectopic beats. We have unfortunately had complications. In about 150–200 patients, we had five cardiac complications and those cardiac complications meant a worsening of rhythm in four. In one a rapid ventricular response developed in a patient with atrial flutter and was misinterpretated as a ventricular arrhythmia, and the patient went into profound shock and had to be cardioverted. We have had two convulsive episodes but without any other complicating sequelae.

Dr Oliver. Did these complications occur after a considerable amount of lignocaine or early on in the infusion?

Dr Lown. Those arrhythmias which worsened were early on. The convulsive episodes occurred after a considerable amount of ligocaine was given and when the drip opened up and ran free.

Dr Oliver. If we are going to try to give an anti-arrhythmic drug at the earliest possible point after acute infarction, it could be argued that the family doctor should carry lignocaine in his bag and give 50 mg. at home. Is this reasonable?

Professor Shillingford. We have made observations on the effect of this drug on haemodynamics. The effect on the cardiac output of a dose of 1 mg./min. is very small. It is depressed in the region of between 5 per cent. and 10 per cent. and associated with this there is a very slight fall in pulse pressure. In some, cardiac output rises slightly, probably because of the suppression of extrasystoles. The only adverse reaction from a normal dose of this drug is a certain amount of cerebral confusion and sleepiness after 12 hours or so. Certainly after 24 hours this is a commoner feature.

Dr Pantridge. Dr Lown, what dose of lignocaine do you use? If you do not get ventricular fibrillation, then there must be situations in which you use relatively large doses. What is the incidence of asystolic arrest and complete pump failure?

Dr Lown. The initial starting dose of lignocaine is 50 mg. If that does not work then we go to 100 mg. If that does not work, we will then resort to the use of other drugs or combinations. We have not had any asystole as a result of this method nor did we induce any ventricular fibrillation. Have you studied the effect on cardiac output of 2–3 mg./min. lignocaine Professor Shillingford?

Professor Shillingford. No.

Dr Killip. I would like to reiterate that this whole business of studying the haemodynamic effects of cardiac drugs is confused by primary and secondary action. As Dr Shillingford indicated, in some patients the minute volume actually went up and one could easily work out a whole sequence of events with a striking improvement in cardiac function in one patient and considerable deterioration in another. General statements must be backed up by specific examples.

PHENYTOIN SODIUM (DILANTIN) AND PROPRANOLOL (INDERAL)

GRAEME SLOMAN

Royal Melbourne Hospital, Melbourne

Phenytoin sodium (dilantin) has been shown to be effective in controlling cardiac arrhythmias (Leonard, 1958; Conn, 1965). Beta adrenergic blockade has also been shown to be of value in the management of certain cardiac arrhythmias including those associated with acute myocardial infarction. This subject has been reviewed by Epstein and Braunwald (1966). Both drugs have been used in patients with arrhythmias and infarction despite a lack of knowledge of their effects on the cardiovascular system under these circumstances. We report here our observations on some of the haemodynamic effects of phenytoin sodium and propranolol combined with atropine in patients with acute myocardial infarction. All patients who received intravenous propranolol were also given atropine sulphate because Johnston (1964) had shown that the bradycardia which followed the intravenous administration of propranolol could be reversed by atropine.

METHODS AND MATERIAL

The effect of an intravenous injection of 250 mg. of phenytoin sodium was studied in 11 patients, while the effect of intravenous propranolol with atropine (propranolol 0·1 mg./kg. body weight together with atropine sulphate 1·2 mg.) was studied in six patients. All patients selected for study had been admitted to the Coronary

115

Care Unit with evidence of a definite transmural myocardial infarction which had occurred within the previous 24 hours. Patients with cardiogenic shock, complete heart block or a past history of bronchial asthma were excluded from the study. The patients were classified as having ' mild ' or ' severe ' infarction according to the criteria of Robinson *et al.* (1964). In the phenytoin sodium group, five patients had ' mild ' infarction and four ' severe ', while the remaining two had been admitted to the Unit following resuscitation from cardiac arrest. In the propranolol with atropine group, four were classified as being ' mild ' and two as being ' severe '. Papaveretum (Omnopon) was used as the analgesic where indicated and all patients received oxygen by face mask.

Bedside cardiac catheterisation was carried out using fine plastic tubing (PE50) inserted percutaneously. Flow guided catheterisation was performed as described by Dotter and Straube (1962). After brachial artery cannulation, intracardiac pressures were recorded with the patient lying in bed with the head elevated on one pillow, the manubrium sterni being used as the point of reference.

The cardiac output was determined using a dye dilution method with indocyanine green (cardio green). The dye solution was injected into the right atrium and arterial blood was withdrawn from the brachial artery at a constant rate through a Waters X301 densitometer coupled to a potentiometric direct writing recorder. The drugs under study were injected over a five-minute period, the completion of the injection being taken as zero time.

RESULTS

Phenytoin sodium

There was little change in the heart rate, the maximum decrease at any time over the 15 minutes of observation being 7 beats per minute (Table 1). The blood pressure showed a tendency to decrease at 5 minutes with a gradual return to the resting level by 15 minutes. The maximum decrease was 35 mm. Hg. systolic from 140 mm. Hg. The mean decrease at 5 minutes after the injection was 18·7 mm. Hg., the mean decrease at 10 or 15 minutes was 6·2 mm. Hg. At 5 minutes, four patients had a decrease in the cardiac output greater than 10 per cent., the maximum decrease being 27 per cent. In another three patients, the cardiac output at 5 minutes had decreased slightly; however, in these, it was not beyond the level of experimental error. In four patients there was an increase of cardiac output at 5 minutes, but only in one was this increase

116

Table I. *Some haemodynamic effects of phenytoin sodium (dilantin) in acute myocardial infarction*

	Blood pressure in mm. Hg.				Heart rate		Cardiac output in litres/min.			Pressure in pulmonary artery or right ventricle in mm.Hg.	
	Rest	5 min.	10 min.	15 min.	Rest	15 min.	Rest	5 min.	15 min.	Rest	5 or 10 min.
1.	170/90	135/75	155/85	—	93	—	5·8	5·0	—	38/18	33/17
2.	—	—	115/75	—	—	—	4·3	3·1	—	—	—
3.	120/85	100/70	—	—	93	90	3·3	3·5	—	32/18	32/18
4.	180/100	145/80	—	—	82	80	5·1	4·9	4·3	28/11	24/3
5.	170/95	140/80	—	165/95	73	72	2·9	—	3·1	33/1	34/5 (15 min.)
6.	100/65	80/55	85/55	90/60	112	105	3·9	3·6	4·5	18/-2	23/-1
7.	150/95	140/95	—	175/100	130	140	3·5	2·6	3·1	—	—
8.	120/85	110/85	—	110/75	128	126	3·4	2·9	6·4	38/3	—
9.	140/85	150/100	—	105/55	92	87	5·7	5·3	4·6	17/10	—
10.	110/	—	—	—	67	70	4·0	—	6·1	12/2	12/2
11.	100/60	—	—	95/55	75	70	5·3	5·8	—	—	—

Phenytoin sodium was administered in an intravenous dose of 250 mg. given over five minutes.

117

beyond that of experimental error. In seven of the eight cases studied at 15 minutes, the cardiac output had returned to the resting value or better. Statistical analysis of the cardiac output 5 minutes after the injection of phenytoin sodium showed that there was no significant change. Right ventricular systolic and pulmonary artery systolic pressures were measured where possible. No systematic change was noted.

The incidence of side effects was low. Two patients vomited immediately after the injection of phenytoin sodium. Coughing was not a problem. Of the 11 patients studied, nine were alive when reviewed six weeks after the acute episode. Neither of the two deaths could be attributed to phenytoin sodium. One patient developed complete heart block two days after the study. In spite of endocardial pacing, he died on the 23rd day. The other patient died of a ruptured heart 10 days after the study.

Propranolol with atropine

Table II summarises the results obtained before and after the administration of propranolol with atropine. The heart rate increased in all but one patient and the increase approaches a significant level. There were no statistically significant changes in the systemic blood pressure and in those patients where there was a fall in blood pressure the effect was transient. The difference in cardiac output was not statistically significant. The mean cardiac output before propranolol and atropine was 3·9 litres per minute and, after propranolol, 4·4 litres per minute. In only one patient was there a decrease in cardiac output beyond the limits of error of the investigation (Case 5). In this patient there was a slowing of the sinus tachycardia. In five of the six patients, the right ventricular systolic pressure was lower after the administration of the drugs.

The incidence of side-effects was low. One patient developed incomplete heart block with episodes of Wenckebach phenomenon of short duration. There was no change in the clinical state of the patient and no treatment was necessary. None of the patients in the 'mild' group developed cardiac failure following administration of propranolol and those in the 'severe' group were given a diuretic (frusemide 80 mg. intravenously) after the completion of the haemodynamic studies and the signs of cardiac failure were neither severe nor prolonged. One patient in this group died three weeks after the study. All other patients survived six weeks.

Propranolol was also used as the treatment of choice in six

118

Table II. *Some haemodynamic effects of propranolol and atropine sulphate in acute myocardial infarction*

	Blood pressure in mm. Hg.		Heart rate		Cardiac output in litres per minute		Stroke volume		Systolic pressure in pulmonary artery or right ventricle in mm. Hg.	
	Before	After	Before	After	Before	After	Before	After	Before	After
1.	170/–	100/–	87/min.	97/min.	4·2 L/min.	3·9 L/min.	48 ml.	40 ml.	24 mm.	20 mm.
2.	100/–	135/–	72/min.	96/min.	3·1 L/min.	4·8 L/min.	43 ml.	50 ml.	23 mm.	24 mm.
3.	140/75	170/95	53/min.	97/min.	4·3 L/min.	6·1 L/min.	82 ml.	62 ml.	23 mm.	18 mm.
4.	120/70	130/80	72/min.	85/min.	3·6 L/min.	4·3 L/min.	50 ml.	51 ml.	27 mm.	18 mm.
5.	135/85	75/50	113/min.	95/min.	5·0 L/min.	3·6 L/min.	44 ml.	38 ml.	25 mm.	16 mm.
6.	125/70	135/75	79/min.	90/min.	3·6 L/min.	3·9 L/min.	46 ml.	43 ml.	35 mm.	29 mm.

Propranolol was administered in an intravenous dose of 0·1 mg./kg. body weight with atropine sulphate 1·2 mg.

patients with various arrhythmias associated with acute infarction (Table III). In five of the six patients, propranolol appeared to assist in the management of the arrhythmia. In eight additional patients, it was decided to use propranolol because of prolonged or recurrent cardiac arrest. The length of time of massage in these eight patients varied from 20 minutes to 120. All the patients were successfully resuscitated initially, but one died three hours after resuscitation. A further three patients died within three days. However, four patients survived to leave hospital.

Table III. *Propranolol. Treatment of arrhythmias in acute infarction*

No.	Sex & Age	Arrhythmia	Outcome
1.	M. 65	Atrial flutter.	Controlled and reverted.
2.	M. 57	Paroxysmal ventricular tachycardia.	Controlled.
3.	M. 52	Recurrent nodal tachycardia and atrial fibrillation.	Rate slowed. Reverted later.
4.	M. 49	Ventricular tachycardia. Supraventricular tachycardia. Atrial fibrillation.	Arrhythmia controlled. Patient died from a ruptured heart.
5.	F. 63	Ventricular tachycardia associated with myocardial aneurysmal and new infarction.	*NOT* controlled with propranolol alone or in combination.
6.	M. 59	Paroxysmal atrial tachycardia.	Propranolol and dilantin did *NOT* control alone. Digoxin added and arrhythmia ceased.

Propranolol was administered intravenously or orally depending on the clinical situation.

DISCUSSION

It has been shown that phenytoin sodium when administered intravenously in a dose of 250 mg. does not cause a significant haemodynamic change in patients with acute myocardial infarction. There was a tendency for the cardiac output to fall a little at 5 minutes after the administration of the drug, but by 15 minutes the cardiac output had returned to the resting value. This finding is not in keeping with Vasko *et al.* (1966) and Mixter *et al.* (1966) who studied dogs. We still lack knowledge on the effect of phenytoin sodium on the myocardium and blood vessels and its role in the prevention and treatment of many forms of cardiac arrhythmias following acute infarction. However, this study suggests that should phenytoin sodium be indicated, then its effects on haemodynamics are not deleterious.

Propranolol with atropine may be given intravenously following acute infarction without causing a decrease in cardiac output. This is unlike the effect of propranolol when given alone when it does cause a decrease in cardiac output (Bay et al., 1967). The relative importance of the negative inotropic effect, bradycardia or decrease in venous return to the heart, in producing a drop in cardiac output is unknown. Bay et al, (1967) suggested that the fall in output is entirely rate dependent, although Sowton and Hamer (1966) showed a decrease in cardiac output following the administration of propranolol in subjects with a fixed ventricular rate. Atropine has been shown to cause an increase in cardiac output (Berry et al., 1959; Gorton et al., 1961) but the mechanism of its action in preventing the decrease in cardiac output which results from the administration of propranolol is not clear. Atropine sulphate may prevent the concomitant bradycardia or it may overcome a negative inotropic effect of propranolol. The decrease in pulmonary artery pressure, although not statistically significant, suggests that atropine also prevents the increase in pulmonary artery pressure which has previously been described following the administration of propranolol (Sowton & Hamer, 1966).

Propranolol has been used in the treatment of certain arrhythmias associated with acute infarction and it appears that there is a special place for the drug in patients with prolonged or recurrent cardiac arrest.

SUMMARY

The haemodynamic effects of phenytoin sodium and propranolol combined with atropine have been studied in patients with acute myocardial infarction. Neither caused an important change in the haemodynamic situation and we conclude that both may be used in this situation for treatment of arrhythmias. There were no significant side-effects.

Acknowledgements

The authors thank Sister N. Downey and the Nursing Staff of the Coronary Care Unit. Mrs N. Charleston, Mrs Linnet Sangster and Miss J. Miles are thanked for their technical assistance.

121

REFERENCES

Bay, G., Lund-Larsen, P., Lorentsen, E., Sivertssen, E. (1967). Haemodynamic effects of propranolol (Inderal) in acute myocardial infarction. Br. med. J. 1, 141.

Berry, J. N., Miller, D. E., Thompson, H. J. & McIntosh, H. D. (1959). Changes in cardiac output, stroke volume and central venous pressure induced by atropine in man. Am. Heart J. 58, 204.

Conn, R. D. (1965). Diphenylhydantoin sodium in cardiac arrhythmias. New Engl. Med. J. 272, 277.

Dotter, C. T. & Straube, K. R. (1967). Flow guided cardiac catheterisation. Am. J. Roentg. 88, 27.

Epstein, S. E. & Braunwald, E. (1966). Beta adrenergic receptor blocking drugs. New Engl. J. Med. 275, 1106, 1175.

Gorton, R., Gunnells, J. C., Weissler, A. M. & Stead, E. A. (1961). Effects of atropine and isoproterenol on cardiac output, central venous pressure and mean transit time of indicators placed at three different sites in the venous system. Circulation Res. 9, 979.

Johnston, M. (1964). Beta receptor blockade during anaesthesia. Congr. mund. Anaesthesiol. 111, 38.

Leonard, W. A. (1958). The use of diphenylhydantoin (Dilantin) sodium in the treatment of ventricular tachycardia. Archs intern. Med. 101, 714.

Mixter, C. C., Moran, J. M. & Austen, W. C. (1966). Cardiac and peripheral vascular effects of diphenylhydantoin sodium. Am. J. Cardiol. 17, 332.

Robinson, J. S., Sloman, G. & McRae, C. (1964). Continuous electrocardiographic monitoring in the early stages after acute myocardial infarction. Med. J. Aust. 1, 427.

Sowton, E. & Hamer, J. (1966). Haemodynamic changes after beta adrenergic blockade. Am. J. Cardiol. 18, 317.

Vasko, J. S., Elkins, R. C., Fogarty, T. J. & Morrow, A. G. (1966). Effects of diphenylhydantoin on cardiac performance and peripheral vascular resistance. Surg. Forum, 17, 189.

Discussion

Dr Sowton. I would like to suggest an alternative approach to the use of propranolol in patients with myocardial infarction. We have used the dextro-isomer of propranolol without the laevo-isomer. Now the laevo-isomer has the beta-blocking activity which is responsible for most of the deleterious effects of myocardial function. We studied the effects of 20 mg. of the dextro-isomer intravenously. There was very little depression of cardiac function and the heart rate, cardiac output, pulmonary artery, aortic pressures, ejection time and calculated tension-time index were all unchanged by this relatively large dose. Now d-propranolol has anti-arrhythmic activity and so I suggest it as an alternative to the combined use of propranolol and atropine.

Dr Oliver. Are you equating 20 mg. of dextropropranolol with approximately 2 mg. of the racemic compound?

Dr Sowton. No, this has the same anti-arrhythmic activity as

122

20 mg. of the racemic compound, but it has virtually no depressent effects on the myocardium.

Professor Shillingford. What are the indications for the use of this drug?

Dr Sowton. We use it for supraventricular and for ventricular arrhythmias. We do not use it prophylactically. We use it in treating individual patients. Our main interest at present is in its clinical assessment and comparison with l-propranolol.

QUINIDINE

Lawrence E. Meltzer

Presbyterian University of Pennsylvania Medical Center, Philadelphia

As one who has repeatedly confessed a strong preference for the use of electrical methods (rather than drug therapy) to terminate or control arrhythmias associated with acute infarction, I am somewhat chagrined to find myself now discussing the use of quinidine. I was undoubtedly assigned this subject solely because of my association with the co-operative trial involving prophylactic quinidine therapy that has just been completed in the United States.

Although quindine is a satisfactory anti-arrhythmic agent in many situations, it has very limited use in the active treatment of those acute arrhythmias associated with cardiac infarction. When administered orally, its action is much too slow to combat critical arrhythmic disturbances. While this problem could be solved by using the intravenous route, experience has shown that this practice is extremely dangerous in this setting and should not be attempted. Secondly, quinidine is less effective than the 'caine' derivatives in controlling ventricular arrhythmias and would seldom be the drug of choice for *active* treatment of these disturbances.

That quinidine might be valuable for the *prophylactic* treatment of arrhythmias related to myocardial infarction presents an interesting possibility. Of the 80–90 per cent. of all patients with infarction who show evidence of some arrhythmic disturbance, at least 50 per cent. develop these disturbances *after* admission. The question arises as to whether the prophylactic use of anti-arrhythmic agents might not prevent these latter arrhythmias. If such prevention was possible, the incidence of late catastrophic arrhythmias could perhaps be grossly reduced as well as the morbidity of circulatory failure (by preserving the haemodynamic effectiveness associated with sinus rhythm).

This premise has been specifically considered in a multi-centre co-operative study during the past four years. The trial was originally designed as follows.

Patients with suspected acute infarction who did *not* present with shock, overt failure or a major rhythm disturbance were included in the study. Once admitted to the trial (conducted in five hospitals), a sealed envelope (randomly sorted) was opened to learn the treatment programme for the patient. One group of patients received quinidine 200 mg. by mouth four times a day after a priming dose. The second group was treated with procaine amide orally, 250 mg. every six hours. A third group was given no treatment. The end point of the original investigation was mortality.

After approximately 800 randomly selected patients were studied, it became apparent to the investigators that the mortality was essentially the same in the three groups and that no benefit was apparent from prophylactic therapy with quinidine or procaine amide when used in the described dosages.

The question then arose as to whether the dosages employed in the study were adequate. (The original dosage schedule was selected with the belief that lesser amounts of a drug are required for prophylactic therapy than for therapeutic use.) In studying the blood levels of quinidine obtained with the original schedule it became evident that the dosage of quinidine must be adjusted according to body weight if adequate levels were to be achieved. Patients who weighed more than 150 pounds usually had blood quinidine levels of only 2 mg. litre or less—a concentration that was deemed ineffective even prophylactically. Procaine amide blood levels (measured as PABA) behaved similarly. It was decided that the trial should be continued with the dosage schedule individualised for each patient according to blood levels measured twice daily.

While the wisdom of relying on blood quinidine (or procaine amide) levels as a guide to dosage may be challenged (because of the belief that only the unmeasurable tissue levels would be meaningful), I am personally convinced that blood quinidine levels are valuable in this regard. As evidence of this premise, I will cite our experience with the use of quinidine to maintain sinus rhythm after successful cardio-version for atrial fibrillation. In studying our high failure rate we noted that a vast majority of reversions to atrial fibrillation occurred during the sleeping hours

124

when the blood quinidine levels were at their ebb. By adjusting dosages to maintain therapeutic blood levels (about 5–6 mg. litre) the incidence of reversion to atrial fibrillation has been markedly reduced.

Those who deny the value of these quinidine levels usually describe reversions that occurred in the face of normal or even high blood levels. I believe that most of the examples are the result of levels that are *spuriously* high. Blood quinidine levels are falsely high in the presence of elevated blood urea nitrogen and when concomitant drug therapy is employed. Particularly misleading results are obtained when patients receive certain diuretics and antibiotics (Table I).

Table I. *Drugs which produce spuriously high blood quinidine levels*

(Precipitation Method)

Dyrenium (Triamterene)
Diuril (Chlorothiazide)
Polycillin (Ampicillin)
Gantrisin (Sulfisoxazole)
Thiamin HCL
Vistaril (Hydroxyzine)
Tofranil (Imipramine)

The trial with prophylactic quinidine and procaine amide has recently ended. I do not know the statistician's conclusion at this time. It is clear that with customary dosages neither of these drugs reduced the mortality. We will know shortly whether weight-adjusted dosages designed to achieve therapeutic levels are beneficial.

DISCUSSION

Dr Oliver. You have correctly emphasised something which I think is in the mind of us all. That is the responsibilities of existing coronary care units, particularly those with any research component. I believe that coronary care units in major teaching hospitals and those with an academic setting should have a research component. It is their responsibility to try to derive an effective and safe anti-arrhythmic drug regime and, indeed, this may be their main responsibility for the future. It is of course satisfying and has been a considerable advance to be able to control various arrhythmias and to pace the asystolic heart, but from the long-term point of

125

view, the development of a drug regime to be given by the practitioner is a major responsibility. We certainly have not got any drug that is more than 70–80 per cent. safe and yet effective and we have not got one that can be used on a long-term basis. It is up to existing CCUs to try to derive such drug regimes. Of course there are great difficulties in doing this and we have examined some of the statistics concerned with the design of clinical trials to test the effectiveness of these drugs. I do not propose to go into this other than to support you in saying that any trial has to be very large. A trial conducted in the early stages after acute infarction is dependent on the end-point to be taken as proving the drug to be effective. Should V.F. be the only end-point? Should suppression of VPB be the end-point? If V.F. occurs despite suppression of VPB, does it matter if you suppress them? Presumably not. The design of these trials is difficult enough. Their conduct is even more difficult and the end-point critical.

Dr Killip. I would just like to reinforce what Dr Meltzer said. Despite the fact that quinidine is the prototype of all these agents, it is not a very good drug to put a patient on for long. We had a large series at a time when we were converting electrically a number of patients. 150 consecutive patients who were put on quinidine after successful reversion to sinus rhythm from atrial fibrillation, we found that roughly one-third of the patients stopped quinidine because they did not like the side-effects, be they minor or severe. One-third of the patients would not take pills over a prolonged period of time and did not tell the physician that they were not taking them; we only found out through blood levels. Only the most passive dependent patients continued taking their medication. This is a problem with any drug which would require multiple doses during the day. The other point which I think is worth reiterating is that all arrhythmic agents have essentially the same effect. Diphenylhydantoin may be an exception although this is becoming less certain. There was great interest in propranolol as being a new approach to anti-arrhythmic therapy but in point of fact, its electrophysiological effect on the action potential is essentially the same as that of quinidine. I think that one can raise the question as to whether we are going in the right direction in looking for another drug. Personally I wonder whether electrical techniques may be not more fruitful.

Dr Meltzer. As said by Dr Lown before, maybe we are looking in the wrong direction and ought to do something very simple. We have been studying ventricular tachycardias and our experiences are identical to those of Dr Lown. We have not seen any of these

126

incidents of rapid tachycardia. The incidence of slow tachycardia is high. In 90 people that we have looked at, we found there was a very low incidence from 11 o'clock at night to 7 o'clock the next morning, but a very high incidence from 7 o'clock the next morning till 4 o'clock that afternoon. Of course, there may be a lot of metabolic things going on and it may be that patients should be more sedated with something simple that does not work on the heart. It would be very interesting for others to look at their experience with ventricular tachycardia and look for this rather unusual distribution of arrhythmias. Dr Lown has noted the same thing. It might be an interesting problem not to work on the heart but to work on the nervous system, which may be almost as much involved.

Dr Nixon. I would like to support that. In my own unit we have tried all sorts of different drugs and the main line of attack has been to put the patient to sleep with phenergan and pethidene when arrhythmias have cropped up. We have been very happy with this and it has rarely been necessary to use the more powerful drugs. It is not irrelevant that Lauder Brunton about 100 years ago, when he was investigating deaths under chloroform anaesthesia, pointed out that when the mind was in distress or in pain, death was much more likely than when the patient was tranquil and sleeping.

Dr Gearty (Dublin). Might we suggest then that the progressive general practitioner should give his patient 100 mg. of lignocaine intravenously, 500 mg. of procaine amide orally and pain suppressants as he waits for the cardiac ambulance?

Dr Meltzer. Yes, unless the heart rate is slow.

HEART BLOCK AND PACING

Chairman: Dr D. G. JULIAN

MODES OF PACING AFTER ACUTE MYOCARDIAL INFARCTION

XAVIER DALLE

St Elisabeth Hospital, Antwerp, Belgium

ALTHOUGH there has still been no satisfactory controlled study of the efficacy of short-term endocardial pacing after myocardial infarction, the multiplicity of reports on the beneficial effects of the method in individual cases is sufficient proof of its value.

The most important changes and developments pertaining to this technique concern the still growing number of indications for its use as a prophylactic or as a therapeutic measure in cardiac arrhythmias, with or without congestive heart failure, complicating acute myocardial infarction, rather than pacing techniques themselves; the vast majority of the modes of pacing currently used in coronary care units have been available to us for several years and we are only learning very slowly how and when to apply them. It is in the light of these changes in philosophy that I will consider the various modes of pacing used after acute myocardial infarction—details of techniques have been reported recently by others (Siddons & Sowton, 1967).

Modes of pacing suited for routine clinical use

Most of the early successes obtained with electrical stimulation of the heart after acute myocardial infarction concern patients with severe bradycardia complicated by congestive heart failure, cardiogenic shock or repeated Stokes-Adams attacks, treated with *conventional or set-rate pacemakers.* This fact proves sufficiently that the vast majority of the cases can be efficiently treated with this mode of pacing. There are however a few drawbacks to conventional pacing. When ventricular pacing is applied in patients with intermittent heart block, 'competitive pacing' is seen during the periods of conducted supraventricular rhythm; in this parasystolic type of iatrogenic arrhythmia, pacing impulses are frequently seen to hit the vulnerable period of previous supraventricular beats. When a ventricular premature beat interrupts the paced rhythm the next pacing impulse may also hit its vulnerable period; ventricular fibrillation may easily result, particularly in acute myocardial infarction (Fig. 1). In addition, such interference, due to competition or ectopic beats, creates marked irregularity of the

131

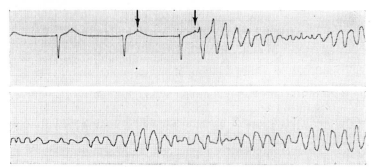

FIG. 1. Induction of ventricular fibrillation by a barely supra-threshold
stimulus in a patient with acute myocardial infarction.

ventricular rhythm and this may not only be accompanied by
troublesome palpitations but also be deleterious to cardiac
haemodynamics.

All these disadvantages and potential dangers are completely
obviated by the use of the *demand pacemaker* (Lemberg *et al.*,
1965). This stimulator, also called ' ventricular inhibited ' pacemaker is programmed to detect the electrical activity of the ventricle
and to release a pacing impulse only if a preset interval is exceeded
without detection of a QRS complex; this mode of pacing is
inherently dependent upon a QRS signal without artifacts and the
intraventricular ECG from the bipolar catheter itself is optimal in
this regard. As shown in Figure 2 the function of a properly
utilised demand pacemaker is remarkable; it behaves as an artificial
ventricular escape mechanism which will never hit a vulnerable
period of a previous beat and the improvement in regularity of the
ventricular rhythm is most probably beneficial to the cardiac output.
Demand pacing has substantial advantages over conventional
pacing and it is our feeling that it should be used in all cases of
ventricular pacing after myocardial infarction.

Whereas complete heart block still remains an unquestionable
indication for endocardial pacing, the technique is now being used
for a growing number of other rapid- and slow-rate arrhythmias—
sinus and nodal bradycardia, sino-atrial block, sinus arrest, slow
atrial fibrillation, refractory ventricular irritability and to abolish
recurrent ventricular tachyarrhythmias. In most of these arrhythmias *atrial pacing* is indicated whenever the atrioventricular conduction is normal and this certainly constitutes more than 60 per cent.
of the cases in whom electrical stimulation is required in the present

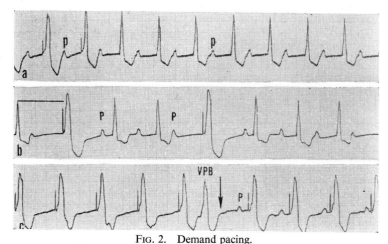

FIG. 2. Demand pacing.
(a) when conducted supraventricular rhythm recurs
(b) in the presence of 2° AV block
(c) in presence of ectopic beats

concept of better intensive coronary care. Atrial pacing has indeed many advantages over ventricular pacing: the normal sequence between atrial and ventricular systole is maintained; the importance of the atrial contraction for end-diastolic ventricular filling and subsequent contraction is well known. This atrial ' booster ' effect is particularly important when ventricular function is already compromised and when rapid stimulation rates are applied; such rapid rates are not infrequently necessary to ' overdrive ' the heart in an attempt to abolish ventricular irritability (Greenfield & Orgain, 1967).

The danger of inducing ventricular fibrillation by means of A.C. stray currents and mechanical or electrical stimulation is abolished or at least very considerably reduced. Sometimes, however a pacing impulse may induce atrial fibrillation by activating the atrial vulnerable period; a loss of atrial capture ensues.

Paired and coupled pacing of the atrium constitute the only presently available means of reducing the electrical *and* mechanical rate in ' excessive ' sinus tachycardia and probably also in refractory cases of atrial tachycardia.

With a straight pacing catheter it may be more difficult to find a stable position in the atrium, but a catheter with a curved tip generally solves this problem. This increasing use of atrial pacing

133

in short-term electrical stimulation constitutes one of the major changes in this technique in recent years.

Methods for experimental use

1. As an attempt to maintain the normal sequence of atrial and ventricular contractions, *short-term atrial synchronised* and *paired atrioventricular pacing* may become of value in the future, provided the technical difficulties concerning insertion of atrial and ventricular catheters can be solved; in this regard, a tetrapolar catheter (with two poles in the atrium and two in the ventricle) may prove useful in that it will allow the use of every mode of pacing. The atrial catheter is used to provide a synchronising pacemaker* with a clear, high voltage ' P ' wave signal: after a preset interval the pacemaker stimulates the right ventricle through a bipolar catheter. This method seems indicated in patients with complete heart block and power failure of the heart, provided the heart rate is satisfactory. Should the atrial rate be too slow and in cases of atrial standstill (sinus arrest or sino-atrial block) the same catheters (or a tetrapolar catheter) can be used to stimulate the atrium and the ventricles in a sequential fashion at an interval of about 150 msec., by means of a paired-pulse stimulator* (paired atrioventricular pacing, Fig. 3).

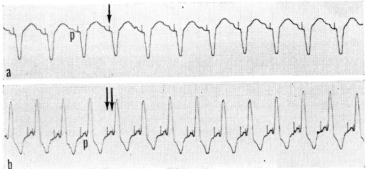

FIG. 3. Artificial atrial synchrony in short-term pacing.
(a) Atrial synchronised pacing
(b) Paired atrio-ventricular pacing

At the present time, these methods are still technically too intricate for routine clinical use, but some very promising results have already been obtained.

* R-wave coupled pulse generator, Model 5837, Medtronic Inc., Minneapolis, Minn., U.S.A.

2. *Paired* and *coupled stimulation of the ventricle* have not generally yielded the expected results in clinical practice and they have been particularly disappointing after acute myocardial infarction (Goetz *et al.*, 1967). Not only are these modes of pacing contra-indicated theoretically in view of the serious increase in myocardial oxygen consumption—proportionally greater than the increase in contractility and coronary perfusion—but the haemodynamic results obtained in coronary patients are poor. In addition, there is abundant experimental and clinical evidence that the risk of inducing ventricular repetitive firing or fibrillation is particularly great in such patients. From a practical point of view we think that the only indication, after acute myocardial infarction, consists of refractory life-threatening tachyarrhythmias unresponsive to other electrical or pharmacodynamic modes of therapy. In such cases, significant reductions in the mechanical heart rate can generally be achieved and the resulting increase in diastolic perfusion time may compensate for the higher myocardial oxygen consumption so that the net result may be beneficial. These cases are rare. This is fortunate since the technique may be difficult to apply after acute infarction because of the frequent induction of bouts of ventricular repetitive firing and even fibrillation. As a rule these complications are less frequent with coupled pacing than with paired pacing (Han *et al.*, 1967).

3. Still more experimental are paired and coupled stimulation of the atrium with the purpose of slowing down ' excessive ' sinus tachycardias electrically *and* mechanically. After a first spontaneous (coupled) or induced (paired) atrial beat, an atrial premature beat is generated which should be timed sufficiently early so that the depolarisation reaches the AV node during its refractory period and will not be conducted to the ventricle; the electrical and mechanical rate of the ventricle may thus be reduced by as much as 30–45 per cent. Indeed the ' blocked atrial premature beat ' recycles the sinus mechanism and delays the occurrence of the next sinus or atrial depolarisation. Sometimes it may be difficult accurately to time the artificial premature beat (Fig. 4) so that drug therapy has to be used to prolong the duration of the AV nodal refractory period.

Whether or when it will prove valuable to slow down sinus tachycardia is unknown at the present time. Sinus tachycardia is generally a compensatory arrhythmia occurring in the presence of power failure of the heart where there is a fixed and low stroke volume; only an acceleration of the heart rate will then improve cardiac output. On the other hand, a rapid heart rate is accompanied

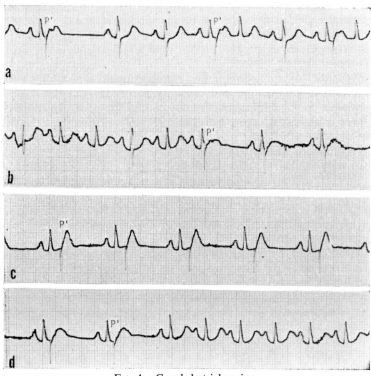

Fig. 4. Coupled atrial pacing.

(a) Prior to digitalisation: some impulses occur early, in the refractory period of the atrium and others, occurring later, induce premature beats which are conducted to the ventricle.

(b) Onset, (c) continuation and (d) end of effective coupled atrial pacing, after administration of digitalis; the ventricular rate is reduced by almost 45 per cent.

by an increase in tension-time index and, thus, myocardial oxygen consumption, and may thus be deleterious on the long run. It will certainly be hard to determine when the tachycardia ceases to be beneficial and becomes self-defeating.

There are enormous differences of opinion concerning the indications for endocardial pacing after acute myocardial infarction. Facilities for insertion of pacing catheters will certainly greatly increase the use of the method when fluoroscopy is used or insertion is under intracavitary electrocardiographic guidance. The clinical condition of the patient also plays an important role; bradycardia should never be tolerated in patients suffering from congestive heart failure, and the heart rate must be increased as soon as possible. To achieve this goal, cardiac pacing is much more efficient and reliable than drug therapy and probably safer in experienced hands. The personality of the physician in charge is crucial. Whereas many of us are reluctant to insert a catheter electrode before the occurrence of an arrhythmic or haemodynamic complication it is becoming more and more evident that endocardial pacing can be a valuable adjunct in the prevention of ventricular asystole or severe bradycardia and in the prevention of overt congestive heart failure when bradyarrhythmias or refractory tachyarrhythmias are present. Such a decision may need courage.

These indications for the use of electrical stimulation of the heart proceed directly from the failures of conventional intensive coronary care, namely the ineffectiveness of the external pacemaker and the still important morbidity and mortality from overt congestive heart failure and cardiogenic shock. There is no doubt that active therapy of all rapid and slow rate arrhythmias is of paramount importance in this regard.

REFERENCES

GOETZ, R. H., JALLAH, E. M. & GOETZ, V. M. (1967). Circulatory dynamics of paired pacing in hypovolemic and cardiogenic shock. *Am. Heart J.* **73,** 506.

GREENFIELD, J. C. & ORGAIN, E. S. (1967). The control of ventricular tachyarrhythmias by internal cardiac pacing. *Ann. intern. Med.* **66,** 1017.

HAN, J., MALOZZI, A. M. & LYONS, C. (1967). Ventricular vulnerability to paired-pulse stimulation during acute coronary occlusion. *Am. Heart J.* **73,** 79.

LEMBERG, L., CASTELLANOS, A. & BERKOVITS, B. V. (1965). Pacemaking on demand in AV block. *J. Am. med. Ass.* **191,** 12.

SIDDONS, H. & SOWTON, E. (1967). *Cardiac Pacemakers.* Springfield, Ill.: Thomas.

ARTIFICIAL PACING IN THE MANAGEMENT OF COMPLETE HEART BLOCK COMPLICATING ACUTE MYOCARDIAL INFARCTION

BENJAMIN LASSERS

Royal Infirmary, Edinburgh

THE development of intensive coronary care has provided both improved treatment of individual patients with acute myocardial infarction, and an opportunity for the clarification of the natural history of this condition and its complications. In addition it has produced an environment in which new and specialised methods of management can be developed and evaluated. The purpose of this communication is to describe the experience of the first 45 patients with complete heart block (CHB) complicating acute myocardial infarction admitted to the Coronary Care Unit of the Royal Infirmary, Edinburgh, with particular reference to the role of artificial pacing in the management of this disorder of conduction (Lassers & Julian, 1968).

ONSET OF COMPLETE HEART BLOCK

In our experience CHB usually developed early in the course of acute myocardial infarction. In 42 of the 45 patients both the onset of symptoms of infarction and the onset of CHB were accurately known. Figure 1 shows that 14 patients (33 per cent.) developed CHB within three hours of the onset of symptoms of infarction and 25 patients (80 per cent.) within 48 hours.

On admission to the CCU 18 patients had CHB. All of the remaining 27 patients had some disorder of conduction, rate or rhythm detected before CHB developed (Table I). In 23 patients CHB was preceded by a premonitory disorder of conduction. The commonest of these premonitory disorders was complete bundle branch block which occurred in 14 patients. These patients with bundle branch block were particularly liable to develop CHB with ventricular asystole suddenly and to die before resuscitative measures could be instituted. Lone partial AV block occurred in seven patients. Two patients had atrial flutter and atrial fibrillation respectively with slow ventricular rates in the absence of digitalis therapy, indicating a high degree of AV block. Lone sinus brady-

138

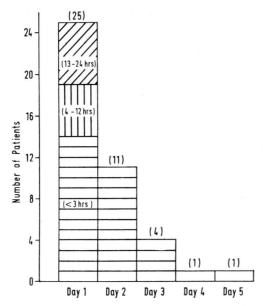

Fig. 1. Time of onset of complete heart block after development of symptoms of acute myocardial infarction.

cardia occurred in only one patient. The remaining three patients had either lone ventricular tachycardia or ventricular fibrillation.

Nine of the 23 patients with premonitory disorders of conduction died. Three of these deaths might have been prevented had pacing electrodes been introduced when the disorder was first detected. In two cases the preceding disorder was complete bundle branch block. In these patients CHB with ventricular asystole developed suddenly and death occurred before a transvenous electrode could be inserted. The third patient had a transient episode of CHB one and a half hours before suddenly developing CHB with asystole which led rapidly to death. Although this had been recorded on the ECG monitor, it had not been detected by the medical staff.

PACING: POLICY AND TECHNIQUES

Our present policy is to introduce pacing electrodes in all patients with 2nd degree heart block and all patients with complete bundle branch block as well as all patients with CHB. We have found the best technique of insertion to be the percutaneous supra-clavicular subclavian vein route. An antecubital vein was found to

Table I. *Disturbances of conduction, rate and rhythm preceding the development of complete heart block*

Preceding disorder	Patients	Deaths	Preventable deaths
Bundle Branch Block: Lone . . . . . 7⎫ Partial heart block . . . 6⎬ Sinus bradycardia . . . 1⎭	14	8	2
Lone Partial AV Block: First degree . . . . 2⎫ Second degree . . . . 5⎭	7	1	1
Slow Ventricular Rate with atrial flutter or fibrillation.	2	0	0
Lone Sinus Bradycardia	1	0	0
Lone Ventricular Tachyarrhythmias .	3	1	0
Total . .	27	10	3

be too unstable a position to guarantee constant and effective pacing for any length of time, and the external jugular vein route was found to be time consuming and often technically difficult. In our experience right ventricular outflow tract pacing has been unstable and unreliable. The electrode tip is, therefore, manipulated to the apex of the right ventricle under fluoroscopic control using a portable image intensifier (Watson ' Cardiovision ') designed for use in a Coronary Care Unit (p. 65).

HAEMODYNAMIC STUDIES

To a certain extent our policy with regard to pacing has been guided by haemodynamic studies carried out in 13 patients. In 11 of the 13 patients circulatory measurements were made both in AV block and during pacing within a few hours of the onset of CHB. Four of the patients had nearly normal mental function and clinical evidence of good skin circulation in CHB. All of these patients were found to have cardiac indices of greater than 2·20 litres per min. per sq.m. The remaining patients, who all had cardiac indices of less than 2·00 litres per min. per sq.m. had, without exception, varying degress of mental apathy, inattention, confusion or restlessness and poor skin circulation. These clinical features were better correlated with cardiac output than either heart rate or systemic blood pressure. Thus in the patients with lower cardiac outputs the heart rate ranged between 40 and 61 per minute and the mean systemic blood pressure between 45 and 100 mm. Hg, while in the patients with higher cardiac outputs the rate ranged between 41 and 60 per minute and the blood pressure between 69 and 104 mm. Hg. However, the systemic vascular resistance was considerably higher in the patients with lower outputs averaging 3,643 dyne sec.cm.$^{-5}$ per sq.m. compared with 2,166 dyne sec.cm.$^{-5}$ per sq.m. in the patients with higher outputs.

The mean pulmonary arterial pressure was mildly elevated in five patients and the mean right atrial pressure was elevated in all but one patient in CHB. The arterial oxygen tension was reduced to an average of 70 mm. Hg and there was an increased alveolar-arterial oxygen tension gradient in CHB. Both physiological dead space and venous admixture were increased in CHB.

Figure 2 shows the effect of increasing ventricular rate by pacing on cardiac index, mean systemic arterial blood pressure, stroke index and systemic vascular resistance. Only those patients who were studied at three or more pacing rates are included. In six cases there was a progressive rise in cardiac index with incressing rates, even with rates above 100 per minute. In two patients (J.D. and C.C.) who were paced at 125 and 130 per minute respectively, the cardiac index fell. Systemic blood pressure changes tended to parallel cardiac index changes at least until high rates were reached. Stroke index fell progressively in seven patients, but in one (C.C.) it rose with an increase in rate suggesting improved ventricular performance. There was little overall change in systemic vascular resistance except at high pacing rates.

Pacing had no significant effect on mean pulmonary arterial pressure, mean right atrial pressure, arterial oxygen tension or pulmonary ventilation/perfusion abnormalities. Arterial oxygen tension was not related either to pulmonary arterial pressure or to cardiac output during CHB, during pacing or after return of sinus rhythm.

Pacing resulted in a progressive and steep rise in the tension-time index with increasing ventricular rates (Fig. 3). If the tension-time index is considered a reliable correlate of myocardial

141

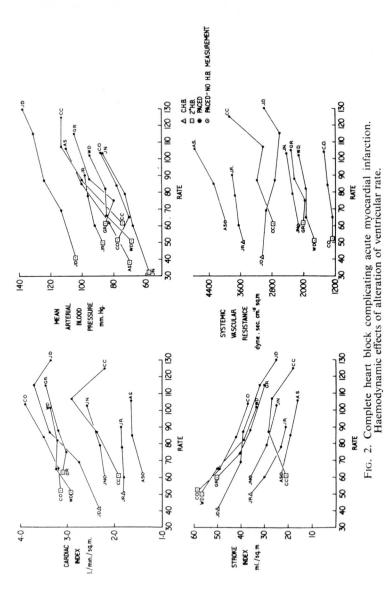

FIG. 2. Complete heart block complicating acute myocardial infarction. Haemodynamic effects of alteration of ventricular rate.

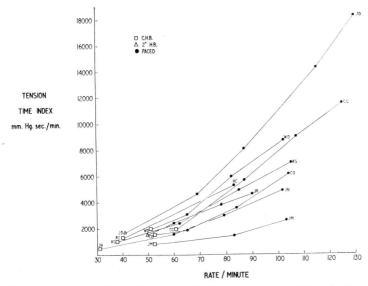

FIG. 3. Complete heart block complicating acute myocardial infarction effect of alteration of ventricular rate on tension-time index.

oxygen consumption, then pacing—especially at high rates—is an expensive procedure in terms of myocardial energetics. It is possible that under the circumstances of acute coronary occlusion where the blood supply to at least part of the myocardium is restricted, pacing is increasing the energy requirements of the heart beyond the availability of oxygen and this could result in a decline in myocardial performance.

EXPERIENCE WITH PACING

In three patients early in our series of 45 patients electrodes were electively not inserted. Two of these patients subsequently died. There was inadequate time for the introduction of transvenous electrodes in two patients admitted to the CCU moribund and in three patients who developed CHB and ventricular asystole suddenly while being monitored. Transthoracic electrodes (Elecath) were introduced in these five patients, but all died. In the remaining 37 patients transvenous endocardial electrodes were inserted. In 13 of these patients the onset of CHB was not associated with any deterioration in the clinical state and pacing was not required. All

143

13 patients survived. Of the 24 patients who were paced, 14 died. In the entire group of 45 patients, 21 (47 per cent.) died. In the 24 survivors, CHB was transitory and sinus rhythm returned although one patient required DC shock for conversion of atrial fibrillation. The duration of CHB ranged from a few minutes to 7·7 days with a mean of 2·5 days.

It is difficult to assess the exact benefits of pacing for heart block complicating acute myocardial infarction. In many patients CHB is not associated with deterioration in the clinical state and specific treatment for this complication is not required. In others, in whom the cardiac lesion is severe, death occurs despite treatment. In the remainder, therapy may be effective by abolishing ventricular asystole or by increasing ventricular rate. In our series of 37 patients with transvenous electrodes, 13 did not require pacing and all survived. Among the 24 patients who were paced, 14 died and 10 survived. Of the 10 survivors, one patient developed angina and dyspnoea with pacing which had to be discontinued and he was not benefited. In the remaining nine patients, pacing abolished attacks of ventricular asystole and produced clinical as well as haemodynamic evidence of increased cardiac output—marked improvement in cerebral function and skin circulation and correction of hypotension. Although these nine patients were thought to have been substantially benefited by pacing, it is possible that some of them might have survived without it.

COMPLICATIONS ASSOCIATED WITH PACING

Patients with CHB have an increased likelihood of developing ventricular fibrillation (Han et al., 1966) and this risk is increased by the insertion of electrodes and by the danger of competition between the patient's own rhythm and that of the pacemaker when AV conduction returns. Ventricular fibrillation was the most serious complication encountered in the present series and occurred in seven patients. In one patient it was mechanically induced during manipulation of the electrode across the tricuspid valve. This patient was immediately defibrillated and survived. Ventricular fibrillation associated with competition, which is the principal disadvantage of conventional set-rate pacemakers, occurred in four patients. Two of these patients died and these deaths were, therefore, probably pacemaker induced. Ventricular demand or stand-by pacemakers reduce the likelihood of competition. This type of instrument is, therefore, now routinely used in our Unit. In two patients repeated episodes of ventricular fibrillation occurred during pacing but these were not considered to be due either to the presence of the electrode or to pacing itself.

The remaining complications consisted of one case of pneumothorax induced during insertion of the electrode in the subclavian vein, three cases of myocardial perforation, one case of atrial flutter which occurred when the electrode was withdrawn from the right ventricle into the atrium, and one failure to pace due to a faulty electrical connection. In addition there was the one patient who developed angina and dyspnoea with pacing and one late recurrence of CHB requiring reinsertion of an electrode. With the exception of the faulty electrical connection, none of these complications had serious consequences.

CLINICAL APPLICATION OF PACING

In our experience of the practical management of CHB complicating acute myocardial infarction, the principal clinical problems which must be faced are: (1) Which patients should have pacing electrodes inserted? (2) Which of these patients should be paced? (3) What is the best rate at which to pace them? (4) How long should the electrode be left *in situ*?

On the basis of our experience we insert endocardial electrodes in all patients with 2nd degree AV block and all patients with complete bundle branch block as well as all patients with CHB. First degree block and sinus bradycardia, which seldom progress to CHB without intervening 2nd degree block, are not regarded as indications for insertion of electrodes.

Since the advantages of an improved systemic circulation which can be achieved by pacing must be balanced against the increased work it requires of a myocardium impaired by ischaemia, we pace only those patients with advanced AV block in whom a low cardiac output is suggested by clinical evidence of diminished cerebral or skin blood flow.

In determining the best rate at which to pace it is reasonable to aim for the lower limits of normal for cardiac output and not to exceed these. The cardiac output cannot usually be measured at the bedside, but with pacing at increasing ventricular rates the blood pressure usually rises *pari passu* with cardiac output at least until the rate exceeds 100 per minute. It may be assumed that the cardiac output has reached adequate levels if the blood pressure has done so and this is accompanied by improved mental function and by evidence of increased skin circulation. On the other hand the provocation of angina or dyspnoea is an obvious indication that

145

the optimum rate has been exceeded. In practice, therefore, this rate can be determined by clinical trial, but in most cases it will prove to be between 80 and 90 per minute.

We have removed electrodes after there has been a period of 72 hours without greater than 1st degree block. Employing this policy we have had only one late recurrence and no deaths. In the case of the patient in whom an electrode is inserted for bundle branch block and who does not subsequently develop CHB, we do not as yet know how long the electrode should be left in place.

SUMMARY

Complete heart block is usually an early complication of acute myocardial infarction. Although it is almost always transient in those who survive, many patients, particularly those with pre-monitory bundle branch block, die within minutes of its development and before any form of therapy can be instituted. In a large number of patients pacing is either not required or the patients die despite pacing. In the remainder pacing is of substantial benefit, either by abolition of attacks of ventricular asystole or by increasing cardiac output, and in a few patients it is life-saving. Against these unquestionable benefits must be balanced the fact that pacing increases myocardial oxygen consumption and is a potentially hazardous procedure which requires continuous electrocardiographic monitoring and staff familiar with pacing problems.

REFERENCES

HAN, J., MILLET, D., CHIZZONITTI, B. & MOE, G. K. (1966). Temporal dispersion of recovery of excitability in atrium and ventricle as a function of heart rate. *Am. Heart J.* **71,** 481.
LASSERS, B. W. & JULIAN D. G. (1968). Artificial pacing in management of complete heart block complicating myocardial infarction. *Br. med. J.* **2,** 142.

DISCUSSION

Dr Sloman. We must all be indebted to Dr Lassers for his very clear description of this common and as yet unsolved problem. The incidence of complete heart block in most published series varies between about 5 or 6 per cent. and in the first 300 patients in our CCU the incidence was also 5 per cent. The mortality in untreated patients is difficult to get at because there are few published series but it would seem to be between 60 and 80 per cent. In an attempt to estimate our own local situation we obtained the figures from four teaching hospitals in Melbourne. In the period from

1964 until July 1967 there were 1,422 patients who were referred to the cardiac departments of these four hospitals. This is not, of course, the total experience of myocardial infarction, but only those seen by cardiologists in these four hospitals. From this group of patients, 30 patients who developed complete heart block were treated with drugs alone. Of those 30 patients there were only 6 survivors, giving a mortality rate of 80 per cent. There is probably some prejudice here because we used to prefer drugs such as atropine and isoprenaline in the patient who was not in cardiogenic shock or in heart failure and whom we thought might survive. There were 48 patients who were paced using endocardial electrodes by the antecubital or femoral routes. Of these 48 patients paced there have been 22 survivors—a mortality rate of 54 per cent. We have favoured the femoral vein as an easily accessible route for placing an endocardial catheter with the additional advantage of being well away from the top of the patient where other forms of resuscitation may be going on. I have found that the femoral vein is quite a useful route for approaching the apex of the right ventricle and we have not had a very high incidence of electrode instability. So, I think we are probably justified in saying that pacing does appear to have a distinct advantage over drug therapy alone. However, I do not think this matter is completely solved by any means. We are rather worried by the fact that those patients who do die are found at autopsy to have severe coronary disease. In general, they have large myocardial infarctions. Furthermore, to my knowledge, there has been no adequate follow-up study of those patients who have survived heart block and pacing after acute myocardial infarction to see what is the long term economic value of this form of therapy.

Dr Leatham. St George's is a very small hospital. Most of our cases are referred, often late, from other hospitals. Our total experience from 1961 to 1967 is 46 cases with a 45 per cent. mortality. We used a fixed-rate pacemaker up to two years ago and there were 20 cases with a mortality at 55 per cent. Low power was used all the time. Thresholds were measured every morning and we only paced just above threshold and the catheter was impacted well in the right ventricle. Displacement was rare. In the last two years we have been using ventricular-inhibited pacemakers. In the last 26 cases, the mortality was 38 per cent. but I do not know whether this difference is statistically significant. When the deaths with fixed-rate units were analysed half of these were probably due to ventricular fibrillation. This appears to have been reduced to about one-third with the use of ventricular-inhibited pacemakers. We continue, therefore, to use the ventricular inhibited unit.

We use the arm and we do not get trouble with displacement provided fluoroscopy is used to impact the catheter properly in the right ventricle—we would not dream of trying to do it without fluoroscopy. The portable image intensifier you have developed in Edinburgh is a break-through because we have lost a number of patients between the ward and the X-ray room. The next point is that if you are going to use the arm it must be fixed to the patient's side; we have lost patients through displacement of the electrode but not since we fixed the arm properly. We do not like cementing it to the chest because this tends to produce hypostatic pneumonia. The best method is probably a special pair of pants with the arm secured to the top of them. Since the pants cannot ride up I don't think there is any problem with displacement. However, I find Sloman's femoral vein approach interesting. The final point I would like to make is the duration of pacing. In Edinburgh you cannot afford to do it for much more than 72 hours. In South London we manage three weeks. We had a reason for this. We had one death at 19 days and another about four weeks after the return of sinus rhythm. At autopsy these patients had not had further thrombosis or infarction, so almost certainly these were electrical deaths. Although these were only two cases, it is our policy at the moment to continue pacing for three weeks—not after infarction but after the return to sinus rhythm.

Dr Julian. I must take the privilege of the chair to make a few comments. First, would Dr Dalle tell us the indications for pacing of patients with sinus bradycardia? As Dr Lassers indicated our policy has been rather different. When we reviewed our records of sinus bradycardia without other forms of arrhythmia we found there was no mortality. We would like to know whether people have had better results than that with pacing! With regard to Dr Leatham's comments, we are exceedingly unhappy with the arm. I think anybody who thinks about nursing a patient with his arm stuck to his pants for four weeks would be too, and I cannot see why he does not prefer a more humane route such as the subclavian vein.

Dr Lassers. I think, Dr Leatham, that our patients and mortality figures are really not comparable to yours. As you pointed out, your patients were often late referrals from other hospitals—that is they had survived long enough to get to you. You will remember that 9 per cent. of our patients developed complete heart block and died before we were able to insert an electrode. I agree with

Dr Julian with regard to the site of electrode insertion. At first we also used the arm because this was the route with which we were most experienced. We found, however, that the patients were very uncomfortable. Furthermore, as many of our patients were at times restless and confused we just could not keep the electrode position stable. However, using the subclavian route we have not yet had to reposition an electrode. My final point concerns the duration for which electrodes should remain *in situ*. This again is to some extent an economic question, as Dr Julian has mentioned. Our aim in the CCU is to have a rapid turnover of patients and to bring the advantages of coronary care to as many people as possible. We believe that patients with pacing electrodes *in situ* should be managed in an intensive care unit. If electrodes are to be left in patients for three weeks, many valuable CCU beds will be blocked and other patients denied intensive care. Moreover, in our experience late recurrences are rare.

Dr Ranzi (Milan). Our results in Milan are nearly the same as those described by Dr Lassers, especially with regard to the haemodynamic findings. However we did need to put permanent pacemakers for persisting heart block in 3 of our 15 patients. Our mortality using a standby pacemaker in acute infarction is 26 per cent.

Dr Cross. Of a number of new cases studied in five coronary care units, there was an incidence of 2nd degree heart block of 4 per cent. and 8·2 per cent. of 3rd degree heart block. The mortality in the patients with 2nd degree block, none of whom were paced, was 50 per cent. The mortality in the patients with 3rd degree block, who were treated with both drugs and pacing, was 51 per cent. I think it is important that the 2nd degree heart block fatality was almost as great as that of the 3rd degree heart block, with varying types of treatment.

Professor Bouvrain. We have had 118 patients with heart block in our Coronary Care Unit during the last five years and among these about one-third were paced. I quite agree with Dr Lassers about the reduction in mortality. Ours has been reduced from 60 to 32 per cent. and has improved with our increasing experience and knowledge of pacing. With regard to the indications for pacing, we put pacing electrodes with demand pacemakers into all patients with anterior infarction and right bundle branch block and in all patients with AV block associated with Adams-Stokes seizures or slow ventricular rates. The relationship of drugs to pacing presents an interesting and sometimes difficult problem. For example, we have seen a patient with complete heart block who developed ventricular tachycardia during an isoprenaline infusion. Pacing was instituted and produced a good response but then episodes of ventricular tachycardia recurred. We continued pacing and gave this patient procaine amide and abolished these episodes. The next day sinus rhythm returned. We removed the electrode but forgot to stop the procaine amide and the next day heart block recurred and the patient died. This case illustrates the difficulties of using isoprenaline and also the problems of combining procaine amide and pacing.

Dr C. S. McKendrick (Liverpool). I disagree strongly with the suggestion made by Dr Dalle that there is uncertainty in deciding whether to use drugs or pacing in this situation. The reason why we pace, surely, is because there are few procedures more difficult than inserting a pacemaker catheter in cardiac arrest. Once the catheter is sited then you are at liberty to try drugs. As far as duration of pacing is concerned in 25 patients we have had to go back in again twice. Our initial idea was to get the catheter out as soon as we felt the situation had calmed down, but our policy has now changed and now quite arbitrarily we are leaving the pacemaker catheter in, switched on for two or three weeks after the patient has returned to sinus rhythm. So far we have had no trouble with this procedure. We also strongly recommend the subclavian route as being by far the easiest and quickest method. However, I am afraid our results are as poor as those of everybody else.

Dr Dalle. I do not think that I said that I would wait for complications to arise before inserting a catheter. On the contrary, we would insert a catheter during the morning or afternoon rather than have to come in at night and do an emergency measure which is nearly always unsuccessful. There is uncertainty in many minds about whether to use drugs or pacing—but not in ours.

Dr Frommer. Did you suggest that there has been no successful experience with coupled pairing?

Dr Dalle. No I did not. But I do not think it is advisable to use coupled pacing with the sole purpose of achieving post-ectopic potentiation in patients with congestive heart failure. It might be indicated in refractory tachy-arrhythmias where one might by decreasing the rate compensate for the increase in oxygen consumption, but it would not be fair at the present time to advocate paired pacing if the patient with infarction has intractable congestive failure.

Dr McDonald. Dr Lassers said that he was unhappy in Edinburgh about pacing outside the unit, but in hospitals in

London there are many patients being paced in wards. What is your problem?

Dr Lassers. You remember that we had seven episodes of ventricular fibrillation, four of which were unquestionably associated with competition. These occurred before we were using demand pacing units and the episodes occurred during the night. There were doctors in the unit at the time, but they were relatively unfamiliar with pacing and they left the set-rate pacemakers on after sinus rhythm had returned. Competition then resulted in ventricular fibrillation. Two of these patients were defibrillated immediately but the other two died. I am reasonably sure that outside the unit all four patients would have died. The other problem is electrode stability. Even with the arm strapped to the side, I think you will find that there are electrodes that move out of position. If the patient then develops complete heart block and requires immediate pacing, it is not available without repositioning of the electrode. We think that this is a real problem.

Professor Harris (London). It seems to me that we have seen a lot of percentages given in the guise of statistics, but I would not have thought that any of them held any statistical water whatever. I strongly suspect, as an uncommitted observer, that you have all occupied yourselves in spending a lot of intellectual energy on tiny marginal changes.

Dr Leatham. I am willing to support Professor Harris's contention as a distinct possibility. I am surprised that in Edinburgh you put in pacing systems which are expensive and time consuming in bundle branch block. We are agreed that 2nd degree block and complete heart block should probably be paced. But should we be putting in pacemakers for a long PR interval and bundle branch block in order to find out what we want to know?

Dr Lassers. We don't put them in for long PR intervals. We found that all but two of our patients, who had 1st degree heart block, went on to 2nd degree heart block before developing complete heart block. The bundle branch block patients are a peculiar group because they tend to develop complete heart block suddenly, then ventricular asystole and often die within minutes. These were the patients in whom we had to use transthoracic electrodes. Reviewing our series we think there were three patients whom we might have saved had we inserted electrodes when we first recognised bundle branch block. Our early belief was that pacing probably had a very limited application in acute infarction. Our present feeling is that it does have a small but definite place. As I tried to point out, I don't believe that the figure of a reduction of 20 per cent. in

151

mortality is anything more than an estimate of the upper limit of benefit which can be achieved with pacing. Our clinical impression was that these nine patients would have died without pacing. Whether they would have survived with drugs alone, I cannot say. Nine patients, or even six patients, out of 45 is not an insignificant reduction in mortality. I think perhaps you are overstating the case against pacing.

Dr Sowton. I agree that the improvement in mortality is small, but let us not forget that 10 per cent. reduction in mortality in the patients who develop acute ischaemic AV block represents about 10,000 lives a year in the United States. Small percentages are important. We do not have trouble with competition at our hospital, because we have used a demand pacemaker in all acute ischaemic heart blocks for the past five years.

Dr Meltzer. In our study we compared arrhythmias and the state of the heart one hour after admission in people who lived and in people who died, and noticed that the major difference was in conduction disturbances. In those in our coronary unit, there was a 27 per cent. incidence of conduction disturbances among those who died against 14 per cent. among those who lived; in those treated in the ward, there was a 30 per cent. incidence of conduction disturbance in those who died against 13 per cent. in those who lived. The problem is to improve the treatment of conduction disturbances and I think pacing is certainly the answer.

Dr Frommer. I agree completely with Dr Dalle that we should think of coupled pacing for the purpose for which it was originally intended, namely, a method of slowing tachycardias which are refractory to other methods of slowing the rate. I think in that context it has been used by several groups with sketchily reported, but apparently favourable results.

Dr Lown. The problem resides not in whether pacing is employed, but in the significance of the underlying arrhythmia. Arrhythmias such as VPB's and ventricular tachycardia may not reflect extensive myocardial damage. Therefore, once they are treated, mortality ceases to be different between those who have them and those who don't. On the other hand in complete heart block there is frequently extensive myocardial damage and the arrhythmia is an indicator of this. Under these circumstances the therapeutic device is not as effective as it is in other arrhythmias. Our results with complete heart block, which we have consistently paced, has been a mortality of about 40 per cent. and this is no different from the mortalities which Drs Lassers, Leatham and Sloman reported.

As regards 1st degree heart block, a quarter of these patients go on to complete block. Everybody agrees, I believe, that 1st degree heart block does not require pacing. As regards 2nd degree heart block, half of our patients went on to complete heart block. Our policy has been to initiate therapy with drugs, while we are getting ready to undertake pacing. Surprisingly atropine and isoproterenal have been effective in many patients with 2nd degree block and in a small percentage of patients with 3rd degree block—about 4 of 25 patients with 3rd degree block did not require pacemakers. The practical problem is that in the majority of small hospitals where the most patients are managed the introduction of pacemakers is a formidable undertaking. I agree with Dr Lassers's formulation of the problem: patients with pacemakers must be observed in an intensive cure unit. With demand pacing, competition has not been a problem, but there are other complications which need to be observed. We remove pacemakers after 72 hours and have had no late recurrencies. Your policy is a sound and economic one.

One other problem is the arrhythmias that develop in conjunction with heart block. Once you have a pacemaker in, the dangers of using anti-arrhythmic drugs are significantly decreased. Therefore one can resort to additional agents. We have used procaine amide and lignocaine without worry for such patients in order to suppress arrhythmias. The major hazard of utilising these drugs in bradycardias is the strong pre-disposition of bradycardia to ventricular fibrillation. But once you have rate control, this ceases to be a danger.

OVERDRIVING OF DYSRHYTHMIAS FOLLOWING ACUTE MYOCARDIAL INFARCTION

EDGAR SOWTON

Institute of Cardiology and National Heart Hospital, London

THE problem of recurrent ventricular tachycardia or fibrillation is not uncommon following cardiac infarction, and the use of anti-dysrhythmic drugs is not always successful in preventing recurrences. Furthermore the dose of such drugs may be limited at ineffective levels because of their depressant effects upon ventricular function. It is well recognised clinically that patients with multiple ventricular ectopic beats are very liable to such episodes and that the risks are particularly high when ' R-on-T ' ectopics occur. The technique of reducing ventricular irritability by electrically increasing the heart rate has been successfully applied to patients after acute myocardial infarction for several years (Sowton *et al.*, 1964; Heiman & Helwig, 1966) and may be used in addition to the usual anti-dysrhythmic drugs. When the heart is overdriven in this way the rate is increased until no spontaneous ectopic beats occur and a regular, stable rhythm is obtained (Fig. 1). This involves driving the heart above a ' critical rate ' which is different for each patient and may vary from time to time in the same patient, since it is affected by many factors, including the irritability of the heart and any concomitant drug therapy. Electrical control of the cardiac rhythm in this way also minimises many of the depressant actions of antidysrhythmic drugs and removes the risks of sudden ventricular asystole from this cause.

The technique of overdriving involves placement of a trans-venous electrode in the heart and this can be done either under fluoroscopy or by monitoring the cavity lead electrocardiogram (Kimball & Killip, 1965). If the patient has developed heart block, pacing must be from the right ventricle; but if AV conduction remains intact, pacing from the right atrium is more satisfactory. In this way, the mechanical irritation of the electrode in the ventricle is avoided and correct atrioventricular synchronisation is maintained. Atrial pacing can be carried out successfully when the electrode tip makes contact with the lateral wall of the right atrium, but a more satisfactory arrangement is for bipolar electrodes to be positioned medially in the region of the SA node. Although the electrode can be passed from an arm vein, the use of the jugular, femoral or sub-

154

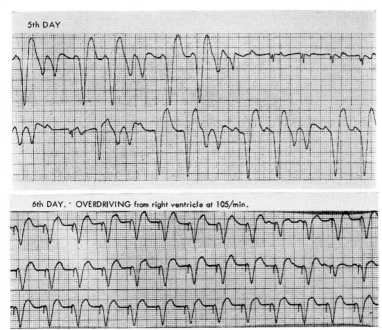

FIG. 1.   Upper panel.   ECG on 5th day following transmural infarction.
The patient had been resuscitated from ventricular fibrillation on 4 occasions
(continuous record).
Lower panel.   Stable rhythm produced by overdriving from the right ventricle
at 105/min. (continuous record).

clavian is recommended as arm movements are then less likely to
cause displacement. Pacing is started at a sufficiently fast rate to
result in ventricular capture and the rate is then further increased until
all non-paced ectopic beats have disappeared. A cautious attempt
is then made to reduce the rate and in some instances the pacemaker
can be slowed considerably, or even withdrawn, without ectopic
beats recurring. This is unusual and in most cases pacing must
be continued at a rapid rate to suppress ectopic ventricular activity;
the most suitable rate is the minimum which prevents recurrence of
ectopic beats.

Overdriving at above the critical rate must be continued until
ventricular irritability has diminished and this may involve continued pacing for several days; the longest continuous period of
overdriving following myocardial infarction carried out at the
National Heart Hospital in London to date was for 23 days. Pacing

must be stable and close supervision of the patient is essential throughout the whole time the technique is in use, but in this respect overdriving does not differ from conventional pacing for the haemodynamic relief of complete heart block. Frequent attempts to reduce the pacing rate should be made in order to detect reduction in ventricular irritability; during these periods there is the possibility that a pacing stimulus may fall during the T wave of an ectopic or a spontaneous conducted beat and, for this reason, a demand pacemaker should be employed whenever possible. The use of this type of pacemaker also provides some protection against iatrogenic dysrhythmias during temporary displacement of the electrode. If pacing is being carried out from the ventricle, rather than the atrium, the use of a demand pacemaker is even more advisable.

Patients in heart block

The critical rate in patients with heart block is often of the order of 70/min. and there is no advantage in faster rates. Indeed, deleterious effects of the artificially produced tachycardia may become apparent at rates only slightly above this. As the pacing rate rises the myocardial oxygen demands are increased and ischaemic pain may be produced if the rate is too fast. At the same time the diastolic filling time is reduced so that the cardiac output may fall significantly as the rate is increased and left ventricular failure may appear.

One complicating effect of ventricular pacing after infarction is the wide variation in systemic blood pressure caused by cyclical coincidence of atrial and ventricular contractions. These swings of pressure may be sufficient for loss of consciousness to occur (Fig. 2). This effect is accentuated as the pacing rate increases

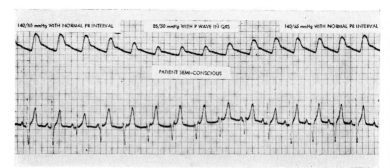

FIG. 2. Ventricular pacing following acute ischaemic AV block. The arterial blood pressure falls from 145/65 to 80/30 mmHg as atrial and ventricular contractions coincide, and the patient becomes semi-conscious.

so that if overdriving at a rapid rate is necessary this phenomenon of varying atrial transport may become particularly noticeable (Fig. 3).

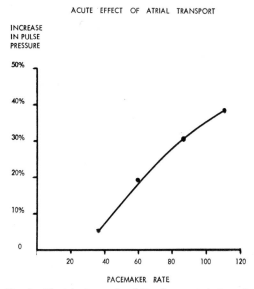

ACUTE EFFECT OF ATRIAL TRANSPORT

FIG. 3. Ventricular pacing following acute ischaemic AV block. Correctly timed atrial systole produces only 10 per cent. increase in systemic pulse pressure at slow rates, but 40 per cent. increase at faster rates. This emphasises the increased importance of atrial transport during tachycardia.

It is apparent that the choice of rate requires careful judgment, but this should not be a deterrent to the use of the technique, since in patients with block it is almost invariably possible to find a rate which suppresses ectopic activity, but does not cause serious deterioration of ventricular function. Further, the presence of the pacemaker makes the use of depressant drugs, such as procaine amide, considerably less hazardous.

Patients without heart block

If the conducting system has not been damaged, overdriving of the heart can be carried out by pacing from the right atrium. Clinical experience indicates that under these circumstances the critical rate may be as fast as 150/min. although most patients are controlled with rates of 120/min. An illustrative case is that of a 54 year old man who was admitted following a large anterior transmural

157

infarction. He had frequent multifocal ventricular ectopic beats, not controlled by lignocaine, and was resuscitated from ventricular fibrillation on three occasions in the first 48 hours. Overdriving was then instituted from the right atrium and a stable rhythm was achieved with a rate of 125/min. (Fig. 4) and this therapy was

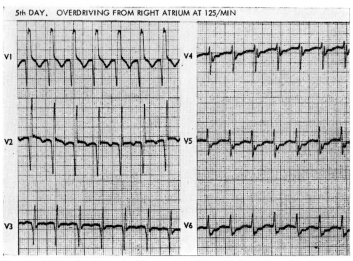

Fig. 4. ECG of a 54 year old man on 5th post-infarct day, showing overdriving at 125/min. from right atrial electrodes.

continued without incident for 10 days. Following this the patient continued to make a good recovery and remains well one year later.

The haemodynamic effects of atrial pacing have been studied in patients with previous infarction and angina pectoris (Sowton et al., 1967) and it seems likely that similar changes occur in subjects with more recent damage. As the rate is increased, the heart size usually decreases and this should result in a diminution of wall tension and so of myocardial oxygen uptake/beat. Nevertheless, pain can be provoked by rapid rates and the left atrial pressure increases sharply at this time. In some patients there is an increase in heart size and this undesirable feature may explain the provocation of pain at low pacing rates in a few patients. As with ventricular pacing, the final choice of rate must be carefully judged and frequently reassessed if this technique is to be of value. The concomitant use of antidysrhythmic drugs, such as lignocaine or propranolol, may allow lower rates of pacing to be used without the return of ventricular dysrhythmias.

The mechanism of suppression of ventricular ectopic beats by this technique is not clear, and it seems likely that more than one type of suppression is occurring. The simple depolarisation of cardiac muscle by the artificial pacemaker before any spontaneous ectopic pacemaker can discharge does not account for the clinical findings that the critical rate may be considerably slower than suggested by the prematurity of spontaneous ectopic beats. Similar observations concerning the suppression, by overdriving, of rapid dysrhythmias from causes other than myocardial infarction have been made by several workers (McCallister *et al.*, 1966; Kastor *et al.*, 1967); the case reported by Schoonmaker and co-workers (1966) is particularly interesting since ventricular tachycardia of 180 beats/min. could be controlled by pacing at 88 beats/min. This represented overdriving above the normal heart rate for this patient and prevented the far more rapid paroxysmal dysrhythmia.

The technique of overdriving should be considered in the control of many repetitive or paroxysmal rapid dysrhythmias but the nature of the method and the circumstances under which it is employed make a controlled trial of its effectiveness meaningless. It should be used as an additional therapy and not as an alternative to drugs. A comparison between these two methods of controlling ventricular irritability has little value. The advantage of overdriving is that it provides a further possibility of handling certain difficult dysrhythmias when conventional drug therapy has proved inadequate. The method is not simple and requires constant attention, so that it is probably not suitable for use outside specialised units. Within the coronary care area, however, it can be rapidly and safely applied.

At the present time suggested indications for atrial overdriving in patients without heart block are:

1. Short periods of ventricular tachycardia or ventricular fibrillation despite antidysrhythmic drugs.

2. Multiple ectopic beats not controlled by drugs.

3. R-on-T ectopic beats.

4. Bradycardia produced by antidysrhythmic drugs in doses which suppress ectopic activity.

5. Sinus bradycardia not responding to atropine.

6. Resuscitation from ventricular fibrillation. (Relative indication.)

REFERENCES

HEIMAN, D. F. & HELWIG, J., Jr. (1966). Suppression of ventricular dysrhythmias by transvenous intracardiac pacing. *J. Am. med. Ass.* **195,** 1150.

Kastor, J. A., DeSanctis, R. W., Harthorne, J. W. & Schwartz, G. H. (1967). Transvenous atrial pacing in the treatment of refractory ventricular irritability. *Ann. intern. Med.* **66,** 939.

Kimball, J. T. & Killip, T. (1965). A simple bedside method for transvenous intracardiac pacing. *Am. Heart J.* **70,** 35.

McCallister, B. D., McGoon, D. C. & Connolly, D. C. (1966). Paroxysmal ventricular tachycardia and fibrillation without complete heart block. Report of a case treated with a permanent internal cardiac pacemaker. *Am. J. Cardiol.* **18,** 898.

Schoonmaker, F. W., Osteen, R. T. & Greenfields, J. C., Jr. (1966). Thioridazine (Melleril R)—induced ventricular tachycardia controlled with an artificial pacemaker. *Ann. intern. Med.* **65,** 1076.

Sowton, E., Leatham, A. & Carson, P. (1964). The suppression of arrhythmias by artificial pacing. *Lancet,* **2,** 1098.

Sowton, E., Balcon, R., Cross, D. & Frick, M. H. (1967). Measurement of the angina threshold using atrial pacing. *Cardiovasc. Res.* **1,** 301.

Discussion

Dr Killip. I think this session on pacing has been very exciting and we have heard three provocative presentations. The last two were so mellifluous and informative that I thought I was listening to the B.B.C.

I agree with Dr Lown's comments. I think there is a tendency for all of us to get so involved in our complex technique that we forget, at least in the States, that some 80 per cent. of the hospitals and the vast majority of patients are in areas where many facilities such as fluoroscopy and so forth are not available and because of this our own group has been working with blind techniques for catheter pacing. There has been a great deal of discussion and argument about these techniques, but for the last three and a half years we have passed several hundred pacemaker catheters, both in patients with heart block associated with infarction and those with arrhythmias and heart block from other causes and we have only, in that period, fluoroscoped three patients.

We are utilising a unipolar electrode which can be passed through an 18-gauge American needle. We have used this almost exclusively in our Coronary Care Unit in the past three years. We have been able to insert the electrode in 90 per cent. of the cases without screening and we have paced without difficulty 90 per cent. of the patients in whom we have inserted the catheter.

We encountered no complications in 87 per cent. In 4 per cent. we induced ventricular tachycardia with cardiac arrest. Stand-by pacemakers were not available at that time. Arrhythmias were always due to competition, and with standby units. I do not believe that we will see this any more. A minor degree of phlebitis occurred in one case, and an episode of septicaemia in one instance done rather carelessly as an emergency procedure. Although the patient subsequently died, it apparently was not directly related to septicaemia. Some groups have been able to emulate our success and some have not. The only point I want to make is that it is entirely possible to insert a catheter quite satisfactorily, be it a soft one or a hard one, into the right ventricle and place it well in the majority of cases. I think this is an important message to carry to the physician in the community hospital. However, there is no question in my mind that when a satisfactory portable image intensifier becomes available we will undoubtedly use this and will utilise a bipolar catheter, since it is more satisfactory for a number of reasons.

I think Dr Sowton's presentation is very exciting. Many groups are beginning to utilise pacemakers for reasons other than for heart block. The importance of the ventricular rate which both he and Dr Lown discussed cannot really be overemphasised. Our own experience has been similar and we find that the haemodynamic results of pacing are rather unpredictable and vary considerably depending upon the circumstances, the patient's cardiac problem and the location of the catheter pacemaker. We believe that one of the key factors in deciding whether or not to pace is the ventricular rate and whether or not there is any irritability of automaticity in association with what appears to be an inadequate ventricular rate. We have measured cardiac function, but I think that we can make too much of a small change in cardiac output, and we do not think a 10 or 12 per cent. change of cardiac output in an acutely ill person is a terribly reliable observation. We have had a few patients in whom there was a steady increase in minute volume as one increased the ventricular rate although, of course, stroke volume always went down. More commonly, if the rate is slow there is a predictable increase in minute volume up to a ventricular rate of somewhere between 60 and 80 per minute, then usually things deteriorate again above that rate. It is difficult to interpret tension-time index data. The term, of course, is unfortunate because one thing that we are not measuring is tension. Perhaps it is correlated with oxygen consumption and perhaps we can draw some conclusions from the fact that again we have a tendency for a rise first and later a fall. Despite the discussion we have had in the previous day and a half about the vigorous use of drugs I think many of us at heart are therapeutic nihilists and we really prefer not to give these patients any drugs at all, because there is no question that on occasion they do confuse the issue. The exciting advantages of the electrical techniques are a combination of judicious use of a small amount of drug and the vigorous application of a technique which can be withdrawn at an instant's notice. I think it is going to be explored even more in the next few years.

I do not know how to evaluate Dr Frommer's comments on paired pacing. We are all excited about the rediscovery of this technique which has been known for some 80 years but certainly in our hands it has not been advantageous, with the exception of three patients with sinus tachycardia and mitral stenosis. In these patients we were successful in controlling the ventricular rate. Our own experience is that it requires almost moment to moment adjustment of the coupling interval, the strength of the impulses and so forth. I am not aware that anyone has shown that paired pacing has been useful in myocardial infarction in a critically ill patient although Dr Cranefield in New York still remains an enthusiast of this technique.

Dr Wallace. I would like to make two comments with regard to Dr Sowton's observations on overdriving—from a physiological point of view. First I think it is going to be important, as we use overdriving, to separate two kinds of response. It is possible in the presence of coupled premature beats or in the presence of ventricular tachycardia to pace at a rate which captures the ectopic activity. In other words, the RR interval of a pacemaker is shorter that the coupling interval of a VPB. I would like to separate this from the phenomenon of suppression by overdriving in which it is not necessary to capture the premature beat by pacing at a faster rate or by an RR interval which is shorter than the coupling interval. I think overdriving may provide certain diagnostic information. There are certain patients with ventricular tachycardia in whom pacing more rapidly than the rate of their ventricular tachycardia leads to disappearance of the particular tachycardia when the pacemaker is stopped. There are other patients in whom fast pacing is followed by ventricular tachycardia when you turn off the pacer. Presumably it has been there all the time and has been captured by the overdrive. I am not sure of the meaning of this but I have an idea that these are fundamentally two different mechanisms of ventricular tachycardia. Once we begin to understand this phenomenon we may be able to use it as a diagnostic tool. The second point I would like to make is that we have been able to confirm in approximately 10 patients the observations that Dr Sowton has made with regard to the relation of atrial transport and heart rate. We have used the technique of measuring stroke volume instantaneously with pressure gradient methods. At slow

162

rates, the atrium appears to play a relatively minor role whereas it can influence stroke volume by as much as 30 to 40 per cent. at rates in excess of 100.

Dr Frommer. In addition to the two proposed by Dr Wallace, I think there is a third mechanism of ventricular tachycardia— that is the re-entry mechanism. There is some evidence that pacing can interrupt this, and some people have used pacing as a diagnostic method for assessing the existence or non-existence of the re-entry phenomena. With regard to Dr Killip's points, I addressed myself strictly to coupled pacing in contrast to paired stimulation. I think there are very important differences. If there are to be beneficial effects, I think they will be achieved by coupled and not paired pacing. The difference is, of course, that with coupled pacing one applies a single stimulus in response to the normally occurring QRS complex, thereby minimising the chance of competition and parasystolic phenomena. It can be used for long periods without readjustment. It is important to remember that at low ventricular rates not only is a 50 per cent. reduction of ventricular rate disadvantageous but also one can provoke ventricular fibrillation. It is known that at very low ventricular rates the dispersion of recovery of refractory periods is sufficiently great to increase irritability.

Dr Cross. It has often been mentioned that if patients have anterior myocardial infarction along with complete heart block it would be impracticable to use temporary pacing and I would like to ask Dr Lown what his experience has been under those circumstances.

Dr Lown. After listening to the points of view of others, I think the general opinion is that the first approach is pacing irrespective of the site of infarction. Friedberg and his group have pointed out that with anterior infarction the mortality is about 80 per cent. and they also pointed out that the site of the idioventricular pacemaker—that is whether it is supraventricular or infraventricular— also indicates prognosis. In the latter case there is extensive infarction of the septum while in the former there is only temporary injury of the AV conduction system.

Dr Lassers. In our series in which all but three patients had pacing electrodes introduced, 80 per cent. of those with anterior involvement died, compared with 30 per cent. of patients with isolated inferior involvement. Thus, if the anterior surface of the heart is involved, the prognosis is very poor whether or not they are paced.

Professor Shillingford. How many of these patients died within

163

the next year or so, how many remain cardiac invalids and how many completely recovered?

Dr Leatham. Of our 24 survivors, two died within three months, two had to go on long-term pacing and 19 remained in sinus rhythm at one year follow-up.

Dr Sandøe. I would like to ask what rates Dr Sowton uses in overdriving?

Dr Sowton. The rate required varies with the individual patient. It depends on a large number of things including concomitant drug therapy. In general, if a patient is in heart block we can control the ectopic beats with a rate of around 70 per minute, but if they are in sinus rhythm we often have to go up to 120 or 130 and we have been up to 160 per minute.

Dr Killip. There is one factor which we have not considered in detail and that is the effect of the pacemaker location on cardiac function. There has been considerable debate in the literature about this, but there is one very convincing paper which clearly showed that in the experimental preparation the more normal conduction is and the less contiguous muscle conduction there is, the better is ventricular function. I would like to ask Dr Sowton in particular whether he has any concrete information on this point? It is hard to believe that in some patients it may not be an important factor.

Dr Sowton. I have no data on the effect of catheter placement but am always happy to find a stable electrode position.

There are many publications of course in animal preparations illustrating on the whole that it is important, but the changes are minor and these were done at relatively slow rates in relatively normal animals. I have been unable to find work carried out at fast rates or in sick hearts, and I am unable to accept it as an important factor.

Dr Wallace. I think the one thing about which there is no debate is that a synchronous contraction initiated through a normal conducting system is better than an asynchronous one initiated from anywhere in the ventricle.

Dr Dalle. Short-term atrial synchronised pacing is feasible—it is a little more difficult, but it is certainly feasible. The one difficulty of course is that you need two catheters. A tetrapolar catheter having two poles in the ventricle and two in the atrium would allow you to do anything you want: ventricular pacing, atrial pacing and sequential pacing. Sequential pacing is rather interesting because it may answer the question as to whether or not normal ventricular conduction is important. This has been studied by comparing atrial pacing with sequential pacing. Atrial pacing allows normal AV conduction, and the normal intraventricular conduction and sequential pacing provide a normal atrial transport mechanism without normal intraventricular conduction. These two techniques are found to give comparable results.

TREATMENT OF HEART FAILURE

Chairman: Dr D. G. JULIAN

CARDIAC GLYCOSIDES IN ACUTE MYOCARDIAL INFARCTION

BERNARD LOWN

Medical Clinics of the Peter Bent Brigham Hospital and the Cardiovascular Research Laboratories, Department of Nutrition, Harvard School of Public Health, Boston

FIFTY-FIVE years have elapsed since Herrick's (1912) classical description of the clinical syndrome of acute myocardial infarction. From the very beginning it was clear that heart failure was a common early complication. It is curious, though, that while digitalis drugs are usually the measures of first choice in chronic congestive failure, when the decompensation, however, results from acute myocardial infarction there is hesitancy, controversy and no clear guidelines to therapy. The controversy revolves around two central questions:

1. Are the digitalis glycosides effective in all cases when heart failure is secondary to acute myocardial infarction?

2. Is the toxic threshold lowered substantially and unpredictably, so that whatever therapeutic value may be derived from the glycosides is jeopardised by the hazard of precipitating major arrhythmias?

PREVIOUS STUDIES

Digitalis efficacy

Though many thousand of patients with myocardial infarction and heart failure receive digitalis preparations, a review of the literature reveals endless impressions and intuitive surmise but no hard facts. Many authors have advised the use of digitalis glycosides beginning with Herrick in 1912 and including Wood (1956), Friedberg (1966), deGraff (1954) and others. Though improvement is commonly reported, it is impossible to dissociate effects derived from the lapse of time itself, the usual employment of an array of other measures, and the action of the glycosides. There are veritably no clinical studies on the subject. Askey (1951) measured circulation times prior to and one week after digitalisation in 17 patients with acute myocardial infarction and compared them with a non-digitalised control group. Both groups showed the same degree of abbreviation in circulation time. A random measurement of circulation time in the course of myocardial infarction obviously cannot provide decisive information.

In the experimental animal with coronary occlusion the results are equally uncertain. In the acute phase following coronary embolisation in the dog, digitalis drugs caused a reduction in both filling pressure of the left ventricle and an increase in cardiac output (Cronin & Zsoter, 1965). This would indicate improvement in ventricular function. In other studies carried out in the subacute phase of infarction, no such improvement was noted (Hood *et al.*, 1967). Following infusion of acetyl strophanthidin, both sham operated dogs and those with coronary artery ligation showed a similar rise in mean arterial pressure and peripheral vascular resistance, as well as a reduction in heart rate and cardiac index. None of the animals showed a fall in left ventricular end-diastolic pressure. Though there was a rise in dp/dt, indicating an increase in contractility, this was not sufficient to offset the increase in afterload to contraction (Hood *et al.*, 1967).

Digitalis toxicity

Clinicians have long viewed with unease the utilisation of digitalis drugs in the early post-infarction period. Experimental studies are extremely meagre. Bellet *et al* (1934) compared the lethal doses of digitalis drugs in coronary-ligated and sham-ligated animals. He found no difference at 30 minutes after ligation, a 20 to 30 per cent. reduction in dose four days after ligation, and a 14 per cent. reduction after six weeks to six months. Travell and his colleagues (1938) re-examined this very problem in cats three weeks following coronary artery ligation. The lethal dose as well as the toxic dose was reduced by 22 per cent. In a recent study Hood and co-workers (1967) found following myocardial infarction a substantial reduction in the dose of acetyl strophanthidin required to produce ventricular tachycardia. There was a rough correlation between the change in toxic threshold and the size of experimentally induced infarction. It is reasonable to question whether the previously healthy dog is a suitable model for such studies; the coronary arteries are free of atherosclerosis and the anatomic distribution differs from that in man.

In the only controlled clinical study relating to drug toxicity changes following myocardial infarction, Askey (1951) found no significant difference in the incidence of sudden death, ventricular premature beats and ventricular tachycardia in patients digitalised as compared to an undigitalised control group. The study was conducted after the first week of infarction and the glycoside employed was digitoxin. However, since there was no electro-cardiographic monitoring of patients, the findings are not conclusive. Thus, the questions of safety and effectiveness of digitalis glycosides in the patient with acute myocardial infarction still await definitive study.

CLINICAL EXPERIENCE

In 300 patients with acute myocardial infarction admitted consecutively to the S. A. Levine Coronary Care Unit in this hospital, 63 per cent. were judged to have had left ventricular failure defined by the presence of moist rales at the lung bases, a third sound gallop at the apex and X-ray evidence of lung congestion. Digitalisation was carried out in 189 patients. In 66 patients (22 per cent) the response to digitalis drugs was inadequate and diuretic measures were additionally employed.

The choice of digitalis

With the availability of potent diuretic drugs, it is pertinent to question whether digitalis is still the initial treatment for heart failure developing after acute myocardial infarction. It is our view that digitalis glycosides are the agents of first choice. Diuretic drugs do not exert a positive inotropic effect. While they may relieve congestion by lowering blood volume, there are a number of hazards. Reduction of blood volume and the associated haemoconcentration may decrease cardiac output, favour hypotension and predispose to thromboembolism. The not infrequent occurrence of electrolyte derangements may result in arrhythmias already a significant problem in the patient with myocardial infarction.

Selection of a cardiac glycoside

In selecting a digitalis drug, we have chosen the short-acting agent ouabain. It affords a number of advantages such as immediate onset of action, ease in achieving rapid digitalisation, possibility of employing small frequently repeated increments, and rapidity of dissipation in case of toxicity. In the early phase of infarction, diverse arrhythmias are frequent. There is no simple way to differentiate between the arrhythmias due to infarction and those resulting from the toxic action of digitalis drugs. With ouabain, onset of action is within one to five minutes. Peak action develops within 20 to 30 minutes and the effect begins to wane in about six hours. This time course of drug action frequently permits determination of whether or not an arrhythmia is related to glycoside administration.

Ouabain is given intravenously in increments of 0·1 mg. to a

171

total dose of 0·4 to 0·8 mg. in 24 hours. The spacing between successive increments varies from 20 minutes to four hours and depends on the gravity of the clinical situation. After two or three days of ouabain therapy, or when the patient's condition stabilises, a longer-acting digitalis preparation such as digoxin is substituted. Ouabain is especially useful in treating patients with moderate and severe heart failure resulting in lung congestion and pulmonary oedema. At the extremes of the pump failure spectrum, namely in cardiogenic shock and in incipient left ventricular failure, benefits have been less obvious.

Toxic effects

Alteration in the toxic threshold to digitalis in the presence of myocardial infarction has been difficult to assess. Although ventricular premature beats and ventricular tachycardia are somewhat more common in patients receiving digitalis drugs, it is also true that seriously ill patients are more likely to exhibit arrhythmias. However, patients with profound heart failure, with hypoxia or acidosis, or with advanced renal or hepatic disease often appear to be unusually sensitive to ouabain and the drug is accordingly administered with great caution and in reduced dosage.

Two of three cases of ventricular fibrillation observed among the 300 patients occurred in relation to digitalis therapy, within 20 minutes after intravenous ouabain administration. These two patients were critically ill with severe pulmonary congestion, atrial fibrillation, rapid heart action, and both had been on chronic digitalis therapy prior to the acute infarction.

Animal experiments indicate that about 1 per cent. of the peripheral toxic dose of glycoside will result in ventricular tachycardia if the drug is administered directly into a coronary artery (Roberge et al., 1967). In the critically ill patient the peripheral tissue uptake of glycoside is impaired. The administration of ouabain by a single bolus may present to the myocardium a toxic quantity of the drug. Because of the two serious complications following bolus injection in patients who were seriously ill, we now give the 0·1 mg. increments of ouabain by a slow drip in a period of 5 to 15 minutes. To date no ventricular arrhythmias have followed this method of administration.

Remaining problems

A number of problems remain to be solved. The presence of early left ventricular failure is frequently overlooked. A simple test is required to identify this stage of cardiac decompensation. Will treatment of this stage of heart failure with digitalis drugs prevent further complications? The increased cardiac output after digitalis is the result of a positive inotropic action and generally occurs when the heart is enlarged and congestion is present. Are the cardiac glycosides of value in the early stages of heart failure in the absence of cardiomegaly, as is true in the majority of patients with myocardial infarction? Is the patient with infarction more susceptible to digitalis toxicity? In animal experiments, coronary artery ligation resulted in a 20 to 30 percent. reduction in the toxic threshold. Is this the case in man? Our experience would suggest that it is not the presence of myocardial infarction which sensitises the heart to toxic action of glycoside, but rather the presence and extent of pump failure.

REFERENCES

ASKEY, J. M. (1961). Digitalis in acute myocardial infarction. *J. Am. med. Ass.* **146**, 1008.

BELLET, S., JOHNSTON, C. G. & SCHELTER, A. (1934). Effect of cardiac infarction on the tolerance of dogs to digitalis: experimental study. *Arch. intern. Med.* **54**, 509.

CRONIN, R. F. P. & ZSOTÉR, T. (1965). Hemodynamic effects of rapid digitalisation in experimental cardiogenic shock. *Am. Heart J.* **69**, 233.

DEGRAFF, A. C. (1934). Digitalis intoxication. Circulation, **9**, 115.

FRIEDBERG, C. K. (1966). *Diseases of the Heart*. Philadelphia: Saunders.

HERRICK, J. B. (1912). Clinical features of sudden obstruction of the coronary arteries. *J. Am. med. Ass.* **59**, 2015.

HOOD, W. B., Jr., McCARTHY, B. & LOWN, B. (1967). Myocardial infarction following coronary ligation in dogs: hemodynamic effects of isoproterenol and acetyl strophanthidin. *Circulation Res.* **21**, 191.

ROBERGE, G., HOOD, W. B., Jr. & LOWN, B. (1967). Digitalisation of the myocardium in the intact animal by direct coronary artery drug administration. *Am. J. Cardiol.* In press.

TRAVELL, J., GOLD, H. & MODELL, W. (1938). Effect of experimental cardiac infarction on response to digitalis. *Archs. intern. Med.* **61**, 184.

WOOD, P. (1956). *Diseases of the Heart and Circulation*, vol. 1. London: Eyre & Spottiswoode.

DISCUSSION

Dr Nixon. There are obviously many questions and very few answers to the problem of treatment of heart failure in myocardial infarction. However, with respect to giving digitalis in the early hours of acute infarction, the work of Allison and his colleagues in Birmingham suggests that for the first few hours after a cardiac infarction occurs, there is a glucose intolerance and a delayed insulin response; then fairly suddenly at the end of three or four hours—perhaps longer in severe cases—there is a sudden shift in the blood sugar and potassium. It is possible, therefore, that this is when ventricular fibrillation occurs, and digitalis may be dangerous at that time. If we are going to learn from our experience about the value of digitalis in heart failure we have to define and categorise the cases in a way that we can understand and which will allow us to make comparisons. One pathway to this is to examine the mechanical functions, not by catheterising which cannot be done repeatedly in acute infarction, but by the impulse of the heart against the chest wall.

In mild infarction, the ' a ' wave in the apex cardiogram gets larger and the fourth sound which may be so close to the first as to be inaudible appears. Now that patient does not need intensive care in my opinion, nor does he need digitalis either to preserve rhythm to help the function of the ventricle which is not severely disturbed. These patients appear to have uncomplicated infarction and to survive. In these patients the left atrial pressure has been found to be normal.

In the rather more severe case the ' a ' wave becomes larger and more prominent, and the left atrial mean pressure is higher—10 or 12 mm. of mercury. This patient may be coming into the area where digitalis may be useful in preserving atrial transport function and where one thinks the ventricular dysfunction is more marked, calling for a more powerful atrial contraction. In the patient with severe infarction, I think the greater disturbance of the ventricular muscle is shown by the fact that the ' a ' wave becomes really dominant and there is little movement outwards of the ventricle except under the influence of atrial contraction. The fourth sound that corresponds with it is very quiet and may be undetectable, but atrial contraction can be palpated with the fingers. Such a ventricle is severely disturbed and may be helped by the inotropic action of digitalis. In acute infarction and in aortic stenosis with muscular hypertrophy of the left ventricular outflow tract, I have disturbed atrial contraction with a catheter. This resulted in sudden cardiac arrest and I think this is a sign that the ventricle is in a condition when it needs a powerful atrial booster pump for its function. If it loses suddenly, it ceases to fill effectively and, therefore, ceases to pump effectively and ventricular fibrillation occurs.

If in addition to this huge atrial contraction with its fourth sound there is a rapid filling peak as well, in my experience the patient's ventricle is at a mechanical disadvantage and there is either an aneurysm or mitral insufficiency—presumably from papillary muscle dysfunction. The ventricle is severely afflicted and at a mechanical disadvantage and I think it is reasonable to give digitalis for its inotropic action.

Now with a ventricle which is in the worst condition of all, there appears to be ' atrial failure '. The apex cardiograms show just a rapid filling wave but although there is sinus rhythm, atrial contraction is not detectable at all. With digitalis and rest atrial contraction may become detectable when the ventricle appears to be improving. The left atrial pressure in these people who have severely afflicted ventricles with acute infarction is usually about 23 to 25 mm. Hg. I consider the apex cardiogram is valuable in categorising the patients who need digitalis.

Dr Julian. I would like to ask Dr Lown about the use of cardioversion in the digitalised patient.

Dr Lown. The teaching has been that digitalis should be withheld for 24 hours or more because it produces increased sensitivity to electrical discharges. I do not think that this is good teaching however. If digitalis is stopped for 24 hours or more while the patient is in atrial fibrillation and when one is giving quinidine simultaneously, there is a tendency for the development of a rapid heart rate because of quinidine's vagolytic action as well as its tendency to reduce the number of F-waves and even convert fibrillation to flutter, with a rapid ventricular response. This may initiate heart failure which is a potent factor in the restitution of atrial fibrillation. Our present policy based on experience with 300 patients is to maintain digitalis therapy throughout the cardioversion. The only exception to this is the presence of digitalis intoxication in which it is mandatory to stop it. Our technique of cardioversion is, however, modified and we start with low energies of discharge to test whether digitalis toxicity can be evoked. We begin with 5 to 10 watt-seconds as our initial shock and, if no arrhythmias ensue, we proceed to energies of 50 to 100 watt-seconds. If ectopic beats occur after 10 or 50 watt seconds we then use lidocaine in a dose of 25 mg. to subdue the arrhythmia and proceed to higher energies. Utilising this method we have had no difficulties and we have had fewer reversions to atrial fibrillation than previously. Thus the titration of energy becomes, in effect, an important tactic in avoiding the effects of over-digitalisation by allowing them to be detected and subdued with antiarrhythmic drugs.

Dr George (Edinburgh). I agree with Dr Nixon that the apex cardiogram has considerable use in assessing atrial and ventricular function, and his records display diastolic events very well. However I have difficulty in understanding how he assesses the size of the ' a ' wave when he severely limits the systolic peak—since the ' a '

175

wave is normally expressed as a percentage of the total deflection.

Dr Nixon. I take the size of the 'a' wave in relation to the diastolic excursion, and not to systole at all. In the normal heart, most of the outward movement is early diastolic and atrial movement is insignificant. As the heart becomes abnormal the rapid filling phase gets less and less until it almost disappears and there is no detectable movement until the atrium contracts.

Professor Harris. Does Dr Nixon seriously mean that he can judge the amount of blood pushed into the ventricle at each atrial contraction by the movement of this 'bump' on the praecordium?

Dr Nixon. No, that is not what I meant. What one can do is to analyse this and empirically correlate the various patterns and appearances with disease. The only clear-cut association I have obtained with flow are studies I did with Humphries and Criley. These were cases with severe subaortic muscular obstruction. The apex cardiogram recorded virtually no movement until the atrium contracted and, cine-radiologically, it looked as though the ventricle scarcely filled until the atrium contracted. I have also recorded in about 100 patients the apex motion or displacement simultaneously with the left atrial pressure pulse and if you can detect a rise in left atrial pressure then you can detect an increased displacement. This is important, for example, after conversion of atrial fibrillation where you may be interested in the electrical and mechanical activity of the left atrium. If under these circumstances you have a catheter in the left atrium and can detect a left atrial pressure rise, you can detect atrial function from the displacement curve. If on the other hand you cannot detect any pressure rise, you cannot get an 'a' wave of displacement. Therefore, although I think its uses are limited, one of them may be to categorise left ventricular or congestive failure.

Dr Kreuzer (Dusseldorf). We have found no correlation between mean left atrial pressure and the 'a' wave in the context of myocardial infarction but only in the context of aortic stenosis.

Dr Semple. I think one reason why so many of us are shy of using digitalis in patients with acute infarction left heart failure with sinus rhythm is that we really are not certain how to use it. We all find it easy enough to judge the effective dose in congestive cardiac failure with atrial fibrillation but, in infarction it is often difficult to balance the harm from toxicity with the good from the positive inotropic effect. I would like to ask Dr Lown how he approaches it.

Dr Lown. I have just spent 30 minutes showing how I do not know how to do that. Our investigative approach to this problem

176

has been to utilise a very short acting preparation, like acetyl strophanthidin that permits you to assess rapidly whether there is an enhancement of the toxic threshold. If this is coupled with certain haemodynamic variables we should be able to start deciphering any clinical correlations that exist. Perhaps we would be able to provide some data, if this conference were to be held six months hence.

Dr Wallace. I want to ask Dr Lown if he has any experience of β-adrenergic blocking agents with counter-shock induced arrhythmias in digitalised patients.

Dr Lown. Three patients out of 800 whom we have cardioverted had been on propranolol, in the hope of averting recurrences of arrhythmia. In each of the three, we encountered sino-atrial standstill and cardiac arrest after cardioversion and they required isoproterenol to initiate cardiac action.

Dr Julian. I wonder whether anybody has been using propranolol as a protective drug in association with digitalis.

Dr Lown. We have used it in that setting for recurrent atrial arrhythmias—the type of arrhythmia that repeatedly recurs over years of atrial fibrillation, atrial flutter, atrial tachycardia. The arrhythmia of choice is atrial fibrillation and what we do now is induce atrial fibrillation deliberately in these patients but these are not patients with acute infarction.

Dr Sloman. We have used it as routine premedication prior to cardioversion and I agree with Dr Lown that results have not been any better. Nor have we found it of value in preventing reversion to atrial fibrillation after cardioversion. However we have not experienced the problem of sino-atrial block, with doses of 10 mg. four times a day, without atropine for two to three days prior to cardioversion.

Professor Shillingford. I think that a further haemodynamic problem is that of disco-ordination of the contraction of the ventricle following an infarction as Gorlin, in particular, has shown. There is an area of the ventricle which is being pushed out while the rest of the myocardium is contracting normally, thereby disturbing the function of the heart. In some of these cases the action of an inotropic drug might be to increase this disco-ordination and produce a fall in the output of the heart. I would like to ask Dr Lown his views on this.

Dr Lown. I think this is one of the many problems that has to be investigated within the context of acute myocardial infarction. Dr Gorlin's studies were in patients who had previously had coronary occlusions and this asynchrony with its mechanical disadvantage was the result of residual damage. However, such a deficit must also occur in the early stages because in 30 per cent. of cases of acute myocardial infarction you can detect these aneurysms by palpating the chest wall.

Dr McDonald. A further drawback in the use of digitalis in cardiac infarction is that we have seen asystole develop in two patients with right bundle branch block when treated with digitalis.

Dr Marquis. I wonder if Dr Lown or any others would support this idea of categorising patients in failure by apex cardiography in deciding on the use of digoxin.

Dr Lown. I have no experience of this.

Dr Meltzer. We are using this method and I think it is quite valuable. The ' a ' wave ratio can be related to left ventricular end-diastolic pressure but not as an absolute number. If the relationship of the ' a ' wave size to the E–O height changes, it seems to go hand in hand with left ventricular end-diastolic pressure changes. I think it is a very valuable method on the same patient; I do not think it has any value in comparing different people but if you take one person and follow him through, the relationship from hour to hour is important.

Dr Leatham. When you mention end-diastolic pressure, most people are thinking in terms of heart failure, but a lot of people measure end-diastolic pressure just before the systolic wave, which is, in other words, the ' a ' wave, and this is nothing to do with heart failure. I am sure you do not mean that, but perhaps we should talk about pre-end-diastolic pressure or something like that.

Dr Oliver. We have seen several cases who have had atrial tachycardia with block, which has occurred after relatively small doses of digoxin, soon after acute infarction. The digoxin has then been stopped; these patients require digoxin because they are in failure. The atrial tachycardia with block has continued with a relatively fast ventricular rate—maybe at a one to one ratio—needing digoxin for its control. What do we do?

Dr Lown. P.A.T. with block is in 70 per cent. of instances due to digitalis toxicity. But there is another variant—I do not know what its incidence is in acute myocardial infarction—where it is not an expression of digitalis toxicity at all. It is a variant of atrial flutter, and in such cases we have used digitalis to slow the ventricular rate without any untoward effects. In your instance probably digoxin or some cardiac glycoside is still the drug of choice.

Dr Marquis. Rather than cardioversion?

Dr Lown. I have not had this problem in acute myocardial infarction frequently. We have had one patient with P.A.T. with block whom we digitalised as we do for these arrhythmias initially. It reverted to sinus rhythm.

Dr Oliver. My problem is more related to the fact that I can think of three patients who have had P.A.T. with block developing when on digoxin and, because of the well-known association, we have stopped digoxin. The P.A.T. with block may have disappeared but it then returned again. In one patient it certainly did not disappear, and in all three of these patients we required, because of other reasons, to give digoxin and we found this a very embarrassing decision.

Dr Lown. So would I! One possibility in dealing with this problem is to try and get them cardioverted but to start with very low energies; if they are deeply digitalised when you give a shock of 5 watt seconds, ventricular bigeminy develops. You give them lidocaine and it abolishes it. This would indicate the mechanism is due to digitalis overdosage; it is dangerous to proceed with cardioversion; it is dangerous to use digitalis; other techniques and perhaps anti-arrhythmic drugs should be employed, such as potassium and procaine amide, in order to control the rhythm disorder. This becomes a modality of deciding definitely whether digitalis toxicity does or does not exist.

DIURETIC THERAPY

LAWSON MCDONALD

The London Hospital, the National Heart Hospital and the Institute of Cardiology, London

SOME months ago our interest was focused on the possible role of diuretic therapy in precipitating ventricular fibrillation after cardiac infarction. This problem inevitably led to a reconsideration of the diagnosis and treatment of left ventricular failure following cardiac infarction.

In our experience (Restieaux *et al.*, 1967) of treating patients after cardiac infarction, in a coronary unit, there appeared to have been an improvement in mortality (from 28 per cent. in 1964 to 14 per cent. in 1966), which could not be solely explained by the effective treatment of potentially fatal cardiac dysrhythmias. This betterment seemed likely to be associated with the early detection and treatment of other complications of cardiac infarction, including left ventricular failure. Slight evidence of left ventricular dysfunction, often without breathlessness, may be overlooked.

179

Clinical evidence of left ventricular dysfunction is common in ischaemic heart disease, and earlier studies on patients with ischaemic heart disease (Seymour *et al.*, 1965; Agnew *et al.*, 1967) helped to define important auscultatory features of it. These include atrial and ventricular gallop rhythm, and reversed splitting of the second heart sound. Systolic murmurs due to papillary muscle dysfunction, to mitral regurgitation occurring otherwise, and to rupture of the ventricular septum will not be considered.

In 100 consecutive patients with ischaemic heart disease, who were referred to an outpatient clinic at the National Heart Hospital, 68 per cent. had at least one of these abnormal auscultatory features; 13 per cent. had an atrial gallop, 53 per cent. a ventricular gallop, and 25 per cent. reversed splitting of the second heart sound (Fig. 1). In only 2 of the 25 was reversed splitting of the second heart sound due to the electrical delay of left bundle branch block.

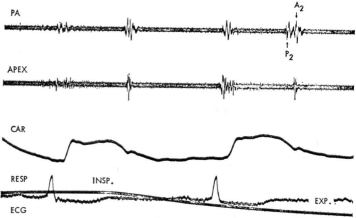

FIG. 1. Phonocardiogram (medium frequency) showing reversed splitting of the second heart sound. PA, pulmonary area; P_2, pulmonary valvar closure; A_2, aortic valvar closure; CAR, carotid trace; ECG, electro-cardiogram; RESP, phase of respiration; INSP, inspiration; EXP, expiration.

Gallop rhythm has long been associated with ventricular dysfunction and it seems likely that reversed splitting of the second heart sound, in the absence of left bundle branch block, is similarly related. Thus 30 per cent. of patients with reversed splitting of the second heart sound showed pulomnary venous congestion on chest radiographs, as opposed to 8 per cent. in whom the second heart sound was normal.

These findings on careful auscultation, with or without phono-cardiography, and chest radiography therefore seemed very important in the early diagnosis of left ventricular dysfunction following cardiac infarction, at a time when left heart catheterisation is usually inadvisable, as well as the grosser clinical and radiographic features of left ventricular failure (Wood, 1961).

Of 150 consecutive patients studied after recent cardiac infarction, who were admitted to a coronary unit, 61 per cent. had abnormal auscultatory features associated with left ventricular dysfunction; there were 31 per cent and 46 per cent. with atrial and ventricular gallop rhythm, respectively, and 2 per cent. with reversed splitting of the second heart sound. The considerably lower number with reversed splitting of the second heart sound, than was found in the out-patients, may be due to the circumstances of the patient's illness after cardiac infarction, which mitigate against such a precise observation. In considering these observations, which were made on admission to the coronary unit, the times of admission after the onset of pain are relevant (Table I).

Pulmonary venous congestion was present in 57 per cent. of the patients who were admitted to the coronary unit, and localised pulmonary oedema (Fig. 2) without clinical signs was not uncommon. Abnormal auscultatory features of left ventricular dysfunction without pulmonary venous congestion occurred in 23 per cent.

It appears, therefore, that in patients after cardiac infarction gallop rhythm, reversed splitting of the second heart sound in the absence of left bundle branch block, and pulmonary venous congestion should all lead to the consideration of the use of diuretic therapy, which will usually be indicated. This may be with digitalis, a mercurial diuretic, frusemide, or a chlorothiazide.

The importance of meticulous bedside examination and of chest radiography, in the diagnosis of early left ventricular failure after cardiac infarction cannot be overemphasised.

The use of diuretics, other than digitalis, after cardiac infarction may obviously lead to undesirable depletion of serum and myocardial cellular potassium. It appeared initially that there might be a correlation between the use of diuretics and the occurrence of ventricular fibrillation in some patients who had recurrent ventricular fibrillation.

Ventricular fibrillation occurred in 15 of 150 patients after cardiac infarction (Restieaux et al., 1967); resuscitation was initially successful in nine, and of these six had several episodes of ventricular fibrillation. All had an extensive transmural cardiac infarction

181

and were in left ventricular failure. Their levels of serum-glutamic-oxaloacetic-transaminase were amongst the highest which were recorded. Four of these patients left hospital, but two died from increasing left ventricular failure while in the unit. After defibrillation the patients rapidly regained consciousness and their clinical state seemed to be little altered by the recurrent ventricular fibrillation. Patient 1 (Fig. 3) had 105 episodes of ventricular fibrillation in 19 days. He was subsequently discharged from hospital and

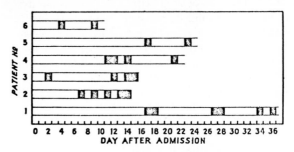

FIG. 3. Incidence of recurrent ventricular fibrillation after cardiac infarction. Each black square represents a day on which one or more episodes of ventricular fibrillation occurred. Patients with extended lines recovered and left hospital.

returned home. In some patients, intravenous propranolol, a mixture of potassium, insulin and dextrose (Sodi-Pallares et al., 1962; Sodi-Pallares et al., 1963), intravenous 2 per cent. lignocaine, and procaine amide, appeared to be effective in maintaining sinus rhythm. The use of lignocaine and procaine amide, particularly, have led to a satisfactory reduction in the incidence of ventricular fibrillation.

The aetiology of recurrent ventricular fibrillation in these patients remains obscure; none had preceding pain, anoxia, acidosis, or electrolyte imbalance. In one patient the R-on-T effect (Smirk & Palmer, 1960) was identified, and in four patients there appeared to be an association with the administration of diuretic therapy in that ventricular fibrillation developed on the days that diuretics were given. It has not been possible to prove this relationship, and from the available data it cannot be assumed that it was other than a chance association. However, diuretics should certainly be used with caution after cardiac infarction, and those which produce a relatively slight loss of sodium and potassium, with an adequate loss of water seem preferable, and supplemental potassium should be given.

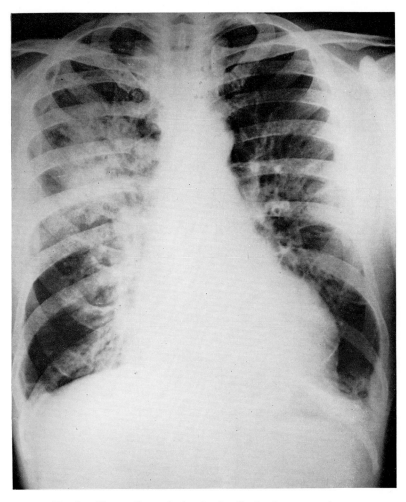

FIG. 2. Chest radiograph showing localised pulmonary oedema.

To face page 182.

It is concluded that a high percentage of patients after cardiac infarction have evidence of left ventricular failure and are likely to benefit from diuretics, but that proper precautions must be observed in their use.

REFERENCES

AGNEW, T., BUCHER, H., McDONALD, L. & SEYMOUR, J. (1967). Delayed closure of the aortic valve in ischaemic heart disease. *Br. Heart J.* **29**, 775.

McDONALD, L. (1963). In *International Symposium on Etiology of Myocardial Infarction*, p. 496. Ed. Keyes, J. W. & James, T. N. Boston: Little, Brown.

RESTIEAUX, N., BRAY, C., BULLARD, H., MURRAY, M., ROBINSON, J., BRIGDEN, W. & McDONALD, L. (1967). 150 patients with cardiac infarction treated in a coronary unit. *Lancet*, **1**, 1285.

SEYMOUR, J., BUCHER, H. & McDONALD, L. (1965). Reversed splitting of the second heart sound in ischaemic heart disease. *Br. Heart J.* **27**, 952.

SMIRK, F. H. & PALMER, D. G. (1960). A Myocardial Syndrome. *Am. J. Cardiol.* **6**, 620.

SODI-PALLARES, D., TESTELLI, M. R., FISHLEDER, B. L., BISTENI, A., MEDRANO, G. A., FRIEDLAND, C. & DE MICHELI, A. (1962). Effect of an intravenous infusion of a potassium-glucose-insulin solution on the electrocardiographic signs of myocardial infarction. *Am. J. Cardiol.* **9**, 166.

SODI-PALLARES, D., BISTENI, A., MEDRANO, G. A., TESTELLI, M. R. & DE MICHELI, A. (1963). The polarising treatment of acute myocardial infarction. *Dis. Chest*, **43**, 424.

WOOD, P. (1961). *Diseases of the Heart and Circulation*. London: Eyre & Spottiswoode.

YURCHAK, P. M. & GORLIN, R. (1963). Paradoxical splitting of the second heart sound in coronary heart disease. *New. Engl. J. Med.* **269**, 741.

DISCUSSION

Dr McNicol (London). The diagnosis of left heart failure obviously presents extreme difficulty, with some people feeling that it requires sophisticated techniques. I believe the simple method of listening to the lung bases is very reliable and, if there are persistent crepitations after taking a deep breath, we diagnose heart failure. It is interesting that using this method we find the same incidence of heart failure as do those using advanced techniques. Basal crepitations correlate well with arterial hypoxaemia. All patients with persistent basal crepitations are given diuretics and we only give digoxin to the severely ill. Frusemide 80 mg. intravenously invariably produced a diuresis of considerable magnitude in patients with acute heart failure. The mean urine flow increased from 60 ml./hour to 440 ml./hour after two hours. After a further two hours it was 210 ml./hour and thereafter it returned to control levels. We had found that in the more seriously ill patients with venous admixture of over 20 per cent., there was a substantial reduction in the venous admixture and in two out of three there was a rise in oxygen tension. There were no adverse effects from this treatment. In the last 50 of our patients, 35 had evidence of mild heart failure. Only 26 of these received oral diuretics. Oral diuretic therapy produced a diuresis in only eight, but none of these patients were in gross failure.

In another study, a group of 15 patients with crepitations were followed with daily observations by two students. They were all treated with diuretics and 12 of the 15 still had crepitations at the time of discharge from hospital. In conclusion, we believe that left heart failure can be diagnosed simply by the presence of basal crepitations, that it responds well to intravenous frusemide but unpredictably to the drug orally and that the crepitations and ventilation perfusion abnormalities may persist for some considerable time.

Dr Sloman. I would like to ask Dr McDonald a question regarding reversed splitting of the second sound. Some workers have stated that this is very common in acute myocardial infarction. Our findings in a series of about 60 patients in whom we did careful phonocardiographs, resulted in an incidence similar to his—about 2 per cent. I think most of the studies in which a high incidence has been recorded have not been supported by phonocardiography, I would suggest to him that perhaps if he did phonocardiographs in all of his patients he would still only have a low incidence of reversed splitting. Dr McDonald, I understand, suggested the use of a diuretic in those patients who have left ventricular failure and then, I believe, he said that he thought digitalis was the diuretic of choice. I would also like him to clarify, in referring to those patients who developed ventricular fibrillation on the day that they had their diuretic therapy, whether these patients were also receiving digitalis, and whether they were having potassium supplements at that time? I agree with Dr McNicol in that we have used the same sort of diuretic regime in those patients who have crepitations at their lung bases, and we have not, to the best of our knowledge, induced ventricular fibrillation in those patients who had a diuresis. We still prefer to use this type of intravenous therapy in an attempt to clear the crepitations at the lung bases and we have evidence, as he has, that there is an improvement in the oxygen tension, but I would add that this improvement, which is never more than about 10 mm. of mercury, can be equally well brought about by the administration of oxygen intranasally or by mask.

Dr McDonald. I think that if you are going to treat somebody with evidence of slight left ventricular dysfunction, it seems to me that digitalis is probably the drug of choice, but if there is more overt evidence of fluid retention then one should probably go on to a diuretic. In that it produces a better water diuresis and less sodium and potassium depletion, I would have thought that a mercurial might be the best of the diuretics. Those patients with ventricular fibrillation on the day of the diuretic therapy were all having digitalis, but they had been having this for some time. They were all having considerable potassium supplements and all had normal serum potassium.

Dr McKendrick. I support Dr McDonald very strongly in his views on the importance of X-rays, because of the frequency of localised venous congestion, and patches of pulmonary oedema. We do serial daily X-rays on all patients in the intensive care unit and feel that it is most necessary to watch what is going on radiologically.

Dr Lown. We have utilised glycosides in 63 per cent. of our patients. In 22 per cent. of these patients we had to resort to diuretic measures—that is, we could not achieve full compensation. Another problem we have encountered is the patient who comes in acutely ill with pulmonary oedema. The house-staff in the emergency ward may respond by what is current fashion in giving ethacrynic acid or frusemide intravenously. In two or three of these patients who did not have hypotension initially, low blood pressure developed by the time they had got through with the first diuresis. My question, therefore, is have those who are utilising diuretics encountered any drop in blood pressure?

Dr Wallace. A couple of relatively simple points; one is that we have been impressed with the undesirable phenomenon of fever in patients with acute myocardial infarction, and on a number of occasions have found that gallop rhythm disappears by lowering the temperature with aspirin or with indomethacin. The other thing is I am really disturbed by the common association of basal crepitations with the phenomenon of heart failure. I am not impressed that this is as frequent as has been implied; I rely more on the X-ray. My finding is that patients with an average age of 70 who are put to bed and sedated will develop atelectasis and that getting them up and using breathing exercises under the guidance of a physotherapist is more effective in clearing the bases than the diuretic is.

Dr Mounsey. There are about six speakers in this room emphasising that daily X-rays are vital if you are really going to follow what is going on. We started doing this about two years ago, and the first thing that struck us was the dissimilarity between our preconceived notions of what the symptoms of left ventricular failure should be and what we saw on the X-ray. We were so surprised

185

to find that patients with fairly gross signs of oedema on the X-ray could lie flat and were not breathless. We then did a planned study of trying to assess what was going on indirectly in the left heart by measuring pulmonary arterial pressures. We found, of course, the pulmonary arterial pressures were raised in all these patients who were not breathless but who had the evidence on X-ray of pulmonary oedema. We followed the pulmonary arterial pressure, its changes day to day and also the X-ray. The first thing to return to normal was the pulmonary arterial pressure. There was a lag of about two days or more before the radiological signs cleared.

Dr M. B. Matthews (Edinburgh). I would like to ask Drs McDonald and McKendrick whether or not they have observed any influence of the position in which the patient is nursed on these changes in the X-ray appearances. I think patients who have to be horizontal because of poor cerebral circulation may develop the appearance of pulmonary oedema on X-ray more rapidly than others do.

Dr Mounsey. If you put the patient's head downwards, the oedema develops at the top.

Dr M. B. Matthews. I have no wish to place the patient's head below the horizontal because I see no advantage in doing this.

Dr Lown. We have followed the teachings of Dr Levine who believed in the armchair treatment of acute myocardial infarction. During the initial 24 hours, at the latest 36 hours, we get patients into an armchair and nurse them in this fashion throughout their stay in the Coronary Care Unit; as you walk in you can see the patients sitting up and quite comfortable. The ancillary need in carrying out an armchair treatment is to utilise the bed in the reverse Trendelenberg position. This becomes extremely important in the patient who is elderly because there is rapid maladaptation to the erect sitting posture and we found initially, that when we started getting patients out of bed, they developed hypotension. Now, we keep them sleeping at an angle of about 10 to 15 degrees. We have found that one can get them nearly all out of bed, and I believe this may be an important way of treating left ventricular failure. We have not encountered untoward effects or vasovagal reactions in this manoeuvre which has now been carried out in close to 400 patients.

Dr Lassers. I am sure that Dr Nixon can give better information than we, but we have certainly seen patients who have normal pulmonary arterial pressures and persistent basal crepitations. If this what you are treating with diuretic therapy then you may in fact not be very successful. We have also seen patients who have had no basal crepitations but have had pulmonary venous congestion on the chest X-ray and elevated pulmonary arterial pressures. I think the two are quite distinct.

Dr Nixon. I deliberately never listen to the lung bases. What I believe is this, if you have got an erection of the pulmonary venous system from left atrial hypertension—left ventricular diastolic hypertension—then you breathe faster. The pattern of breathing monitored by the nurse is very important and this correlates well with the X-ray. I believe there is another sort of pulmonary oedema which is hypostatic or dependent, and when you put the patients' head downwards all the water which should be round the sacrum runs into the thorax. Now this sort makes the patients equally blue and anoxic but the breathing rate does not change. In other words, one looks clinically to see if there is stiff-lung breathing or not stiff-lung breathing and takes an X-ray.

Professor Shillingford. Perhaps I may add something here and that is, that we were interested in the haematocrit following infarction. I think it is known that you find that the haematocrit is raised in the majority of cases for the first four or five days following an infarction. We have used radio-active albumen to see where the plasma protein was going and found that the albumen in the blood fell, and we found that it went to a large extent into the lungs. If the lungs were squeezed at autopsy there was the radio-active albumen. It looks a though, following an infarction with or without left ventricular failure, there is some exudation of albumen into the alveoli. This seems to remain for some time. In fact, if at autopsy you make sections of the lung, you can see the albuminous material on the surface of the alveoli. This is one added factor which leads to crepitations in the alveoli although there may not be actual fluid there.

Dr McNicol. Can I dispute Dr Nixon's contention about the pattern of breathing. We have looked at this, and this is in fact not so. The pattern of breathing does not correlate with other indices of lung function.

Dr Oliver. I do not think the discussion should end without mentioning sodium regimes. Has anybody any objective evidence about the more rapid reduction of pulmonary venous congestion if low sodium regimes are implemented early? Is there any reason to have a low sodium regime or do we not need to trouble about low sodium in the management of failure in the first 48 hours?

Dr Meltzer. We have kept people on a set sodium diet, about 30 m.Eq. sodium per day, and measured their excretion rates in an attempt to predict heart failure. I think that people who are going

187

into failure show a decrease on a set sodium diet. Whether they benefit by reducing this below 30 m.Eq. I don't know, but the pattern of excretion differs in people who are about to fail compared to people who are not failing. It is worth measuring this sodium excretion, if one controls the intake.

CIRCULATORY AND RESPIRATORY EFFECTS OF ACUTE MYOCARDIAL INFARCTION

Chairman: Professor K. W. DONALD

OBSERVATIONS ON CARDIOGENIC SHOCK

PETER NIXON

Charing Cross Hospital, London

CARDIOGENIC shock is a mystery, and the purpose of this communication is to define useful questions rather than to provide answers.

The subject of this paper is the condition of the patient suffering from acute cardiac infarction who looks as though he is dying by the hour. Consciousness is impaired and there are brief periods of restless confusion. Peripheral cutaneous blood flow is undetectable. The ears and fingers are cold and blue, and the trunk is mottled with cyanotic patches. There is anuria and metabolic acidosis. The jugular venous pressure is raised and the arterial pressure usually low. We are satisfied that he is not syncopal from the effect of drugs; tachyarrhythmia is not present and, in the case of heart block, the heart rate has been controlled with intravenous pacemaking apparatus. The deterioration continues.

The first question concerns the pathological condition of the heart. Is the destruction of the left ventricle so extensive that the illness must be regarded as the act of dying? Or is it so slight that the patient may if he recovers, return to his normal activities? Experience suggests that either condition is possible.

The second question concerns the clinical diagnosis. How may the hopeless condition be distinguished from the recoverable?

At present I am attempting to answer this question with a trial of intravenous 5 per cent. dextrose infusion in doses of 100 ml. The trial was suggested by an experience of the treatment of patients in a low output state at the end of heart-lung bypass operations where recovery may depend upon transfusion raising the venous pressure to a point far above its preoperative level.

In the coronary patient it is possible to judge the effect of the infusion when 300 or 400 ml. have been given. If it is ineffective, the patient continues to die, and digitalis and sympathetic amines are equally ineffective. Autopsy shows extensive destruction of the left ventricle. Six patients were in this group. Each had one or more previous infarctions and, in most, death occurred in the second or third week in hospital.

Where the infusion was effective, the arterial pressure improved within minutes and the infusion was continued until the patient

191

recovered a stable and adequate circulation. Six patients were in this group and in each the shock developed within a few hours of the first known infarction. Four had heart block but pacemaking did not halt their deterioration.

The amount and the rate of infusion varied with the case, ranging from 4 litres in 16 hours to 11 litres in seven days.

The third question is concerned with the physiological differences between the hopeless and the recoverable groups. What physiological distinctions can be made?

The immediate and striking differences lie in the response of the central venous pressure to infusion. In the patients who die, the venous pressure rises with each dose of 100 ml. dextrose solution, and remains at the level to which it is raised. In the patients who recover, the response is different. Here the venous pressure, usually about 10 cm. water, rises steeply with the infusion. In a few minutes it drops, and, as it drops, the arterial pressure rises (Fig. 1).

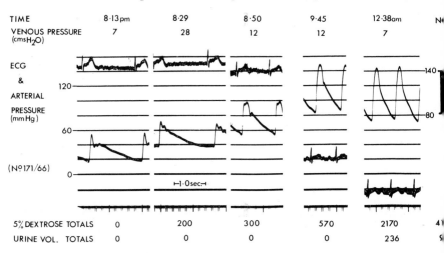

FIG. 1. The effect of intravenous infusion on venous pressure, ECG, arterial pressure and urinary volume.

As the circulation improves a stage is reached where, within the attempted limits, the arterial pressure may be adjusted upwards or downwards by chosen alterations in the venous pressure (Fig. 2).

In the later stages of recovery, when the extremities are pink and warm and the urine flowing generously, 200 ml. dextrose solution may be added to the circulation without a detectable rise in the venous pressure (Fig. 3).

192

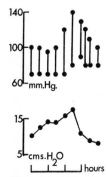

FIG. 2. The effect of variations in venous pressure
on arterial pressure.

The fourth question concerns the nature of the venous pressure responses. What are the underlying conditions that determine the two varieties of response?

In the hopeless patients with a greatly destroyed left ventricle, the failure to improve when the venous pressure is increased suggests that the heart has reached or passed the peak of Starling's curve.

In the patients who recover, the improvement in the circulation which follows the raising of the venous pressure suggests that the heart is on the upward slope of Starling's curve and that elevation of the venous pressure has a beneficial effect. The abnormally high initial level of the venous pressure may well result from venous constriction; this is suggested by the great increase which occurs when 100–200 ml. of fluid are first infused.

If it is accepted that infusion may be beneficial in certain cases, the fifth question must concern its mode of action. How does it act?

Ross (personal communication, 1966) has shown that the recently injured dog's ventricle needs to be distended before its output can return to a normal level; and in cardiogenic shock the infusion may act by distending the left ventricle to the point where it can achieve an adequate output.

This hypothesis points to a reason for the resemblances between oligaemic and cardiogenic shock. In oligaemic shock there is an absolute reduction in the circulating blood volume. In cardiogenic shock the normal blood volume, probably reduced by the intense sweating, may be too small for the needs of the recently injured heart.

This finding of the different venous pressure responses in the hopeless and the recoverable case raises a question of practical

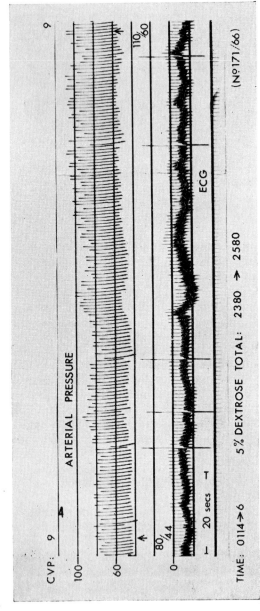

FIG. 3. The arterial pressure in response to venous infusion in a patient in the later stages of recovery.

CVP: 9

100—

60—

ARTERIAL PRESSURE

110/60

80/44

0—

ECG

T

20 secs

5% DEXTROSE TOTAL: 2380 → 2580

(N°171/66)

TIME: 0114→6

194

importance in this age of powerful diuretics. Before we use them in an acute coronary case, can we be sure whether their lowering the venous pressure will help the patient or whether it will deprive the heart of the filling pressure that venous constriction is attempting to maintain?

Whenever infusion in acute cardiac infarction is discussed, the question of pulmonary oedema is raised. In acute infarction without infusion there appear to be two chief varieties. One, the ' batswing ' type, may be seen as it was in a case with a ruptured papillary muscle, where the peak left atrial pressure reached 90 mm. Hg. The breathing is consistent with stiffness of the lungs from pulmonary venous hypertension. The other, dependent oedema, may be seen where the patient has been nursed with the foot of the bed raised high. Here the pattern of breathing does not suggest pulmonary venous hypertension. Neither variety presented in the patients who were resuscitated by infusion. Pulmonary oedema did occur in a dying patient when the infusion was continued far beyond 400 ml., but even then it was not worse than in similar cases dying without infusion.

With regard to the choice of infusion fluid, I have found no indication to change from 5 per cent. dextrose solution. Its use as an expander of the extra-cellular volume in acute cardiac infarction and heart-lung bypass may depend upon the fact that glucose metabolism is greatly reduced in these conditions (Allison et al., 1967).

REFERENCE

ALLISON, S. P., PROWSE, K. & CHAMBERLAIN, M. J. (1967). Failure of insulin response to glucose load during operation and after myocardial infarction. Lancet, 1, 478.

DISCUSSION

Professor Donald. These are challenging concepts. Most of us agree that in severe cardiogenic shock the patient is in a mortal condition. You are, in essence, proposing that you can sort out the mortal from the non-mortal by putting them under stress by raising the filling pressure in a Starling way—that is by raising the filling pressure by putting more fluid or pressure behind the heart. The real Starling Law is concerned when the heart is failing and its residual volume increases and the diastolic pressure and the filling pressures rise. Nevertheless you make this claim and it should be very seriously considered. The blood volume problem has perhaps been too easily passed in Mackenzie's work, and other people have reported on this matter. The blood volumes are sometimes lowish but within the normal range, although recently in America it has been reported that a number of people who have been in shock for days and survived have had a fall in blood volume. I would seek views from the audience about this matter.

Professor Shillingford. I think you can achieve exactly the same result without infusing sugar or anything else—by simple posture. If first of all you have the patient propped up and then you lay the patient flat and lift up his legs, you will have the same result. At one time we looked into this and used it as a test for residual failure of the L.V. If you raise the legs and the output rises that is fine—the heart is performing normally. If you raise the legs and the output and pressures fall, then there is something wrong with ventricle. Maybe I could have Dr Nixon's views on this method rather than infusing fluid.

Dr Nixon. It took me two or three years to get enough courage to give anyone an infusion. Once the patients had reached the advanced stage in spite of posture change, there was really nothing else to try and it really did work.

Dr Rossi (Rome). I used the same technique as Dr Nixon in eight cases of cardiogenic shock and in two of these cases I noticed that when the central venous pressure increased pulmonary congestion appeared. I used also small doses of acetylstrophanthidine and isoprenaline—5 micrograms per minute. The central venous pressures went down and the pulmonary congestion was decreased with very good results on the urine output and systemic blood pressure.

Dr Nixon. With regard to that, the ideal answer may be not to use a solution like dextrose alone, but to give a certain amount to distend the left ventricle a little bit and then add digitalis or an inotropic agent. But I did not want to do that in these patients because then everybody would have said ' Well, the digitalis would have enabled them to get better in spite of the infusion '. I really just wanted to see the effect of this alone.

Professor Donald. I think the majority experience so far is that these mortally wounded hearts, or near mortally wounded hearts do not respond to digoxin.

Dr. Wallace. In the United States there are a large number of patients who have been hypertensive and on diuretic therapy or on severe salt restriction through a rice diet. We have often seen in this group—and by the way they do have low blood volume prior to their infarction—a picture of shock or hypotension. In these patients, volume expansion works very effectively to correct their hypotensive shock state, I think because of the setting of low volume to begin with. I am concerned about volume expansion, however, because we have recently adopted your technique of infusion of 5 per cent. glucose in water and have seen three patients who went into acute pulmonary oedema with central venous pressures of less than 8 cm. of water. I think that the phenomenon of acute left ventricular failure without right ventricular failure is a real one. Patients can go into pulmonary oedema without an elevation of central venous pressure. This is overt pulmonary oedema.

Dr Lassers. I am wondering, Dr Nixon, if you know what the arterial oxygen tension and pH was in those patients who survived. I note that one of the patients was in complete heart block. We found that some patients with complete heart block, although apparently shocked, did not have the severe metabolic abnormalities described by Mackenzie.

Dr Muir. I wonder if I could ask Dr Nixon if he ventilated his patients at this time.

Dr Nixon. The first patient came to the casualty department, had a cardiac arrest due to ventricular fibrillation, was resuscitated and then was found to be in heart block with hypotension. We put a pacing catheter in and paced him at rates varying from 70 to 120, which at that time did not make any difference to his general condition. I was using artificial ventilation for bad coronaries rather more then than I am now so that he was intubated and put on positive pressure and was ventilated to try and oxygenate him as well as possible, but it made no difference. One other patient had artificial ventilation. This was a woman whose X-rays showed pulmonary oedema, and she had a second or third infarct. She had been in hospital for three weeks when she collapsed. The autopsy showed massive destruction of the left ventricle. Deliberately in that case I went on beyond 400 ml. of 5 per cent. dextrose. I thought I would be able to control the pulmonary oedema with artificial ventilation but I was unable to do so.

Dr Muir. In Mackenzie's series we had great difficulty in raising oxygen tension. I wonder when you ventilated, what happened to oxygen tension?

Dr Nixon. I cannot tell you.

Dr Sloman. I would like to ask Dr Nixon his views on the aetiology of this interesting condition of cardiogenic shock. Pathologists have drawn our attention to the changes in the microcirculation of the systemic circulation of the lungs and of the coronary circulation. There have been some suggestions that drugs which prevent intravascular coagulation may have a place in the management of cardiogenic shock.

Dr Nixon. I really do not know. These patients were nursed on the X-ray table which is in the intensive care suite so that one could watch for the development of pulmonary oedema during infusion. You can often palpate the paradoxical ' flopping out ' movement of the heart and, in experimental infarction in animals, there is a very large paralytic area. I have wondered, as there is quite a large part of the ventricular wall just not contracting, whether the reason why inotropic agents are not much good is that if the healthy part of the myocardium contracts more forcibly it has nothing to act against. If you increase the volume of the ventricle, it may just splint this flopping, ballooning area and enable the functioning muscle tissues to contract and to eject. At that stage, when you have distended the ventricle, digitalis may be useful in aiding its function.

Dr Cameron (Glasgow). Could I come back to the question of arterial hypoxaemia, which is one of the very striking features of this syndrome, and the difficulty found by Mackenzie and his colleagues in raising oxygen tension. We are fortunate in Glasgow in having a hyperbaric chamber and we are trying to do a trial on this desperately ill type of patient. The criteria and the type of patient are very similar to those described by Mackenzie and his associates. In fact death is inevitable in these patients using conventional methods, either within the first few hours or at most within two to three days. We have only treated three patients with this shock syndrome. We have surprisingly been able to raise the arterial oxygen tension reasonably—nothing like you get in the healthy subject or in less seriously ill infarction patients —but up to a level of about 2–300 mm.Hg. This can also be accompanied by certain haemodynamic and metabolic responses which may or may not be beneficial. One patient had dramatic clinical and haemodynamic response and, after removal from the hyperbaric environment, this was maintained for a few hours, but a fatal cardiac arrest developed from which we could not resuscitate him. The second patient had little or no clinical, haemodynamic or metalbolic response and following removal from the hyperbaric environment lingered on for about 48 hours and died in progressive cardiac failure. The third one made absolutely no response at all. I am sorry to be so pessimistic, but so far, although our experience is very small, it is not very encouraging despite the fact that one can raise the arterial oxygen tension appreciably.

Professor Donald. I do not think many people feel that raising the blood oxygen will cure the whole situation. It is just one of the manifestations of a very grave general disturbance which affects the lungs as well as many other important organs. I think we should have views about the concept that one can thrust on the ventricle in this highly lethal state a further load as a therapeutic measure.

Dr Meltzer. We have done this for several years but have given up measuring central venous pressure as the end-point simply because it is influenced by too many other things and now rely on kidney function. The people who die get no response to a sudden load of glucose or, nowadays, dextran given quickly over 15–20 minutes. Those who respond to shock get a diuresis or at least they get a $\frac{1}{2}$ ml. per minute, perhaps 1 ml. per minute, response to this type of load. Central venous pressure does not run parallel to the renal response. There are many factors that can influence central venous pressure in addition to the loading of fluid, but I think it probably does have some merit, although not by itself. It's one method of helping to assess prognosis.

Professor Donald. Would you think, Dr Meltzer, that some of these patients might survive anyhow, and that by loading them you lose some of those who might survive?

Dr Meltzer. I am not sure whether this is a real 'load'. I don't know whether 200 ml. or 300 ml. of dextran is a load. The dextran presumably, as Dr Sloman suggested, may be beneficial in its own right for the micro-circulation and is a therapy in that way. I do not think you are hurting anybody but whether you are doing any good is an entirely different matter; but with those who improve there is a response within 15 minutes of the infusion in terms of urinary output. Those who get none do not live.

Professor Chazov. The problem of cardiogenic shock is very complicated. It cannot be understood if one only considers haemodynamics and the increase in peripheral resistance. Our observations in cardiogenic shock show that hormonal shifts are important—aldosterone, catecholamines and others. In cases of cardiogenic shock we usually have lower aldosterone levels than in patients with acute myocardial infarction with normal pressure. Treatment with hormones is important in cases of cardiogenic shock in myocardial infarction.

199

Dr Oliver. This touches again on the problem which has been raised by Dr Sloman which I think we should try not to avoid. What can we say about the aetiology of shock? We have been talking about how we should treat it and how we support the patient when it occurs. Professor Chazov has been implying that there are hormonal and other disturbances. We cannot, of course, judge whether these are consequential or primary and I doubt if it will be possible to determine which comes first. I think it might be worthwhile referring again to Mackenzie's work because he confirmed what had been shown many years ago—that patients who die in cardiogenic shock have very high blood glucose levels. Interestingly enough, he had, I believe, three other patients who survived who did not have high blood glucose levels. We have looked at this again from another point of view and confirm that all those with cardiogenic shock who died have had high blood glucose levels 150–300 mg. per 100 ml. a few hours before death. It appears that those who are shocked on arrival in the unit and then survive, or at least get out of shock, do not have high blood glucose levels. I do not know what this means but there appear to be two groups—one with elevated blood glucose and the other with normal levels—of severely shocked patients. Perhaps those who die have an adrenaline response greater than those who survive. Maybe those who do not die have more of a noradrenaline response. There appears to be something which might be worth examining from the metabolic point of view with regard to degrees of shock.

Professor Donald. Are there any comments on this matter of blood sugar levels. Does anyone in this audience feel that giving these small amounts of intravenous fluids is worth continuing, or does anybody violently oppose it? I think we are so desperate clinically that we must consider all suggestions.

Dr Killip. I should think we should take the attitude that this is really something very worthwhile investigating, but we should be prepared to accept the consequences, which is precipitation into acute pulmonary oedema. Unless you are equipped to move pretty rapidly, I should think that this could be disastrous.

CIRCULATORY FAILURE FOLLOWING
MYOCARDIAL INFARCTION

JOHN SHILLINGFORD

Royal Postgraduate School for Medicine, Hammersmith, London

CLASSICALLY, the circulatory abnormality following myocardial infarction is a low cardiac output with peripheral vasoconstriction. The concept of low cardiac output and a state of peripheral vasoconstriction is mainly based on studies of groups of patients on whom single haemodynamic measurements have been made during the first few days following acute myocardial infarction. Serial studies in special units have modified this view, however, as the following cases show. Figure 1 shows the haemodynamic changes in a patient with a low cardiac output following myocardial

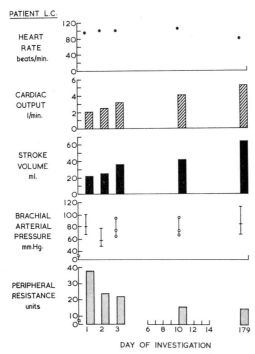

FIG. 1. Haemodynamic changes in a patient with low cardiac output following myocardial infarction.

infarction. This 56-year-old man was first studied 14 hours after cardiac infarction and successful resuscitation following cardiac arrest. At the time of the investigation he was very pale, cyanosed and mentally confused. He was in sinus rhythm, 60 beats/min., with ventricular extrasystoles. Arterial pressure was 100/68 mm. Hg, mean 80. Mean central venous pressure was +5 mm. Hg. The apex beat was not palpable. A third heart sound was present. Râles in the lungs and a pleural rub were present. There was no peripheral oedema but he was anuric. The electrocardiogram showed pathological Q waves and S-T segment elevation in V_2–V_4. Chest radiograph showed cardiac enlargement and pulmonary oedema.

The cardiac output was 2·1 litre/min., and stroke volume 22 ml., with a high peripheral resistance at 38 units. Brachial arterial pressure was 100/68 mm. Hg, with a mean of 80. On the second day the cardiac output rose to 2·5 litre/min. and stroke volume to 25 ml. during the same period; this was associated with a fall of peripheral resistance to 23 units and the blood pressure to 78/48 mm. Hg, with a mean of 57. Urine was passed on the second day and clinical improvement progressed uneventfully. This was associated with an increase in cardiac output and stroke volume. Measurements made during convalescence and after the patient returned to work showed further increases in stroke volume and cardiac output. Arterial pressure rose but the peripheral resistance remained within the normal range.

This patient illustrates how systemic hypotension may be associated with low stroke volume and low cardiac output. An additional fall in arterial pressure on the second day was related to a fall in peripheral resistance, the stroke volume and cardiac output rising slightly. The heart rate remained within a narrow range throughout the acute illness. Clinical improvement with a rise in arterial pressure occurred in association with a rise in stroke volume and cardiac output.

Not all patients show this haemodynamic picture and some may present with a normal or high cardiac output with a low peripheral resistance. Figure 2 shows the haemodynamic changes in such a patient. This 51-year-old man was admitted to hospital following acute chest pain. Soon after admission he was successfully resuscitated following ventricular fibrillation. The first haemodynamic study was made 18 hours later. At the time of the investigation he felt very weak, looked ill but was free from pain. The skin was normal in colour and temperature but was moist. He was in sinus rhythm. The arterial pressure was 98/53 mm. Hg

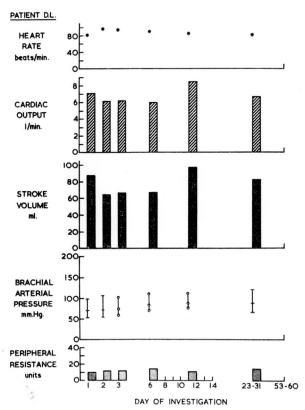

FIG. 2. Haemodynamic changes in a patient with a high cardiac output and a low peripheral resistance.

mean 70. The mean central venous pressure was +2 mm. Hg. The apex beat was abnormally sustained but normal in position. Heart sounds were normal. No added sounds were present. Crepitations were audible in the lungs. There was no peripheral oedema.

The electrocardiogram showed pathological Q waves in leads V_4R-V_4, S-T segment elevation in V_1-V_4. Chest radiograph showed slight cardiac enlargement and pulmonary venous congestion with pulmonary oedema. The cardiac output, however, was 7·1 litre/min., stroke volume 87 ml. and there was a low peripheral resistance of 10 units. The arterial blood pressure rose during convalescence in association with a rise in peripheral resistance. Cardiac output changed but little, as did the stroke volume.

203

This patient illustrates how hypotension may occur in association with a low total peripheral resistance. The rise of pressure that occurred in convalescence was associated with a rise in peripheral resistance.

The factors governing these responses are not clear and we can only speculate on the possible physiological mechanisms that may be associated with these changes. In some patients it seems clear that the primary and most important factor is failure of the myocardium with resultant low stroke output and cardiac output. Although an increase in the patient's temperature is known to be responsible for a lowered peripheral resistance, this does not provide a complete explanation of the low peripheral resistance and high cardiac output found in other cases.

The results of these haemodynamic studies may have some importance in the practical management of patients who have a fall in arterial blood pressure following myocardial infarction. In some, hypotension does not appear to be associated with an adequate regional blood flow. In others it may be associated with intense vasoconstriction and failure of adequate perfusion of the vital organs. More work has to be done to clarify these various mechanisms in the application of rational methods of treatment.

CHANGES IN CARDIAC FUNCTION DURING ARRHYTHMIAS FOLLOWING CARDIAC INFARCTION

So far, changes that may occur in the circulation when the patient is in sinus rhythm have been considered. The development of a cardiac arrhythmia in itself may be responsible for a disordered heart action and consequent disturbance in function. These arrhythmias may vary from extrasystoles with momentary changes in stroke output to ventricular fibrillation with complete cessation of an effective cardiac contraction. Recent work has shown that some form of arrhythmia occurs in 80 per cent. of all patients at some time in the first few days following a myocardial infarction. These arrhythmias are often transient and may last from a few seconds to a few hours. Their unpredictable behaviour, with often spontaneous recovery, thus makes the assessment of the value of drugs in their treatment difficult. The arrhythmias include ventricular fibrillation, supraventricular tachycardias, ventricular tachycardias, supraventricular bradycardias, shortening of the P-R interval and nodal rhythms, ventricular bradycardias or heart block and extrasystoles.

With the development of ventricular fibrillation there is complete cessation of effective cardiac function and failure to maintain the circulation. Until recently the appearance of this rhythm almost always meant the death of the patient; with the development of methods of external cardiac massage and direct current counter-shock, about a third to a half of all patients who develop this rhythm following myocardial infarction may be converted to sinus rhythm and saved.

Either supraventricular tachycardia or atrial fibrillation may lead to a disordered cardiac function especially in the presence of a rapid ventricular rate. In each case there is usually a reduction in minute output of the heart with an even greater reduction in stroke output due to the associated rapid heart rate.

Supraventricular bradycardia or slowing of the heart in sinus rhythm occurs at some stage in about 20 per cent. of all patients following a myocardial infarction and often within a few hours of its onset and can lead to a severe disturbance in cardiac function. The usual finding is that the patient develops slowing of the heart with a falling blood pressure, pallor and sweating, frequently accompanied by nausea and vomiting with clouding of the sensorium. There is a severe fall in the cardiac output. The syndrome may occur spontaneously or at times appears to be related to the administration of morphine or pethidine. It seems likely that this is a form of vasovagal or fainting attack mediated by reflexes from the heart. Further proof of this is shown by the satisfactory response these patients made to the administration of atropine.

A changing position of the P wave in relation to the QRS may often be seen on the electrocardiogram in the first few days following an acute myocardial infarction. This is associated with a disturbance of the normal co-ordination between the contraction of the atrium and ventricle. As a result there is failure of the atrium to deliver the blood to the ventricle during its contraction. Figure 3 shows an example of this and records the electrocardiogram, the right atrial pressure pulse and brachial arterial pressure in a patient following myocardial infarction. It will be seen that there is a very short P-R interval which is varying in length. As this interval becomes shorter the right atrial pressure pulse increases in amplitude due to atrial contraction against a closed atrioventricular valve and decreases again as the P-R interval lengthens. Associated with the increase in the atrial pressure pulse there is a fall in the brachial arterial blood pressure due to failure of the atrium to fill the ventricle at the end of diastole. It is interesting to note that this arrhythmia, associated with a fall in blood pressure, occurs without a signficant change in the heart rate. This irregularity of the heart

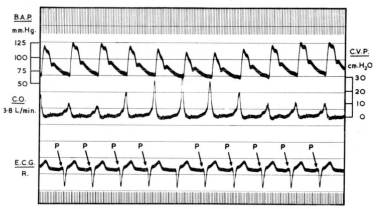

FIG. 3. The effects of changing position of the P wave in relation to the QRS on arterial pressure, central venous pressure and cardiac output.

action is often transient and spontaneously reverts to sinus rhythm in the normal course of the recovery of the patient.

The development of heart block can have a serious effect on the circulation, especially if it occurs in the acute stage following myocardial infarction where there is already impairment of myocardial function in terms of potential stroke output. The minute cardiac output is therefore reduced by the slowing of the heart rate and the disturbance of myocardial function due to muscle damage. Figure 4 shows an example of the considerable fall in blood pressure as a result of the development of heart block following myocardial infarction. Should the heart block persist, the cardiac output can often only be adequately maintained by electrical pacing of the heart.

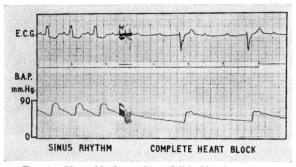

FIG. 4. Heart block causing a fall in blood pressure.

'SHOCK' AND MYOCARDIAL INFARCTION

The clinical syndrome of 'shock' following myocardial infarction is commonly seen. This manifests itself by a falling blood pressure, cold peripheries with sweating, oliguria, irritability or cerebral confusion or, in more severe cases, coma. The underlying causes of this syndrome are varied and it is probably better to abandon the word 'shock' in view of an increasing and more accurate knowledge of the various changes taking place in the circulation which result in this syndrome. New and powerful drugs in many cases may do more harm than good if administered to a severely ill patient without a knowledge of the basic causes for the circulatory disturbance. This is especially so in the case of pressor agents or morphine which are administered on account of the diagnosis of 'shock' or 'cardiogenic shock' having been made.

The more rational approach is to determine the circulatory changes that are underlying the patient's clinical condition. In many cases a disturbance in the cardiac rhythm will be the cause. These include the onset of supraventricular tachycardia, where the treatment may be the exhibition of anti-arrhythmic drugs or direct current countershock, atrial fibrillation where digitalis is indicated, the vasovagal supraventricular bradycardias where raising the legs and the administration of atropine is specific, heart block with a falling output where electrical pacing of the heart will restore the circulation to normal. In other cases, the myocardium itself may be failing as a pump due to extensive muscle injury and the treatment is that of salt restriction, diuretics and oxygen.

Reflex vasodilatation is a cause of hypotension but in itself seldom needs treatment, as vital organ perfusion is usually adequate in these cases. Disturbances in serum electrolytes may lead to disordered action of the heart and circulation. Hypoxia due to pulmonary disturbances may be contributing to the general deterioration in the patient's condition. The infrequent occurrence of pulmonary embolism may cause severe circulatory embarrassment. Finally, the unnecessary administration of drugs, especially heavy sedation by morphia or the allied drugs, may in itself be responsible for impairment and depression of the circulation.

It will thus be seen that it is dangerous, and unscientific, in view of our understanding of the changes taking place in the circulation, to treat symptoms such as hypotension and 'shock' rather than to try to elucidate and treat the underlying circulatory disturbance causing the symptom.

REFERENCES

FLUCK, D. C., OLSEN, E., PENTECOST, B. L., THOMAS, M., FILLMORE, S. J., SHILLINGFORD, J. P. & MOUNSEY, J. P. D. (1967). The natural history and clinical significance of arrhythmias after an acute cardiac infarction. *Br. Heart J.* 29, 170.
MALMCRONA, R. & VARNAUSKAS, E. (1964). Haemodynamics in acute myocardial infarction. *Acta med. scand.* 175, 1.
THOMAS, M., MALMCRONA, R. & SHILLINGFORD, J. P. (1965). Haemodynamic changes in patients with acute myocardial infarction. *Circulation*, 31, 811.
THOMAS, M., MALMCRONA, R. & SHILLINGFORD, J. P. (1966). Circulatory changes associated with systemic hypotension in patients with acute myocardial infarction. *Br. Heart J.* 28, 108.

EARLY DETECTION OF ' PUMP ' FAILURE

LAWRENCE E. MELTZER

Presbyterian-University of Pennsylvania Medical Center, Philadelphia

IT is now clear that the original system of intensive coronary care (designed ostensibly to prevent arrhythmic deaths) has already reached its point of optimal effectiveness and that no further reduction in mortality from myocardial infarction can be anticipated with the existing programme. The basis of this limitation is readily apparent; despite the prevention of all primary arrhythmic deaths in 300 consecutive, unselected patients, we were unable to reduce the mortality below 19 per cent. Of the 57 deaths, 54 were due to power (pump) failure. This death rate is essentially the same as described by Day, Julian and Oliver, Killip, Sloman, and Lown. This similarity of results merely reflects a uniform ability to prevent arrhythmic deaths and a uniform inability to combat death from power failure. Until the problem of circulatory failure can be controlled, it is unlikely that the overall fatality rate will be decreased additionally.

The fundamental question is what can be done about power failure? It is quite evident that existing therapeutic practices are grossly inadequate and that a new approach is necessary.

Perhaps the solution will be found in a superior pharmacological agent, a surgical technique or a mechanical means of assisting the circulation. But certainly none of these methods are in close view and, at best, they remain only potential solutions.

It is our belief that the overall mortality from power failure can

208

be reduced at the present time utilising available methods. The premise is simple: by detecting and treating pump failure at its earliest (incipient) stages, the morbidity and mortality of *overt* power failure might be reduced.

The basis of this approach can be estimated from the following data relating to the incidence of power failure in acute myocardial infarction. Power failure, as used here, refers to the presence of overt clinically detectable signs of left heart failure (i.e., crepitations in lungs and/or third and fourth heart sounds).

Twenty-four per cent. of 240 patients with proven infarction had evidence of decompensation on admission. Forty-eight per cent. of these patients died. Of great interest is that among those patients who did *not* have failure on admission, 38 per cent. developed power failure within 96 hours; the mortality was 40 per cent. In 12 per cent. of the remaining patients, power failure began after the fourth day and one-half of these patients died.

If these data are valid (which now seems apparent from the other reports presented here) about 60 per cent. of all patients hospitalised with cardiac infarction have overt evidence of heart failure. In three out of five instances, the failure is not present on admission. Once left-sided failure develops, the mortality is between 40–50 per cent.

Can ' late onset ' (not present on admission) failure be detected before it becomes overt, and could the mortality be reduced if treatment was initiated at this incipient stage? If our own data, to date, is representative, the answer to both of these questions would appear to be ' yes '.

In attempting to develop a useable system to detect incipient pump failure, it was clear that the techniques employed had to be simple and, above all, *non-intimidating* to the patient. Specifically, the methods had to be well-tolerated, carry minimal risk and arouse little anxiety. The determination of cardiac output, the measurement of a-v oxygen differences, the sampling of coronary sinus blood or other studies that require multiple catheterisations, do not meet these requirements and were considered inappropriate.

May I review some of the methods we are currently using to detect incipient failure and comment very briefly about their value.

Of the methods I now consider of proven value (Table I) radiographic examination of the chest is the one most accurate and dependable means for detecting left ventricular failure in *asymptomatic* patients. At least 70 per cent. of all patients with proven myocardial infarction have radiologic evidence of left-sided failure.

Table I. *The detection of early power failure with non-intimidating methods*

Methods Considered Valuable:

1. Radiographic examination of chest—daily—
   Interstitial oedema, etc.
   Heart size and volume
2. Physical examination by nurse
3. Circulation time—
   Right atrium to ear with an oxymeter
4. Continuous phonocardiography—
   3rd and 4th sounds
   Frequency of sounds
   Time between electrical and mechanical systole

In approximately one-third of these patients this latter diagnosis would not be suspected by physical examination. Although interstitial oedema is the most obvious radiographic sign of incipient left heart failure, it is apparent that there are several earlier, more subtle X-ray changes that permit this diagnosis. A particularly significant finding is dilatation of the pulmonary veins from the upper lobes with paradoxical constriction of the veins from the lower lobes. This sign, reflecting pulmonary venous hypertension, is probably the earliest manifestation of left-sided decompensation.

A second standard practice that we have adopted involves physical examination by *nurses.* Nurses have been trained specifically to observe the patient for symptoms that suggest decompensation, and to examine the patient in terms of crepitations, neck vein distention, hepatojugular reflux, oedema, and even the presence of third and fourth heart sounds. This examination is conducted twice during each nursing shift (every four hours). Those who have been impressed with the remarkable competence of nurses in electrocardiographic monitoring, will not be surprised by their ability to perform this task. Repeated examinations of this type have proven quite valuable and are certainly worthwhile, particularly in those institutions without house staffs.

The circulation time can be used to good advantage in detecting early failure. This measurement is performed by injecting Evans Blue through a central venous catheter and recording the appearance time with an ear oxymeter. (A catheter is positioned in the vena cava at the time of admission in all patients and no other catheterisations or venepunctures are performed thereafter. This catheter serves for infusions, blood sampling, and testing.) Prolongation of the circulation time (performed in this manner) correlates very well with radiographic findings of left ventricular failure.

210

Perhaps the most interesting technique we have studied thus far is that of continuous phonocardiography. A sensitive microphone is anchored to the skin allowing continuous oscilloscopic visualisation of the heart sounds at different frequencies. (A direct write-out device permits recording as well.) We were originally concerned with the detection of transient third and fourth heart sounds and found that more than 60 per cent. of patients with infarction had these sounds. Paradoxical splitting of the second heart sound which Yurchak and Gorlin, as well as Dickerson, have described as very common after infarction was noted by auscultation in only 2 per cent. of patients. Systolic murmurs were recorded in 25 per cent. of our patients. Wide splitting of the first heart sound frequently accompanies early failure.

In addition to the detection of heart sounds, the phonocardiogram may prove valuable as a means of indirectly estimating the rate of pressure rise within the ventricle during the isometric period of contraction since this rate change can be related to the intensity of the first sound. Similarly, the period of isometric contraction can be estimated by timing the period between electrical and mechanical systole.

A second group of methods can be described as potentially valuable in detecting incipient failure (Table II):

Table II. *The detection of early power failure with non-intimidating methods*

Methods of Potential Value:
1. Estimation of LVED pressure from ' a/EO ' ratio of apex cardiogram
2. Measurement of pre-ejection and ejection periods—
    Vibrocardiogram
    Accelerocardiogram
    Carotid artery wave
3. Central venous pressure response to loading, tourniquets and inhibiting venomotor tone
4 Urine volume and osmolality

1. APEX CARDIOGRAM. There is some evidence (Dimond *et al.*) that the a/EO ratio of the apex cardiogram (Fig. 1) accurately reflects changes in the left ventricular end-diastolic pressure and can be used to assess relative (not absolute) variations in this pressure. This ratio has little meaning as an isolated measurement but by comparing the heights of these waves at set periods, the usefulness of the method is enhanced. (This is accomplished with the same ' permanent ' microphone used for phonocardiography. A filter

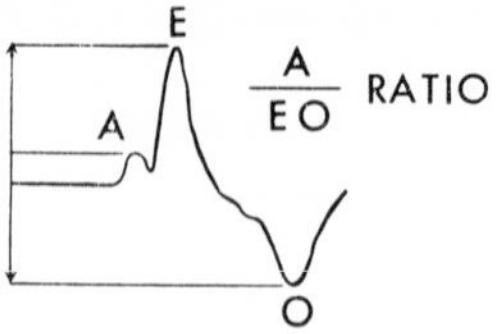

Fig. 1. Apex cardiogram.

system blocks out frequencies above 20 cpm for the purpose of recording the apex cardiogram.)

2. PRECORDIAL VIBRATIONS. One of the most promising of the non-intimidating techniques is the *indirect* measurement of phases of the cardiac cycle by means of displacement curves obtained from the precordium. There are several methods of recording these precordial vibrations including the vibrocardiograph, apex-cardiogram, kinetocardiogram and accelerocardiogram, all of which yield information that seems to correlate with that obtained by direct catheterisation techniques. At the present time of the cardiac phases the ejection time (which is shortened in heart failure) and the pre-ejection time (lengthened in heart failure) command the most interest. It would appear that these intervals can be measured continuously with simple computer timing devices so that variations in the phases can be detected promptly. This may prove to be the most valuable method to assess cardiac function.

3. CENTRAL VENOUS PRESSURE. The measurement of CVP, as such, is of little value in detecting incipient heart failure. Although CVP is high in most instances of *advanced* heart failure, it varies widely with lesser degrees of decompensation and cannot be correlated with positive radiographic findings or prolonged circulation time of early failure. On the other hand, the response of central venous pressure to rapid loading of the cardiovascular system with 200 ml. Dextran may be a pertinent determinant of incipient failure. In the presence of decompensation, the CVP usually rises 15–20 per cent. in response to this infusion. The test, however, is not fully standardised at this point.

Another potentially useful adaptation of CVP measurement is the response to inhibition of venomotor tone. Recognising that increased venomotor tone is an early finding in cardiac decompensation, it is possible that aminophyllin, sodium nitrate or ganglionic blockaders might be used to assess the degree of venous constriction in terms of reduction of CVP. While the CVP falls (about 15–20 mm.) in response to aminophyllin among patients with overt failure, the decrease is not as distinct or predictable in early failure.

4. Urine volume and osmolality. With overt failure, the urinary output is decreased, and there is a reversal of the day-night ratio of urine volume. By measuring the urine volume every four hours (voluntary voiding) a pattern indicative of these alterations may become evident early in the course of decompensation. We have been impressed with the changes in urine osmolality that occur concomitantly with decompensation.

The last group of non-intimidating methods we are exploring can only be categorised as of uncertain value (Table III) because of a lack of evidence up to this time. It may well be that one or more of these techniques will the be useful in ultimate profile of the failing heart that we are attempting to develop.

Table III. *The detection of early power failure with non-intimidating methods*

Methods of uncertain value:
1. Daily sodium excretion
2. Continuous body weight measurement
3. Pulmonary function with impedence plethysmography
4. Ballistocardiogram
5. Oxygen saturation—ear oxymeter
6. Chemical studies—
   pH and CO_2
   haematocrit

Table IV. *Mortality rates in acute myocardial infarction*

Year	Intensive Coronary Care Unit (%)	Regular facilities (%)
1960 . .	—	30·6
1961 . .	—	31·4
1962 . .	21·0	31·0
1963 . .	21·2	29·8
1964 . .	22·4	27·3
1965 . .	19·4	31·9
1966 . .	15·8	31·6
1967 . .	13·9	28·8

213

From our data it would appear that 60 per cent. of patients with myocardial infarction have signs of overt failure, and that another 30 per cent. have evidence of pre-clinical (incipient) failure. Thus 90 per cent. of all patients could be considered to have some form of decompensation. It is our current practice to digitalise all of these patients as soon as the diagnosis is established. The wisdom of this premise remains to be proven; however, the mortality rate in our unit, after remaining at 19–20 per cent. for three years, has dropped to 14 per cent. since we adopted this concept (Table IV).

DISCUSSION

Dr McDonald. I thought that your pragmatic approach was delightful, Dr Meltzer, but I would require a lot of convincing that careful clinical examination with or without phono-cardiography and the chest radiograph are really going to be bettered by any of those tests you have recommended. I like very much the idea of the nurses examination, because we must not be stuffy about this. We should have everybody in the units making all the observations they can.

I don't know really whether heart size is going to be too useful because surely cardiac infarction is the example *par excellence*, in which we have got acute pulmonary oedema with a normal-sized heart. I was interested that you brought the circulation time back. I think this has been a little neglected. I wondered if you had deliberately avoided using the Valsalva manoeuvre. This does not need any equipment—one simply detects a rate change or no rate change with a square-wave response which can be either felt by the finger or recorded on the electrocardiogram.

Nevertheless I think we are approaching this problem in the wrong way, because although all these observations are extremely important, what we really want to know from the beginning is how extensive is this infarction and therefore how likely is frank left heart failure to develop. It would ve very useful in comparing our data if, instead of speaking only of anterior and posterior infarction or whatever it happened to be, we said an infarct with an isoenxyme level of x or y or whatever it is. This might correlate extremely well with the evidence of ventricular failure and ventricular dysfunction. Besides the enzymes and the isoenzymes, Oliver will no doubt tell us about the possible value of free fatty acid release as indicative of the degree of subsequent dysfunction. We have been also studying catecholamine levels in the blood for the same purpose. I am sure we will increasingly be concerned with the degree of damage and its biochemical indicators.

214

Dr Samuel. I was most interested in Dr Meltzer's report on the radiographic findings and I feel they are of the utmost importance in the diagnosis of pulmonary oedema, but I do think that we have been considering advanced stages of pulmonary oedema. My own observations arose out of a very personal and tragic association with a nurse in my own department who complained of breathlessness. Being in an X-ray department she was sent for an X-ray. I, being in charge of the department, did not see the films. They were seen by a junior, and we did not discuss it very much at all that afternoon, but she was seen by a physician who admitted her because of acute breathlessness with a diagnosis of pneumonia. My junior colleague reported back to me that the chest was clear. I saw the plates the following morning in discussion. I went to see the patient, and on the way to the medical ward I was told, ' You need not bother to go, the patient is dead.' The heart was of normal size but when we looked at the chest films there was a curious pattern of lines over it. This young girl had medial necrosis of the aorta and she died from rupture into intracardiac structures around the aorta. In point of facts, she had acute left ventricular failure and pulmonary oedema and had died from this. Subsequently, I looked to see whether these lines could be seen in other cases of left ventricular failure, and we went through our cases in the Coronary Care Unit. They are common in these patients and are what are called A-lines. They are of extreme significance especially when they are associated with a heart of normal size. They are easily mimicked by cloth or dressing on the patient and we tend to disregard them. If there is interstitial pulmonary oedema the case is advanced. The other point I would like to raise is that interstitial pulmonary oedema does not necessarily start at the hilum. It may start peripherally and all you will see are rather unusual thin lines crossing pulmonary veins. Of course, you can see these as well and they are usually, as Dr Meltzer said, in the upper lobes of the lungs and an oblique film may be necessary to see them.

Dr Nixon. In trying to assess how much the ventricle is injured, apex cardiography has been mentioned, as has phonocardiography. There was an earlier comment that both of these could be related to left ventricular end-diastolic pressure, but I want to make it quite clear that enlargement of the ' a ' wave on the apex tracing or a fourth heart sound does not correlate with left ventricular end-diastolic pressure. An apex cardiogram may have a perfectly normal little ' a ' wave when the left ventricular end-diastolic pressure is quite raised.

We had a severely hypertensive patient, in whom the left atrial pressure was quite normal when there was a huge ' a ' wave.

No matter how careful the auscultation that tries to pick up the presence of a fourth heart sound, there will be problems, because the fourth sound may occur after the onset of the Q wave of ECG. It is so close to the first sound that the ear cannot differentiate it from a first sound. Only if you have an apex tracing for reference can you see that there is enlargement of the ' a ' wave, which is a sign of ventricular disturbance. This happens in about 100 per cent. of infarcts. I have not yet seen an acute infarction without enlargement of the ' a ' wave in a displacement curve in the left ventricle. Powerful atrial contraction, which is the give-away of the disturbed ventricle, is not always associated a noise.

Dr McKendrick. I agree with Dr Meltzer. The problem of measuring cardiac performance without adding to the patient's difficulties is a big one. We use an isotope technique with radio-active albumen and external counting. This correlates very accurately both with arterial dye-dilution curves and with the direct Fick procedure. The only snag in this method is that one can only do four or five studies using I^{131}. One of our biochemists has, I hope, tagged albumen with technetium—this is an isotope with a half-life of eight hours. It is a very powerful gamma emitter and might be a marvellous thing for serial bedside measurement.

Dr Marquis. I should like to make one comment on the X-ray diagnosis of pulmonary oedema. This has been emphasised re-peatedly. Localised pulmonary oedema may be associated with no crepitations, but what has not been emphasised is that you may at times get crepitations due to left ventricular failure without radiological signs.

HYPOXAEMIA AND ACIDOSIS

BRIAN J. KIRBY

The Cardio-thoracic Department, Central Middlesex Hospital, London

HYPOXAEMIA

PULMONARY oedema has long been recognised as a common complication of myocardial infarction in man, and animal experiments have shown that myocardial infarction is often accompanied by a rise in left atrial pressure. Changes in respiratory function might therefore be expected and because these changes occur in a previously healthy pulmonary circulation, their study may aid understanding of respiratory function in other forms of heart disease. Arterial hypoxaemia has been demonstrated in pulmonary oedema both in man (Cosby *et al.*, 1957) and in animals (Williams, 1953; Forster, 1957; Said *et al.*, 1964). Since Barcroft's (1920) observations, it has often been regarded as due to impairment of oxygen diffusion but development of the ventilation/blood flow concept and recent observations on the alveolar membrane (Staub *et al.*, 1967) suggest that ventilation/blood flow inequality is more important. The overall efficiency of the lung in gas transfer can be gauged by measurement of the difference between the calculated alveolar oxygen tension and the measured arterial oxygen tension (alveolar-arterial oxygen tension difference). Decreased arterial oxygen tension and increased alveolar-arterial oxygen tension difference have been found in pulmonary oedema (Cosby *et al.*, 1957; Vitale *et al.*, 1954) and more recently in myocardial infarction (Mackenzie *et al.*, 1964; McNicol *et al.*, 1965; Higgs, 1965; Cameron *et al.*, 1966; Valentine *et al.*, 1966). These increases in alveolar-arterial oxygen tension difference and arterial hypoxaemia may be due to:
1. Inadequate ventilation.
2. Ventilation/blood flow inequality.
3. Impairment of diffusion across the alveolar membrane.
4. Veno-arterial shunting.

Inadequate ventilation occurred in only seven patients and therefore could not account for the hypoxaemia observed in the majority. Ventilation/blood flow relationships can be analysed by applying Riley's approach in which alveoli are considered to deviate from normal in one of two ways. In the first, ventilation is reduced in relation to perfusion resulting in failure to oxygenate

217

fully the mixed venous blood with which they were perfused. Venous admixture occurs and leads to arterial hypoxaemia. In the second, perfusion is reduced in relation to ventilation which increases physiological deadspace. Whilst this does not cause hypoxaemia, it does decrease the efficiency of oxygen transfer in the lung. Increases in both indices indicate a ventilation/blood flow abnormality. Recent animal experiments suggest that thickening of the alveolar membrane is unlikely to cause significant hypoxaemia (Staub et al., 1967). Reduction of oxygen tension in poorly ventilated alveoli may however increase the importance of diffusion across the alveolar membrane.

At the Central Middlesex Hospital, my colleagues and I have studied 200 patients since 1963. Arterial blood was taken in all patients and additional studies were made in 50 of these. All observations were made within 24 hours of the onset of symptoms in patients with unequivocal clinical and electrocardiographic evidence of myocardial infarction. Standard laboratory methods for measuring arterial oxygen tension, carbon dioxide tension and pH were used (McNicol et al., 1965; Kirby & McNicol, 1966); plasma bicarbonate was derived from Siggaard Andesen's nomogram.

Hypoxaemia, that is an arterial oxygen tension less than 85 mm. Hg. was present in 88 per cent.; this figure probably represents an over-estimate of the frequency of hypoxaemia as there was a tendency to investigate the more severely ill. A simple clinical classification was adopted in an attempt to correlate the clinical with the cardio-respiratory findings. Forty-two patients (21 per cent.) had uncomplicated myocardial infarction (Group 1). Patients with systemic hypotension, defined as a systolic pressure less than 90 mm. Hg. were divided into two groups according to the presence of left ventricular failure. Thus, there were 9 patients (4 per cent.) with no evidence of left ventricular failure (Group 2), and 42 patients (21 per cent.) with left ventricular failure (Group 3). Group 4 was composed of patients with left ventricular failure alone—107 patients (54 per cent.). Left ventricular failure was diagnosed when crepitations or rhonchi persisted after coughing in patients without a history of heart or chest disease. The high proportion of patients with hypotension and left ventricular failure (corresponding to the concept of ' cardiogenic shock ') was due partly to our interest in this group. It is notable that hypotension without left ventricular failure was the least common group. It should be stressed that the classification was based solely upon clinical criteria.

Using this classification it can be seen from Table I that oxygen

Table I. *Hypoxaemia in Myocardial Infarction*
(190 Patients)

	$So_2 \pm S.D.$ (%)	$Po_2 \pm S.D.$ (mm. Hg.)	$A-aDo_2 \pm S.D.$ (mm. Hg.)
Total	$86 \pm 8\cdot2$	$63 \pm 13\cdot4$	$39 \pm 14\cdot7$
Group 1. M.I. . .	$94 \pm 2\cdot4$	$76 \pm 11\cdot8$	$30 \pm 14\cdot1$
Group 2. M.I+H . . .	$92 \pm 3\cdot5$	$68 \pm 10\cdot2$	$41 \pm 17\cdot4$
Group 3. M.I+H+L.V.F.	$82 \pm 10\cdot6$	$56 \pm 16\cdot2$	$49 \pm 9\cdot2$
Group 4. M.I+L.V.F. . .	$87 \pm 7\cdot2$	$62 \pm 13\cdot2$	$41 \pm 14\cdot3$

tension was reduced in every group but that the greatest reduction was seen in these with left ventricular failure. Although the group means showed this pattern there was considerable overlap between the groups. It is not known whether other signs of incipient left ventricular failure, such as triple rhythm or reversed splitting of the second sound, would have led to the detection of left ventricular failure at an earlier stage and thereby produced better separation of the groups. Equally, severe hypoxaemia was seen, as often in those with a few basal crepitations as in those with more widespread physical signs—a finding in agreement with previous workers (Vitale *et al.*, 1954).

Alveolar-arterial oxygen tension difference was calculated as an index of the efficiency of gas transfer in the lung. This can be represented diagrammatically on an oxygen/carbon dioxide diagram (Fig. 1). The horizontal distance of each point from the respiratory exchange line represents the alveolar-arterial oxygen tension difference. In this age group, alveolar-arterial oxygen tension difference should be less than 20 mm. Hg.; clearly the majority deviate considerably and, furthermore, the greater the deviation, the higher the mortality.

Further studies were undertaken in 50 patients to examine the way in which the changes arose. Simultaneous expired air and arterial blood collections were made in all and in 29 mixed venous blood was sampled from the pulmonary artery enabling calculation

219

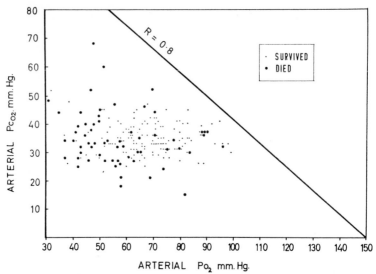

Fig. 1. Alveolar-arterial oxygen tension difference. The horizontal distance of each point from the respiratory exchange line (R) is proportional to the alveolar-arterial oxygen tension difference.

of cardiac output from the Fick equation. Venous admixture was increased in all groups but especially in those with clinical evidence of left ventricular failure. Some patients with severe left ventricular failure and systemic hypotension behaved as if 30 per cent. or more of the cardiac output passed through the lungs without contact with alveolar air. Increased physiological deadspace/tidal volume ratio paralleled the changes in venous admixture and further confirmed the presence of ventilation/blood flow inequality. Although in itself it does not cause arterial hypoxaemia it does decrease the efficiency of gas transfer. The severest hypoxaemia was seen in those patients with the lowest cardiac and stroke indices. Similarly, right atrial pressure was highest in those with severest hypoxaemia. This hypoxaemia can be explained by the observed increase in venous admixture when it is combined with a fall in cardiac output (and therefore a fall in mixed venous oxygen content). Figure 2 illustrates the dependence of arterial oxygen tension on oxygenation of mixed venous blood when venous admixture is increased. With a constant venous admixture of 10 per cent., halving cardiac output from 5·10 l. per min. to 2·51 l. per min. results in a fall of mixed venous oxygen tension. Admixture of this blood of low oxygen tension therefore further reduces arterial oxygen

220

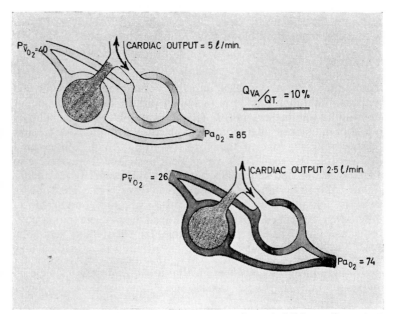

FIG. 2. Effect of cardiac output on oxygen tension. A fall in cardiac output reduces oxygenation of mixed venous blood and when there is increased venous admixture will cause a further fall in arterial oxygen tension.

tension. In other words, when venous admixture is increased arterial oxygen tension reflects changes in the degree of oxygenation of mixed venous blood and therefore of cardiac output.

Venous admixture could have been increased in two ways. Firstly, decreased lung compliance in some regions due to interstitial and perivascular oedema reduces regional ventilation and, if perfusion is unchanged, it will reduce ventilation/blood flow ratio and hence increase venous admixture. Secondly, alveoli may close due to either (a) loss of alveolar surface, as has been demonstrated in experimental pulmonary oedema (Said *et al.*, 1965) or (b) to filling of alveoli with oedema fluid. Mixed venous blood by-passing completely unventilated alveoli behaves as a veno-arterial shunt and may be detected by failure of arterial oxygen tension to rise when 100 per cent. oxygen is given.

In 16 subjects administration of 100 per cent. oxygen showed that whilst there was a rise it was not as great as would be expected in normal subjects; it rose in no patient above 500 mm. Hg. indicating that completely closed alveoli were present and that in

221

the severest cases considerable amounts of the lung behave in this way. In the less severe cases, however, the contribution of areas with a low ventilation/blood flow ratio was important.

Acidosis

Turning to acidosis, acid-base status was examined in the same 200 patients. Metabolic acidosis (a fall in plasma bicarbonate below 22 mEq/l.) was present in 107 (53 per cent.) but in the majority it had been compensated by a fall in arterial carbon dioxide tension thereby restoring pH to the normal range. An uncompensated acidosis (pH less than 7·35) was present in 22 and it was severe in 18, all of whom had systemic hypotension and severe left ventricular failure. Mortality amongst those patients was high. Respiratory acidosis (carbon dioxide tension over 45 mm.) occurred in only seven patients (3 per cent.) who all had severe pulmonary oedema. Group mean results (Table II) show that metabolic

Table II. *Acidosis in Myocardial Infarction*
(200 Patients)

	pH		$Pco_2 \pm S..D$ mm. Hg.	Standard Bicarbonate $\pm$ S.D. mEq/1
	mean	Range		
Total	7·38	7·27–7·52	$34 \pm 6·9$	$20 \pm 4·1$
Group 1. M.I . .	7·41	7·37–7·46	$35 \pm 4·8$	$23 \pm 8·1$
Group 2. M.I + H . .	7·40	7·36–7·44	$32 \pm 7·6$	$21 \pm 3·8$
Group 3. M.I + H + L.V.F.	7·29	7·14–7·54	$34 \pm 9·9$	$19 \pm 5·0$
Group 4. M.I + L.V.F. .	7·40	7·32–7·45	$35 \pm 6·1$	$22 \pm 3·0$

acidosis was commonest in Groups 2 and 3, i.e., in patients with systemic hypotension. The most severe metabolic acidosis was seen with the lowest cardiac index. Poor tissue perfusion leading to tissue anoxia and anaerobic glycolysis would be expected to raise lactic acid levels and measurements in 42 patients have confirmed this (Kirby & McNicol, 1966) especially amongst patients with left ventricular failure and systemic hypotension. A further index of tissue anoxia is mixed venous oxygen tension and the observation that it is markedly reduced in some, further confirms the presence of tissue anoxia. The combined effect of a fall in cardiac output and reduced arterial oxygenation is to reduce the amount of oxygen delivered to the tissues with consequent tissue hypoxia.

The clinical implications of these observations will be briefly considered. Decreased oxygen delivery to the tissues can be treated either by increasing cardiac output or by improving the efficiency of gas transfer in the lung. Administration of oxygen in high concentration will overcome ventilation/blood flow inequality and increase arterial oxygen tension, but fundamentally the disorder is one of cardiovascular function. Treatment directed to improving myocardial performance and counteracting changes in the peripheral circulation would seem rational. The effect of such measures on respiratory function is unknown. Metabolic acidosis is usually compensated by a fall in carbon dioxide tension due to overventilation. Interference with this compensatory mechanism is potentially dangerous. Therefore drugs such as major analgesics which depress ventilation should be used only in sufficient dose to relieve pain. When the patient's condition is grave and metabolic acidosis occurs, its correction would seem rational. This can be done with either sodium bicarbonate or tris buffer but in a small number of severely ill patients although we have corrected the acidosis there was no effect on mortality.

Finally, these changes can be related to mortality. Overall mortality was 34 per cent. but individual groups deviated from this significantly. Thus only one patient classified as having uncomplicated myocardial infarction died, whilst 79 per cent. of those with left ventricular failure and hypotension died. An uncompensated acidosis (pH less than 7·35 but over 7·30) was associated with a 50 per cent. mortality which rose to 89 per cent. when the pH was less than 7·30. Similarly, a plasma bicarbonate between 16 and 22 mEq/l. was associated with a 31 per cent. mortality but this increased to 83 per cent. when plasma bicarbonate was less than 15 mEq/l. Severe hypoxaemia (arterial oxygen tension less than 50 mm.) was associated with a 74 per cent. mortality. Although these changes were marked, they probably simply reflected the extent of the underlying cardiovascular disorder.

In conclusion, much more needs to be known of the respiratory function in all forms of heart disease but it can be concluded that in myocardial infarction there is significant hypoxaemia which can be attributed to a ventilation/blood flow abnormality due to left ventricular failure. Combined with a fall in cardiac output, this leads to tissue anoxia and lactic acidosis.

Acknowledgements

I would like to thank Dr Martin W. McNicol for his active help and interest throughout this study and to my other colleagues in the Cardio-thoracic Department, both medical and nursing, who have helped. Mrs Madeline Hard, B.Sc., helped with the laboratory work. This work was supported by a grant from the Medical Research Council.

REFERENCES

BARCROFT, J. (1920). Some problems of the circulation during gas poisoning. *Jl R. Army med. Cps*, 34: 155.

CAMERON, A. J. V., HUTTON, I., KENMURE, A. C. F. & MURDOCH, W. R. (1966). Haemodynamic and metabolic effects of hyperbaric oxygen in myocardial infarction. *Lancet*, 2, 833.

COSBY, R. S., SOTWELL, E. C., HARTWID, R. & MAYO, M. (1957). Pulmonary function in left ventricular failure, including cardiac asthma. *Circulation*, 15, 492.

FORSTER, R. E. (1957). Exchange of gases between alveolar air and pulmonary capillary blood: Pulmonary diffusing capacity. *Physiol. Rev.* 37, 391.

HIGGS, B. (1965). Respiratory changes in acute myocardial infraction. *Br. Heart J.* 27, 953.

KIRBY, B. J. & McNICOL, M. W. (1966). Acid- base status in acute myocardial infarction. *Lancet* 2, 1054.

MACKENZIE, G. J., TAYLOR, S. H., FLENLEY, D. C., McDONALD, A. H., STAUNTON, H. P. & DONALD, K. W. (1964). Circulatory and respiratory studies in myocardial infarction and cardiogenic shock. *Lancet*, 2, 825.

McNICOL, M. W., KIRBY, B. J., BHOOLA, K. D., EVEREST, M. E., PRICE, H. V. & FREEDMAN, S. (1965). Pulmonary function in acute myocardial infarction. *Br. med. J.* 2, 1270.

SAID, S. I., LONGACHER, J. W., DAVIS, R. K., BANERJEE, C. M., DAVIS, W. M. & WOODELL, W. J. (1964). Pulmonary gas exchange during induction of pulmonary oedema in anesthetised dogs. *J. appl. Physiol.* 19, 403.

SAID, S. I., AVERY, M. E., DAVIS, R. K., BANERJEE, C. M. & EL-GOHARY, M. (1965). Pulmonary surface activity in induced pulmonary oedema. *J. clin. Invest.* 44, 458.

STAUB, N. C., NAGANO, H. & PEARCE, M. L. (1967). Pulmonary oedema in dogs, especially the sequence of fluid accumulation in the lungs. *J. appl. Physiol.* 22, 20.

VALENTINE, P. A., FLUCK, D. C., MOUNSEY, J. P. D., REID, D., SHILLINGFORD, J. P. & STEINER, R. E. (1966). Blood gas changes after acute myocardial infarction. *Lancet*, 2, 837.

VITALE, A., DUMKE, P. R. & COMROE, J. R. (1954). Lack of correlation between rates and arterial oxygen saturation in patients with pulmonary congestion and oedema. *Circulation*, 10, 81.

WILLIAMS, M. H. (1953). Effect of ANTU-induced pulmonary edema on the alveolar-arterial oxygen pressure gradient in dogs. *Am. J. Physiol.* 175, 84.

DISCUSSION

Professor Donald. Thank you very much Dr Kirby for a very impressive series.

Firstly we would like to have a short comment by Dr Cameron on his experiences with hyperbaric oxygen which may perhaps provide an answer to these very severely shocked hypoxic patients.

Dr Cameron. Dr Mackenzie, Dr Kirby and many others have shown that arterial hypoxaemia and metabolic acidosis are frequent occurrences in myocardial infarction particularly in the really ill patient. In the present state of our ignorance as regards the fundamental causes, various empirical strategic measures must be considered of which oxygen under high tension is one.

About eight years ago, my surgical colleagues in the Western Infirmary, Glasgow, showed, in animal experiments, that with hyperbaric oxygen ventricular fibrillation could apparently be prevented following experimental ligation of the coronary artery. Thereafter they got a pressure chamber and I was pressed into trying to see whether this form of therapy had any effect on human myocardial infarction and I think I have been suffering from oxygen toxicity ever since. The first step was to run a full clinical trial on men, all of whom were admitted within 24 hours of onset of infarction. They were divided by random allocation into two groups and were all given continuous oxygen for the first 48 hours, half of them at the ordinary pressure of one atmosphere, and the other half at two atmospheres. The result of this trial was inconclusive. The number was relatively small and in 40 patients divided into two equal groups, the mortality over the first six weeks in hospital was the same.

I decided at that point, for various reasons, to call a halt to this particular trial, partly because it was quite obvious that hyperbaric oxygen alone was certainly not going to make any great impact on the mortality of myocardial infarction in general. Further, if we were going to continue in this, we would require so many patients that it would take all the resources we had. Even with a chamber to which we could get reasonably good access, it would take a very long time to get any answer. Finally, and most important of all, the primary reason for using hyperbaric oxygen at that time was removed by the arrival of coronary care, electrical defibrillation and pacing. In the last two or three years we have been continuing research work with oxygen at one and two atmospheres. First, we investigated the physiological aspects and other haemodynamic and circulatory responses to hyperbaric oxygen with a view to trying to see if it is possible to select some of the more seriously ill patients. For example, we selected those with the shock syndrome and have run another control trial on this group which has an extremely high mortality and from which it might be possible to get a statistical answer very soon. We have not proceeded very far with these trials and I want only to comment very briefly on one or two of the findings in the 35 men with myocardial infarction whom we have managed to investigate, breathing air at one atmosphere, oxygen at one atmosphere and oxygen at two atmospheres absolute. One of the differences found in patients with myocardial infarction is that there is no effect on the heart rate from oxygen at one atmosphere or at two atmospheres. Incidentally, they breathe oxygen at one atmosphere for one hour and then the pressure is increased in the chamber and they breathe 100 per cent. oxygen at two atmospheres for another hour. There is no effect on the heart rate; there is a rise in arterial pressure and in vascular resistance; a drop in cardiac output; and a rise in respiratory rate. The rise in arterial pressure is statistically significant only at two atmospheres. On the other hand, the drop in cardiac output is statistically significant at one atmosphere. These are somewhat different responses from healthy subjects. With one atmosphere there is a 5 to 6-fold increase in oxygen tension irrespective of the initial level and there is a 15-fold increase at two atmospheres. The response varies from patient to patient but nevertheless it is fairly linear.

There is no doubt that oxygen, especially given in high concentration and particularly given at two atmospheres absolute is associated with definite and sometimes quite marked haemodynamic changes and also with some metabolic response. Whether these are good, bad or indifferent as far as the patient is concerned has yet to be decided.

Professor Donald. Did the haemodynamic status improve in any of those with severe shock?

Dr Cameron. Yes, one of them did quite definitely. His mean arterial pressure was in the region of 50 mm. Hg., his cardiac output was less than 1·5 l./min. and his PO_2 was 24 mm. Hg.

His cardiac output responded in a paradoxical way with oxygen and eventually rose. He appeared well, his mental state improved and we took him out after exposure to hyperbaric oxygen of about two hours. However, fatal cardiac arrest occurred about six hours later.

Dr McKendrick. My first point is a technical comment in reply to a question Dr Marquis asked earlier. We have not found floating in P-60 catheters a completely benign experience. We have had spontaneous ventricular tachycardia in one and on withdrawal of a P-60 we have had one ventricular fibrillation. Now this may be due to inferior technical ability, but in view of our experience of first day arrhythmias, it is not altogether surprising that we get some complications and as a result of this we stopped slipping them in on the first day.

The next thing is that its high time that we developed a common coding system so that we could really compare our results. We have been using with satisfaction the old Peel index, which is a very simple method of scoring. It needs modifying with regard to arrhythmias as a result of recent experience with coronary care and it does need relating to the time of onset of symptoms. Nevertheless, we have found it quite useful. Obviously it alters from day to day and you need to do a recoding every morning and in a group of patients this gives you a trend.

We agree with the importance of hidden hypoxia. This is still not widely appreciated among the general practitioners throughout the country. We have not found any startling acid-base changes except in the virtually moribund cases. We are all using more intense therapy of all sorts on the more ill patients and it is an impossible problem to define which component is benefitting them most. One thing, which I think you will agree with, is that the light weight modern masks and nasal catheters are a much more effective way of giving oxygen.

Professor Donald. There would appear little doubt that the deficiency of oxygenation—sometimes moderate, sometimes very severe—is important but it appears that, in the severely ill cases, gross underperfusion of the body is the critical matter. Until this is remedied, raising oxygen is really not going to alter the issue.

Dr Wallace. Well, I think you have touched on the vital question as regards hyperbaria. We played this game in North Carolina too, and I think the really critical question is whether, in the presence of reduced blood supply, oxygen is or is not the critical substrate needed to sustain metabolism and function. We have attempted to approach this question recently in the experimental animal where we have produced a graded and controlled reduction of coronary blood flow until a decrement in cardiac performance was observed and then switched over from one atmosphere of air to two atmospheres of oxygen. The changes that we have observed in mean atrial pressures, dp/dt, left ventricular function curves and contractile force have been totally unimpressive in response to an

227

increase in oxygen with a fixed low coronary blood flow. I think the data are very suggestive that oxygen may not be the critical substrate that is needed by relatively ischaemic myocardium. However, I do not wish to extrapolate from this that oxygen might not be good for the patient who has a reduced cardiac output as a result of the myocardial infarct. The only other point I would make is that the hyperbaric chamber turns out to be a very good coronary care unit because it creates a very high ratio of physician to patient.

Dr Lassers. I would just like to comment on some of Dr Kirby's findings, particularly that the low cardiac output could be attributed to the arterial hypoxaemia. When Dr Anderton and I studied complete heart block in acute myocardial infarction we were unable to alter the hypoxaemia or the ventilation—perfusion disturbances—by changing the cardiac output.

Dr Semple. We still use the so-called Peel coronary prognostic index. We score our patients during the first 24 hours and before discharge. By this method we try to compare our admissions each year and we hope to compare the severity of our patients over the last three years with the severity of admission to our Coronary Care Unit, when we have one. The arrhythmic parameter will have to be altered, but we do feel that the index has a place both for comparing admission severity statistics from year to year, and possibly comparing the severity of patients admitted to different coronary care units. But we hope to change it a little so that the arrhythmic parameter will be of more value. We may have to leave it out altogether as so many patients get arrhythmias, but we wonder whether dividing them into simple and malignant arrhythmias might not be of some value.

Dr Kirby. We have put pulmonary artery catheters into 49 patients with myocardial infarcts and one-third have developed ectopic beats as the catheter traversed the right ventricle. No patients had ventricular fibrillation. Dr McKendrick pointed out our high incidence of acidosis. We did initially look at the more acutely ill patients so the figures were weighted and I am sure if you look at the whole spectrum of myocardial infarction you would find a lower incidence.

THE ARTIFICIAL HEART—MYOCARDIAL INFARCTION PROGRAMME

THEODORE COOPER

National Heart Institute, National Institutes of Health
Bethesda, Maryland 20014, U.S.A.

THE number of patients with myocardial insufficiency is increasing. Despite the magnitude of this problem and the substantial progress in its management there has been general recognition that research in this area has been disproportionately small and inadequate. Large segments of the scientific community with the expertise that could be brought to bear on this problem have not been attracted to it, and too few scientists with this specific interest are being trained. Stemming from the conviction that the rate of acquisition of new knowledge can be accelerated, the National Heart Institute is now providing resources, co-ordination, and direction for a targeted research programme under an Artificial Heart—Myocardial Infarction Programme. Funds have been specially appropriated by the Congress of the United States for this purpose.

The Programme objectives are: (1) The design and application of circulatory assist devices for use in patients with myocardial insufficiency. (2) The reduction in mortality and morbidity in patients with myocardial infarction.

The juxtaposition of these two targets is intentional. At its conception, the Programme had as its goal the development of an artificial heart. However, it was soon realised that the development of hardware must occur concomitantly with the extension of certain biological information. Particularly lacking is knowledge of the physiological effects of artificial circulation. Also, it is apparent that means for temporary mechanical circulatory assistance must be available before perfection of a practical total replacement for the heart. Utilisation of temporary devices requires much more precise definition of the clinical situations in which they will be useful.

Patients with atherosclerotic heart disease form the largest pool of potential recipients of mechanical circulatory support. Of these, the largest number will have suffered myocardial infarction. Serious gaps in knowledge of this complex disorder also exist. It has been decided that a large-scale co-ordinated research effort can close

229

some of these gaps and concomitantly provide information and experience needed in the area of artificial circulation.

Of the several independent experiences recently reported on the use of mechanical devices to support the failing circulation in man, some of these have involved patients with acute myocardial infarction. The experimentalists believed that the survival of some of the treated patients would not have occurred without the intervention of mechanical assistance. It appears then that, as in the instances of valvular heart and congenital heart disease, the cardiologist and the surgeon have found another common ground upon which to evolve new methods to treat heart disease.

It is clear that there is no need to be concerned about the feasibility of mechanical intervention. There is, however, need for new information upon which to formulate indications and operational standards for treatment. The Artificial Heart—Myocardial Infarction Programme is designed to facilitate the generation of this new information.

To accomplish its several related aims, the Programme has been organised into two Branches. One is responsible for developing more suitable devices for circulatory assistance; and the other for co-ordination of research in myocardial infarction. The scientists in these Branches do not conduct experimental work as their primary responsibility. The experimental work is conducted by scientists in university medical centres, non-university hospitals, and in private industry. The principal instrument for their support is the research contract. The contract mechanism was chosen to keep research 'on target'; to permit greater flexibility in the adjustment of workscopes and in the provision of resources in order to take advantage of new findings with as little delay as possible; and to facilitate co-ordination of related activity at various institutions.

The Artificial Heart Branch supports research across a spectrum which extends from basic research to clinical application of hardware. One segment of the Programme concerns itself with research on components and sub-systems such as the materials for basic structural units and for insuring compatible interfaces with blood and other tissues; energy generation, storage, conversion and transmission; blood pumps; and control mechanisms. The components and sub-systems need to meet the requirements for a variety of devices that can permit mechanical assistance by different approaches including arterio-arterial assistance; left ventricular bypass; veno-arterial bypass; intracorporeal ventricular massage; and total heart replacement.

The second segment of the Programme is primarily concerned with the experimental utilisation and testing of the devices. Evaluation will be particularly concerned with determining the effectiveness with which the device can assume part or all of the pumping load of the heart and can reverse functional circulatory abnormalities. This requires the determination of the consequences of application of the instruments not only on the heart but on the rest of the body. In the course of such evaluations, the indications for use of each type of device must be developed.

A third segment of the Programme is concerned with the broad application of the devices to clinical problems. Both the second and third segments of the Programme, but particularly the third, are closely related to the programme goals of the Myocardial Infarction Branch. It is clear that, as single experiments begin to define the individual patients likely to benefit from mechanical circulatory assistance, larger problems, some of them being economic, sociological and ethical will arise. These include acceptance of the therapy by the patient, profession, family and community; the need for skilled manpower to implant and maintain the devices; the requirement of special facilities; and finally, there will be special problems of manufacture and distribution. Obviously, one cannot wait to consider these problems until they have fully materialised.

The Myocardial Infarction Branch is also diversified. A major programme component at present is the clinical investigation of myocardial infarction. A network of Myocardial Infarction Research Units (MIRUs) is being established. A MIRU will provide the setting in which clinical and basic scientists with different skills and interests can converge on the many problems of myocardial infarction. The resources of such units should provide an environment conducive to the most efficient collection of data under conditions of optimal patient care. Not all MIRUs will work on the same problem, but together they will provide systematic coverage of more facets of this problem than isolated investigators are now achieving. The network will provide common ground for inter-institutional communication and collaboration.

Interventions in large numbers of patients with myocardial infarction can also be carried out in coronary care units other than MIRUs. Such 'testing satellites' are envisioned as complementing the major network. They will also provide a source for patients for study, and serve to translate research knowledge to wide clinical application with minimal delay.

The hospital physician does not see one of the important groups of patients with acute myocardial infarctions. These are patients who die suddenly. A segment of the programme will support a close inspection of sudden deaths. Retrospective studies of case histories of patients who die suddenly may contain more clues than heretofore revealed. Prospective studies will also be supported. These may be epidemiologic or therapeutic in approach.

It is imperative that a programme of this magnitude and diversity avail itself of the most expert assistance present in the scientific community. This is true for conception, operation and evaluation of progress. Indeed, the establishment of each of the two Branches was developed from the findings of panels composed of distinguished cardiovascular scientists. There are advisory committees and special consultants for both Branches and for the overall Programme. In order to plan effectively, it is also necessary that the staff have comprehensive analyses of the current 'state of the art' in key areas. Experts are supported to review critically special problem areas, identifying deficiencies in both current information and research activity. The objectives of the Programme are converted to specifications which are advertised to the research community. The responses are evaluated by the Programme Office with the assistance of the consultants and awards are determined on the basis of scientific merit and programme relevance.

The Programme aims to attract more scientists with diverse skills into research in myocardial infarction and circulatory assistance. This is essential to insure the quality of future research in the area and the availability of qualified technical and professional personnel.

Targeted research of the type represented by the AH-MI Programme is not an indictment of current research philosophy. It is not a device for diverting funds from less differentiated research. Rather, it is a source of additional support and resources to permit the scientific community to translate discoveries in diverse disciplines into practical relief for those threatened with disability and untimely death.

DISCUSSION

Dr Kreuzer (Dusseldorf). With arterial counter-pulsation in normal hearts there is a decrease in left ventricular pressure of between 30 and 50 per cent. but the cardiac output and the coronary flow are unchanged; also the mean arterial pressure is not different. In a failing heart during counter-pulsation, the cardiac output and coronary flow increase while left atrial pressure decreases. For

232

this reason counter-pulsation could be an advance in the treatment of myocardial infarction and cardiogenic shock. We have performed two series of experiments. In the first group we ligated the descending branch of the left coronary artery while the pump was running and there was only a small decrease in left ventricular pressure and in cardiac output while the coronary flow in the other branch of the coronary artery increased. After stopping the pump, all our cases developed ventricular fibrillation soon. Perhaps counter-pulsation prevents ventricular fibrillation but, of course, it is impossible from this type of experiment to draw such a positive conclusion. In the second group we tried to produce cardiogenic shock, but I am not certain that this is comparable to cardiogenic shock in the human subject. We also ligated the descending part of the left coronary artery but without pumping and we waited until ventricular fibrillation occurred. After three or four minutes of ventricular fibrillation, we defibrillated and then found in all our cases a low cardiac output, a systolic blood pressure between 50 and 70 mm. of mercury, acidosis and a low oxygen tension. Without treatment all the dogs died in a short time. Giving fluid into the arterial system led to a transistory increase in blood pressure. Using the pump alone, there was only a small effect because it was impossible to pump sufficient volume, but using the pump and giving dextran the blood pressure and cardiac output came up to normal in nearly 60 per cent. of the animals and stayed there. Our impression is that it would be better not to infuse fluid but to restore venous blood volume by reinjecting it into the arterial system with or without an oxygenator.

Dr Cross. I am familiar with the proposal of putting a catheter into the atrium and withdrawing venous blood from the right atrium and then using a bubble oxygenator and reinfusing it into the femoral artery. The question which has caused worry is the possibility of getting pulmonary thrombosis as a result of the low pulmonary flow and deterioration of proteins and of haemolysis. I was wondering whether or not anyone had experience with the so-called sinus pump.

Dr Cooper. We are supporting studies with the so-called sinus pump which is a sort of counter-pulsator originally designed to withdraw from the arterial system during systole and pump it back in during diastole, supposedly to reduce the work load during systole and to provide increased coronary flow during diastole. A variation on this is the veno-arterial phase pumping mechanism. In common with all the techniques at present under study, because of the materials and the characteristics of the pumps, as well as the plastic surfaces, there is haemolysis of varying degrees, denaturation of protein and the danger of emboli. Large sums are being invested in the basic research to try to overcome these barriers. If these important material problems cannot be overcome, we cannot do the necessary physiological studies to test the effects of long-term circulation and therefore the real feasibility of a total replacement. On the other hand there is no question in our minds that patients with circulatory failure, be it myocardial infarction or drug over-dosage, will benefit from any number of these techniques. With the pumps now available, circulating support is practicable for short periods.

Professor Chazov. What do you think about the clinical use of counter-pulsation methods in patients with cardiogenic shock?

Dr Kreuzer. Out of five patients with post-operative low cardiac output there was only one long-term survivor. Four patients died, so I can't really say.

Professor Chazov. Have you any experience in the clinical use of the arterial pump in cardiogenic shock, Dr Cooper?

Dr Cooper. I have no experience personally. I have heard that patients in acute pulmonary oedema could be placed on renal-arterial pumps even without an oxygenator in the line, and within 10 minutes the oedema has cleared. The long-term results were not successful and the surgeons attributed the lack of success to a lack of aggressive cardiological approach!

Professor Donald. Well, this has been quite a day. Although we all feel a great need to have a temporary pump for patients in mild shock who appear to need perfusion and little else, some of us also have grave worries about the future of this sort of thing. One imagines a third of the population handing out pills, a third earning money and a third keeping the graveyard alive!

METABOLIC CONSEQUENCES OF ACUTE MYOCARDIAL INFARCTION

Chairman: Dr M. F. OLIVER

CATECHOLAMINE METABOLISM IN PATIENTS WITH ACUTE MYOCARDIAL INFARCTION

ANDREW G. WALLACE

*From the Department of Medicine, Duke University Medical Center
Durham, N.C., U.S.A.*

ACUTE myocardial infarction is accompanied by chest pain, severe anxiety, alterations of cardiac rhythm and frequently by evidence of heart failure or shock. There is strong evidence to suggest that each of these physiological phenomena is associated with an increase in the activity of the autonomic nervous system, particularly the sympathetic nervous system. It is not surprising, therefore, that a number of investigators have considered it likely that patients with acute myocardial infarction would manifest an increase in the urinary excretion of catecholamines. This study was undertaken to examine the pattern of urinary catecholamine excretion in patients with acute myocardial infarction admitted to a Coronary Care Unit.

Materials and methods

The observations described in this report were made on 26 male patients who were admitted to the Coronary Care Unit of Duke University Medical Center. All of these patients manifested the typical signs of acute myocardial infarction, including chest pain, diagnostic electrocardiographic changes and elevation of the serum enzymes. Nine male patients who were admitted to the Coronary Care Unit with chest pain not due to myocardial infarction served as controls. Patients in this control group had chest pain which was the result of either coronary insufficiency without infarction or pericarditis. In addition, catecholamine excretion was studied in nine normal subjects without cardiovascular disease.

The patients with acute myocardial infarction were admitted to the Coronary Care Unit and remained in the Unit for at least 10 days. During that period of time the electrocardiogram was monitored continuously and the patients remained at bed rest. Twenty-four hour urine specimens were collected in a plastic jug containing 15 ml. of 6 N hydrochloric acid and the urine was kept on ice during the collection period. The protein-free supernatant was titrated to pH 8·5 with sodium hydroxide. Catecholamines were adsorbed on an alumina column and eluted subsequently by

237

the addition of 0·3 M acetic acid. The eluate was then brought to pH 6 and placed in a Technicon Autoanalyzer. In the auto-analyzer, catecholamines were converted to their trihydroxyindoles and fluorescence was determined. Total catecholamines were estimated using ascorbic acid as the stabilizing agent. Norepine-phrine was then determined using thioglycolic acid as the stabilizing agent. Epinephrine was calculated as the difference between total catecholamines and norepinephrine concentrations. Recoveries of norepinephrine and epinephrine were 89 per cent. and 76 per cent. respectively.

RESULTS

In nine normal subjects the 24 hour excretion of norepinephrine averaged 27·5 μg./24 hr. and epinephrine excretion averaged 7·5 μg./24 hr. Twenty-four hour urinary creatinine averaged 1·24 g. in these nine normal subjects. In nine patients admitted to the Coronary Care Unit with chest pain, but without myocardial infarction, the excretion of norepinephrine averaged 22·4 μg./24 hr., epinephrine averaged 7·6 μg./24 hr. and creatinine averaged 1·18 g./24 hr.

In the majority of the 26 patients with acute myocardial in-farction the 24 hour urine collections were complete and the excretion of creatinine was comparable to that observed in normal subjects. Furthermore, the excretion of creatinine did not vary significantly from day to day during the period of hospitalisation. Therefore, in order to compensate for occasional patients in whom isolated urine specimens were lost, each patient's urinary excretion of catecholamines was expressed in nonograms (ng) per milligram (mg) of creatinine.

In the patients with acute myocardial infarction the average excretion of norepinephrine during the first 24 hours of hospitalisa-tion was 76 ng. per mg. of creatinine. In patients with chest pain, without myocardial infarction, the average excretion was 22 ng. per mg. of creatinine and in normal subjects it was 20 ng. per mg. of creatinine. In patients with acute myocardial infarction the average excretion of epinephrine during the first 24 hours of hospitalisation was 18 ng. per mg. of creatinine, and in patients with chest pain, but without myocardial infarction the average excretion was 7 ng. per mg. of creatinine. In the normal subjects, epinephrine excretion was 6 ng. per mg. of creatinine. Thus, during the first 24 hours of hospitalisation, patients with acute myocardial infarction had a significant elevation of both norepinephrine and epinephrine in the urine (Fig. 1). Patients with chest pain, but without acute myocardial infarction, did not differ from normal subjects with respect to either norepinephrine or epinephrine excretion.

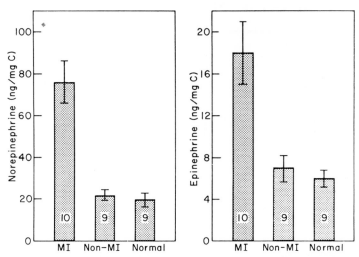

FIG. 1.   Urinary catecholamines during the first 24 hours of hospitalisation.

Twenty-four hour urine catecholamines were measured during the first 10 consecutive days of hospitalisation in the patients with acute myocardial infarction. During this 10-day period catecholamine excretion remained elevated; however, there was a stepwise decrease with each day of hospitalisation (Fig. 2).

Because the 26 patients with acute myocardial infarction comprised a heterogeneous group with respect to the incidence and severity of complications, they were divided into three sub-groups characterised as (1) uncomplicated, (2) those with shock, and (3) those with heart block. In the uncomplicated patients, the highest values for norepinephrine and epinephrine were observed during the first 24 hours of hospitalisation. In patients with shock or with heart block, the highest excretion of catecholamines during the period of the complication was selected for comparison with the uncomplicated patients. Patients with heart block manifested the highest levels of both norepinephrine and epinephrine in the urine. In these patients the average excretion of norepinephrine was 135 ng. per mg. of creatinine and for epinephrine it was 66·5 ng. per mg. of creatinine. In the uncomplicated patients the average excretion of norepinephrine was 32 ng. per mg. of creatinine and of

239

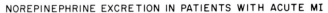

NOREPINEPHRINE EXCRETION IN PATIENTS WITH ACUTE MI

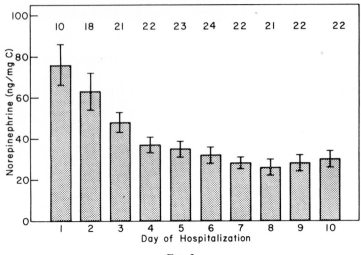

FIG. 2.

epinephrine, 6 ng. per mg. of creatinine. In patients with shock the excretion of norepinephrine was 55 ng. per mg. of creatinine and the epinephrine excretion was 36 ng. per mg. of creatinine. Thus, in patients with shock and in patients with complete heart block epinephrine and norepinephrine were both strikingly elevated, by comparison with uncomplicated patients. The relative increase of epinephrine in both groups of patients with complications, but particularly in those with heart block is of note.

The analysis of daily urinary excretion of catecholamines in individual patients demonstrated repeatedly that psychologically stressful events, such as transfer from the Coronary Care Unit to another ward of the hospital, alterations of the nurse-patient relationship, receiving a bill for hospitalisation, etc. were associated with significant alterations in the pattern of urinary excretion of catecholamines (Klein *et al.*, 1967). Late complications such as post-myocardial infarction syndrome and arrhythmias also were associated with an increase in the urinary excretion of catecholamines on the day of the complication.

DISCUSSION

Valori *et al.* (1967) have recently reported four patients with acute myocardial infarction. Urinary excretion of noradrenaline and

240

adrenaline was examined during the first 15 days of hospitalisation on a Coronary Care Unit. In all patients, the levels of noradrenaline were initially high. The number of patients studied was too small, however, to correlate differences in the pattern of catecholamine excretion with the incidence of various complications.

In our study, we have demonstrated consistently an increase of norepinephrine in the urine in patients with acute myocardial infarction. The majority of patients also demonstrated an elevation of epinephrine. The 24 hour excretion of epinephrine and norepinephrine in patients with acute myocardial infarction decreased in a step-wise manner during the first 10 days of hospitalisation. Patients admitted to the Coronary Care Unit with chest pain, but without acute myocardial infarction, did not demonstrate a similar increase in the excretion of either norepinephrine or epinephrine.

Patients with shock or with heart block had significantly greater excretion of norepinephrine and epinephrine than patients who were initially uncomplicated. In patients with shock and in patients with heart block the relative increase of epinephrine was greater than the increase of norepinephrine. From these observations we can conclude that changes in the activity of the sympathetic nervous system are prominent features of the response to acute myocardial infarction. Norepinephrine and epinephrine tend to be elevated most strikingly in those patients with heart block or with shock. As a group, patients with uncomplicated acute myocardial infarction tend to have only a moderate increase in norepinephrine and little or no increase in epinephrine.

Norepinephrine and epinephrine are most strikingly elevated in the group of patients with acute myocardial infarction who have the highest incidence of serious arrhythmias. These data, coupled with the observation that stimulation of the cardiac sympathetic nerves produces ventricular tachyarrhythmias and fibrillation in animals with experimental myocardial infarction (Harris, 1966) suggest that there may be a cause and effect relationship between the activity of the autonomic nervous system and the incidence of arrhythmias. It is of further interest to note that in experimental animals in which the heart has been denervated, we have observed that the incidence of arrhythmias following acute ligation of a branch of the coronary arteries is markedly reduced.

Our data do not provide definitive evidence for a cause and effect relationship between the activity of the sympathetic nervous system and arrhythmias in patients with acute myocardial infarction. They do suggest that patients can be subdivided into relatively

241

homogeneous sub-groups based on the pattern of urinary excretion of catecholamines. It seems clear that circulatory insufficiency, resulting either from extensive myocardial necrosis or significant disturbances of cardiac rhythm, can initiate a strong adrenergic drive in patients with acute myocardial infarction. It is equally evident that psychological events may lead to a significant change in the pattern of catecholamine excretion in these patients. Our observations indicate that the urinary catecholamine excretion can be useful as a biochemical symptom of ' stress ' in patients with acute myocardial infarction. Future studies might profitably be directed toward the question of whether or not overactivity of the sympathetic nervous system represents a beneficial or a detrimental response to the patient.

Supported by Grants HE-07776-04, 5 TI HE-5242 and PO 1 HE-11306-01 from the National Institutes of Health and from the Fund for Research and Teaching, Department of Nutrition, Harvard School of Public Health.

REFERENCES

HARRIS, A. S. (1966). Genesis of ventricular tachycardia and fibrillation following coronary occlusion. In *Mechanisms and Therapy of Cardiac Arrhythmias*, p. 293. Ed. Dreifus, L. S. London: Grune & Stratton.

KLEIN, R. F., KLINER, V. A., ZIPES, D. P., TROYER, W. G., Jr. & WALLACE, A. G. (1968). Intrahospital transfer and its effects upon patients with acute myocardial infarction. *Am. J. Cardiol.* In press.

VALORI, C., THOMAS, M. & SHILLINGFORD, J. P. (1967). Urinary excretion of free noradrenaline and adrenaline following acute myocardial infarction. *Lancet*, **1**, 127.

Discussion. See p. 258.

FATTY ACID RESPONSE TO TRAUMA

Lars A. Carlson

*Department of Internal Medicine, Karolinska Hospital and
King Gustaf Vth Research Institute, Stockholm, Sweden*

In the care of the acutely ill patient, we must consider the metabolic responses of the body to the disease. In the acute situation, some of these may be purposeful and some harmful and we have very little knowledge about the basic metabolic responses to trauma in man. Acute myocardial infarction is an unusually complicated situation for the body. This trauma subjects the patient to three major acute stresses: pain, tissue damage and serious circulatory disturbances. It would indeed not be surprising if the final result of these conditions resulted in complex, clinically important metabolic aberrations. This area is so far rather neglected; its challenge and virginity invites the clinical investigator.

We became interested in the metabolic aspects of trauma, and especially the metabolism of plasma free fatty acids (FFA) in this regard some years ago. The three major reasons for this interest in FFA were:

1. The importance of FFA in energy metabolism.
2. The increased secretion of catecholamines in trauma.
3. The clinically significant side effects of excessive mobilisation of FFA.

1. FFA are continuously mobilised from adipose tissue. The control of this process is extremely complex in the intact organism. Factors of importance in this regard are nutritional conditions, hormones, nervous activity (sympathetic nervous system) and various metabolites of carbohydrate, lipid and protein metabolism. In the context of acute illness and trauma in man the nutritional condition and catecholamines are probably among the more important factors to be considered; the latter being among the more potent stimulators of the mobilisation of FFA in man. FFA are major substrates for fuel in the body and it is likely that more than half of our energy consumption is covered by oxidation of FFA in different tissues. Of special interest in regard to myocardial infarction is that a very significant part of the energy requirements of the heart is covered by oxidation of lipids delivered to it mainly as FFA. Detailed aspects of the mobilisation of FFA from adipose

243

tissue and energy metabolism have been given recently (Renold & Cahill, 1965).

2. During trauma of various kinds there is an increased secretion of urinary catecholamines. For instance, Forssman and his colleagues (1952) studied 15 patients with acute myocardial infarction. In 14 of these there was a dramatic increase in urinary catecholamine secretion. Dr Wallace has confirmed and elaborated these findings in the preceding paper. This suggested to us that mobilisation of FFA might be significantly increased during the acute phase of trauma.

3. When the amount of FFA mobilised from adipose tissue exceeds the amount needed for energy metabolism, we call this excessive mobilisation (Carlson *et al.*, 1965; Carlson, 1967). Conditions which may be induced by excessive mobilisation of FFA are summarised in Table I. These conditions and their possible role in acute myocardial infarction will be discussed later on.

Dr Oliver will speak later on about FFA specifically during acute myocardial infarction, so I will confine myself to more general aspects of this problem and try to outline present concepts with regard to the metabolism of FFA.

I will first emphasise to you that changes in FFA levels may be regarded as a general body response to traumatic conditions. For instance, data obtained from burned patients admitted to our hospital within six hours of the burns demonstrated this quite clearly (Birke *et al.*, 1965). We followed the arterial levels of free fatty acids in samples taken each morning during several days, and the patients were divided into groups according to severity. The normal level of the free fatty acid is around 0·5 mEq. per litre. All three groups of burned patients had raised levels of FFA during the first two days, above 1 mEq. per litre, and there was a positive correlation between a degree of trauma and free fatty acid response. The most severely injured had pronounced elevations for several weeks, the FFA level being around 1·3 mEq. per litre for the first days and around 0·7 for the ensuing three weeks.

The general pathways for the metabolism of FFA are depicted in Figure 1. FFA are continuously mobilised from adipose tissue into the blood stream. This process is regulated by three major influences: nutritional factors, hormonal factors and nervous factors (Renold & Cahill, 1965). In man the factor which effects this mobilisation most strikingly is the catecholamines which have a very immediate stimulating effect on mobilisation of FFA. Once mobilisation has started, FFA are bound to serum albumin and

244

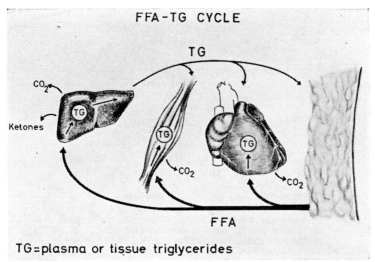

FFA-TG CYCLE

TG

CO_2

Ketones

CO_2

CO_2

FFA

TG=plasma or tissue triglycerides

Fig. 1. General, schematic pathway for the metabolism of FFA. See text.

transported via blood and taken up by various tissues. After uptake into a tissue their fate is in most tissues straightforward as they are immediately esterified to triglycerides. Two things can then happen; as depicted, they can either be stored as triglycerides or oxidised to generate carbon dioxide and energy. There is no other way for FFA to be metabolised, except in the liver. In that organ they may in addition be converted to ketone bodies or they may be recirculated as plasma triglycerides (Fig. 1).

As I see it, the unique feature of this simplified system is that the uptake of FFA into various tissues is directly proportional to the amount of free fatty acids delivered to the tissues. This has been shown by various *in vivo* and *in vitro* studies on different tissues in animals. In man this is true for the splanchnic region as visualised in Figure 2. This means that it is not the tissue itself which determines how much fatty acid should be taken up but the rate of mobilisation from adipose tissue. I think this is rather an important property of this system and from the simplified picture in Figure 1 I will try to discuss and also to illustrate some experimental studies on the side-effects of excessive mobilisation of FFA, excessive in the sense that the mobilisation of FFA from adipose tissue exceeds the needs of the body for oxidative purposes. In our experiments we have often used catecholamines

245

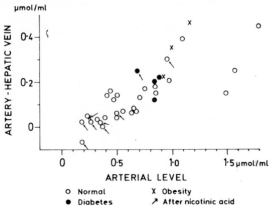

FIG. 2. Concentration dependent on splanchnic uptake of FFA in man. FFA concentration difference over splanchnic region plotted against arterial FFA levels. Data obtained by catherisation of hepatic vein in man (Carlson *et al.*, 1967).

to induce such excessive mobilisation, but you can as well induce excessive mobilisation with other agents and get similar results.

Side-effects of excessive FFA mobilisation (Table I) can be related to tissue triglyceride formation, to increased energy metabolism and to increased ketone body production. FFA have also for various reasons been implicated in the process of thrombogenesis.

Table I. *Conditions of potential interest in myocardial infarction which may be induced by excessive mobilisation of FFA*

Energy metabolism
Increased basal metabolic rate
Increased myocardial O_2 consumption

Carbohydrate metabolism
Decreased glucose tolerance

Lipid metabolism
Fatty infiltration of myocardium
Fatty infiltration other tissues
Increased ketone body formation

Thrombogenesis
Shortened clotting time
Increased platelet aggregation
Thrombo-embolism

After excessive mobilisation of FFA in animals by infusing noradrenaline for eight hours we saw fat droplets in practically all myocardial fibres (Carlson *et al.*, 1965). These droplets were

246

located in close contact with the mitochondria. Similar findings with increased amounts of intracellular lipids were seen in many organs: liver, lungs, skeletal muscle, kidneys and gastro-intestinal tract. Now, of course, one might very well argue that noradrenaline has several effects other than stimulating mobilisation of FFA. In order to settle these possibilities, we have done studies where we have specifically inhibited the noradrenaline induced lipid mobilising effects. Administration of nicotinic acid inhibits this effect of catecholamines but not their cardiovascular effects. (Carlson & Orö, 1962.)

NA was infused for 8 hours into anaesthetized dogs

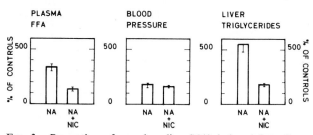

FIG. 3. Prevention of noradrenaline (NA) induced fatty liver in dogs by nicotinic acid (NIC) which inhibits the NA induced stimulation of FFA mobilisation but does not modify NA induced blood pressure changes. Values expressed as percentage of control dogs (Carlson & Liljedahl, 1963).

Two groups of dogs, one receiving noradrenaline and one receiving noradrenaline plus nicotinic acid were studied (Carlson & Liljedahl, 1963). Infusion of noradrenaline raised FFA levels about 400 to 500 per cent. (Figure 3). If at the same time nicotinic acid was administered, this increase was almost completely blocked. The blood pressure response in these two groups was similar, but, as a consequence of the inhibition of the mobilisation of FFA, the increase in hepatic triglyceride content induced by noradrenaline infusion was almost completely inhibited by the simultaneous administration of nicotinic acid. There are several other kinds of evidence which all suggest that it is really the excessive mobilisation of FFA that is responsible for the accumulation of lipids in various tissues.

With regard to energy metabolism, it has been known for quite a long time that catecholamines have something which is called their calorigenic action. We wanted to study to what extent this

247

calorigenic action could be connected with the stimulation of the mobilisation of FFA. Figure 4 shows that infusion of noradrenaline to healthy volunteers increases FFA levels, blood glucose concentration and the oxygen uptake. When the increase in FFA was inhibited by nicotinic acid it could be seen that the calorigenic action was significantly reduced. This suggests that at least part of the calorigenic action of the catecholamines can be related to the lipid mobilising effect. In the context of myocardial

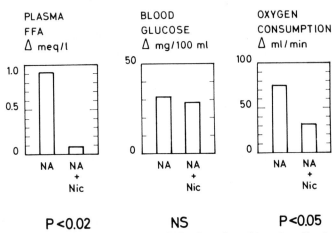

FIG. 4. Demonstration of the calorigenic action of noradrenaline in man and its reduction by inhibition of the stimulation of FFA mobilisation (Havel *et al.*, 1964).

infarction, it may be clinically relevant that O_2-consumption of the perfused heart is stimulated by high levels of FFA in the medium (Challoner & Steinberg, 1966).

Finally I would just touch upon the problems of thrombogenesis. Different types of studies *in vivo* and *in vitro* have suggested that free fatty acids might stimulate various parts of thrombogenic process (Hoak *et al.*, 1967). To study these effects *in vivo*, we injected fibrinogen labelled with ^{125}I into dogs and then followed the turnover for one week and in that way we obtained the half life of fibrinogen under normal conditions (Table II). We then infused noradrenaline for eight hours in order to raise FFA levels (Table II).

We continued to follow the turnover of fibrinogen and observed that this infusion of noradrenaline very dramatically decreased the half life of fibrinogen (Table II) indicating that there was increased fibrinogen consumption. Unfortunately however when we then looked at the control animals receiving only saline in addition

Table II. *Effect of 8-hour infusion of saline (C) or noradrenaline (NA) to nembutal anaesthetised dogs*

Plasma FFA (m.Eq/l.)		Liver TG (μmol/g.)		Platelets (millions)				Fibrinogen half time ($t\frac{1}{2}$) (days)			
C	NA	C	NA	C		NA		C		NA	
				Before	After	Before	After	Before	After	Before	After
0·68	1·58	12	58	201	182	231	194	2·2	0·8	2·5	0·9

to anaesthesia, we observed the same effect! Presumably the increased consumption of fibrinogen was related to the effect of anaesthesia, or other parts of the experimental procedure. This is a hitherto unknown effect, and one which we are trying to explore currently.

SUMMARY

Different kinds of trauma, experimental trauma as well as clinical trauma in man, raise the free fatty acid levels in plasma. This may have the following clinical implications. It may be of importance for energy metabolism, as it may increase the basal metabolic rate, and perhaps more important in myocardial infarction it may also increase the oxygen consumption of the heart. With regard to lipid metabolism, increased FFA levels may result in a very significant fatty infiltration of various tissues, whatever this means for the function of these organs. Excessive mobilisation of FFA may also increase ketone body formation, which is pertinent in the context of metabolic acidosis. With regard to carbohydrate metabolism, which I have not discussed here at all, high levels of FFA may decrease glucose tolerance. An interesting possibility, finally, is that it may influence thrombogenesis but this is at present only based on experimental data.

REFERENCES

BIRKE, G., CARLSON, L. A. & LILJEDAHL, S-O. (1965). Lipid metabolism and trauma. III. Plasma lipids and lipoproteins in burns. *Acta med. scand.* **178**, 337.

CARLSON, L. A. (1967). Recent advances in the metabolism of plasma lipids. *Progr. biochem. Pharmacol.* **4**, 170.

CARLSON, L. A. & LILJEDAHL, S-O. (1963). Lipid metabolism and trauma. II. Studies on the effect of nicotinic acid on norepinephrine induced fatty liver. *Acta med. scand.* **173**, 787.

CARLSON, L. A. & ORO, L. (1962). The effect of nicotinic acid on the plasma free fatty acids. Demonstration of a metabolic type of sympathicolysis. *Acta med. scand.* **172**, 641.

CARLSON, L. A., FREYSCHUSS, U., KJELLBERG, J. & ÖSTMAN, J. (1967). Suppression of splanchnic ketone body production in man by nicotinic acid. *Diabetologia.* In Press.

CARLSON, L. A., LILJEDAHL, S-O. & WIRSEN, C. (1965). Blood and tissue changes in the dog during and after excessive free fatty acid mobilisation. A biochemical and morphological study. *Acta med. scand.* **178**, 81.

CHALLONER, D. R. & STEINBERG, D. (1966). Effect of free fatty acid on the oxygen consumption of perfused rat heart. *Am. J. Physiol.* **210**, 280.

FORSSMAN, O., HANSSON, G. & JENSEN, C. C. (1952). The adrenal function in coronary thrombosis. *Acta med. scand.* **142**, 441.

HAVEL, R. J., CARLSON, L. A., EKELUND, L-G. & HOLMGREN, A. (1964). Studies on the relation between mobilisation of free fatty acids and energy metabolism in man: effects of norepinephrine and nicotinic acid. *Metabolism,* **13**, 1402.

HOAK, J. C., WARNER, E. D. & CONNOR, W. E. (1967). Platelets, fatty acids and thrombosis. *Circulation Res.* **20**, 71.

RENOLD, A. E. & CAHILL, G. F. (1965). *Handbook of Physiology,* vol. 5. *Adipose Tissue.* Washington: American Physiological Society.

Discussion. See p. 258.

THE RELATIONSHIP OF SERUM FREE FATTY ACIDS TO ARRHYTHMIAS AND DEATH

Michael Oliver

Royal Infirmary, Edinburgh

In a previous study (Kurien & Oliver, 1966) we have shown that serum free fatty acids (FFA) are elevated during the first day following acute myocardial infarction. We examined possible explanations of this rise, such as the effects of a preceding fatty or carbohydrate meal, of a prolonged period of fasting and of the stress and anxiety of admission to hospital. In none of these situations were serum FFA elevated to the degree observed after acute myocardial infarction. We also examined the effects of severe pain, as manifested by acute coronary insufficiency and by plain muscle spasm due to acute renal colic, and concluded that severe pain can cause elevation of serum FFA and that it probably contributes to the rise after acute myocardial infarction. However, the degree and the duration of serum FFA elevation in patients with renal colic or acute coronary insufficiency was less than in patients with acute myocardial infarction. Furthermore, the changes observed in these patients were similar to those in patients with acute cerebral vascular occlusion, who had been admitted unconscious and presumably had not experienced any pain. It seemed, probable, therefore that prolonged hypoxia and damage of myocardial and cerebral tissue also contributes to the high serum FFA levels.

During the course of this earlier study, we observed that the response following acute myocardial infarction was not uniform and that there were more deaths in patients with particularly high serum FFA levels. We have therefore studied the relationship of serum FFA levels to arrhythmias and deaths after acute myocardial infarction.

Selection of patients

This study was made on 200 patients admitted to the Coronary Care Unit in the Royal Infirmary of Edinburgh with proven acute myocardial infarction. The diagnosis of myocardial infarction was made on the basis of characteristic ECG changes (Minnesota Code) *and* elevated levels of serum creatine kinase and glutamic oxalacetic transaminase. The patients admitted to the study were consecutive providing that they did not have diabetes mellitus, there had been no prior administration of heparin or catecholamines (which elevate serum FFA levels) or Atromid-S, reserpine, guanethidine or methyldopa (which lower serum FFA levels). In addition, no patient over 70 years has been included since it is not the policy of the Royal Infirmary Coronary Care Unit to admit such patients routinely (Lawrie *et al.*, 1967).

Serum FFA measurements

Patients were admitted to the study providing a serious arrhythmia had not preceded the first venupuncture for serum FFA analysis. If such an arrhythmia had occurred, patients were excluded. The minimal requirements for admission to the study were to obtain one non-fasting or fasting specimen within 24 hours of the onset of symptoms and, unless death intervened, one fasting specimen next morning. Usually the first specimen was not taken in the fasting state since most patients came into hospital during the course of the day or evening and had already had a meal, but when a patient was admitted in the early hours of the morning then the first specimen would be taken later in the morning in the fasting state. This was always followed by another specimen on the following morning, also taken in the fasting state. Usually three specimens were obtained and two of these were taken with 24 hours of the onset of symptoms. The method of analysis was a modification of the colorimetric technique described by Mosinger (1965). The fasting level in 100 healthy men between the ages of 19 and 46 was 525 ± 124 μEq/l. giving an upper 95 per cent. confidence limit of 773 μEq/l.

Results

In Figure 1, the percentage distribution of serum FFA levels is shown for the normal healthy population and for patients immediately after acute myocardial infarction. It should be pointed out that the samples were obtained from the healthy population in the fasting state while those from patients following acute myocardial infarction were seldom fasting specimens, and that the mean age of the healthy men was younger than that of the patients with myocardial infarction; in addition, the patients were of both sexes. A mixed carbohydrate-fat meal will, if anything, tend to

252

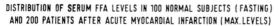

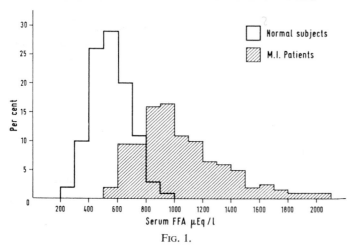

FIG. 1.

depress serum FFA levels and we have not observed any increase in serum FFA with age or any major sex difference.

In Figure 2, an attempt has been made to depict the typical response of serum FFA levels following acute myocardial infarction. This curve has been derived from 50 patients in whom three or more serial blood specimens were obtained during the first 48 hours and in most of these patients four or five specimens were analysed. The figures in the first part of this curve have been designated ' maximum ' serum FFA levels and used for the correlation which will follow. In fact, most of them must be submaximal since it is obviously impossible to determine from an estimation of serum FFA taken within the first 8 or 12 hours whether the resultant value has been derived from the upstroke or downstroke of the curve. The real maximum will often be higher and certainly not lower than the ones given here. This inadequacy in interpreting the results of early samples would of course underestimate the significance of any correlation which might be derived from relating serum FFA levels to another variable. It is difficult to be sure when the serum FFA levels begin to rise since we have obtained comparatively few readings within the first four hours but the shape of this curve suggests that they may be elevated soon after the onset of symptoms.

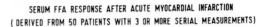

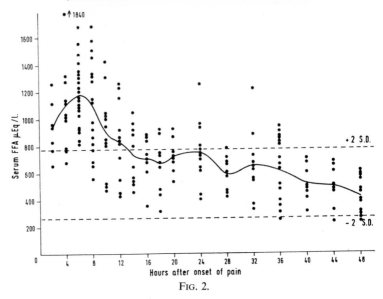

SERUM FFA RESPONSE AFTER ACUTE MYOCARDIAL INFARCTION
(DERIVED FROM 50 PATIENTS WITH 3 OR MORE SERIAL MEASUREMENTS)

FIG. 2.

Table I shows the relationship between maximum serum FFA levels and arrhythmias. The 200 patients have been arbitrarily grouped according to their serum FFA levels in such a way that there are approximately equal numbers in four groups. It can be seen that there is a statistically significant difference in the incidence of all arrhythmias in those patients who have serum FFA levels greater than 1,200 μEq/l., when compared with those who have serum FFA levels between 500 and 1,199 μEq/l. Moreover, there is a significant progression from groups 1 to 4 in all groups with the exception of those who developed primary ventricular tachycardia or ventricular fibrillation.

Table II shows the relationship between maximum serum FFA levels and deaths. A similar grouping of serum FFA levels has been made and it can be seen that there is a significant difference in the number of deaths in patients with more than 1,200 μEq/1. when compared with those with lower levels and that there is also a significant progression from groups 1 to 4. It will also be noted that the principal difference between group 4 and the others occurs in those who died after transfer from the Coronary Care Unit—in other words, high serum FFA levels occurred in the first 24 hours

254

Table I. *Relationship of maximum observed serum FFA levels and arrhythmias in 200 patients with acute myocardial infarction*

Groups	Maximum Serum FFA (μEq/l)	No. of patients	No. without any arrhythmia		No. with atrial arrhythmias		No. with V.P.B.		No. with primary V.T. or V.F.		No. with 2° or 3° block		No. with V.T., V.F. or block	
			No.	%	No.	%	No.	%	No.	%	No.	%	No.	%
1.	500–799	42	12	29	4	10	24	57	8	19	1	2	9	21
2.	800–999	65	21	32	11	17	32	49	10	15	5	8	13	26
3.	1,000–1,199	42	10	24	7	17	26	62	6	14	4	10	7	17
4.	1,200+	51	3	6	16	31	40	78	18	35	11	22	21	41

Significance tests	No arrhythmias	Atrial arrhythmias	V.P.B.	Primary V.T. or V.F.	2° or 3° block	Primary V.T., V.F. or block
Difference between serum FFA of 500–1,199 compared with 1,200+ μEq/l χ_1^2 P values .	<0·01	<0·02	<0·01	<0·01	<0·01	<0·005
Contingency analysis—Groups 1 to 4 (χ_3^2) P values . .	<0·02	<0·05	<0·05	N.S. at 5%	<0·50	<0·05

VPB = Ventricular Premature Beats.　　VT = Ventricular Tachycardia.　　VF = Ventricular Fibrillation.

Table II. *Relationship of maximum observed serum FFA levels and deaths in 200 patients with acute myocardial infarction*

Groups	Maximum serum FFA (μEq/l)	No. of patients	Total No. of deaths*		Deaths in C.C.U.				Deaths after transfer			
			No.	%	All	V.F. or V.A.	Shock	Failure	All	Sudden	Failure	Rupture
1.	500–799	42	2	5	1	0	0	1	1	0	1	0
2.	800–999	65	5	8	5	2	2	1	0	—	—	—
3.	1,000–1,199	42	8	19	4 (10%)	1	2	1	4 (10%)	3	0	1
4.	1,200+	51	17	33	7 (14%)	2	4	1	10 (20%)	9	1	0

* Significance of difference between Groups 1–3 and Group 4 χ_1^2 – P < 0·05.
** Contingency analysis: Groups 1 to 4 (χ_3^2) – P < 0·002.
VF = Ventricular Fibrillation.　　　　VA = Ventricular Asystole.

in those who died suddenly and unexpectedly in the wards two and three weeks later.

No correlation existed in these 200 patients between maximum serum FFA levels and maximum serum CPK or maximum serum GOT levels. There was no correlation between serum FFA levels and blood sugar levels. The only point worth commenting on is that seven of the eight patients who died from shock had blood sugar levels above 150mg. per cent., confirming the findings of Mackenzie *et al.* (1964).

DISCUSSION

There are three possible interpretations of this elevation of serum free fatty acids after acute myocardial infarction. One is that it is a result of increased catecholamine, particularly noradrenaline, activity causing mobilisation of FFA from adipose tissue. Another is that plasma lipolysis occurs with release of FFA from plasma triglycerides; the main cause of plasma lipolysis is activation of lipoprotein lipase and this is unlikely in the absence of heparin. A third possibility is that an abrupt decrease in utilisation of plasma FFA occurs. There is no evidence for this, and, indeed, it has been shown experimentally that profound myocardial ischaemia is associated with an increased extraction of FFA (Scheuer & Brachfield, 1966).

Exactly what sequence occurs following the onset of the first symptoms of myocardial infarction is not clear. Severe hypoxia of myocardial tissues could lead to release of the rich stores of myocardial noradrenaline. The general sympathetic response associated with severe pain might then be expected to contribute further to increasing circulating noradrenaline concentration. In addition, an adrenal component probably comes into operation fairly soon with the release of catecholamines, and also of cortisol.

There are two explanations of the association of high circulating free fatty acid levels with arrhythmias and deaths. One is that both are a result of increased circulating noradrenaline. The other is that there is a cause and effect relationship. Dr Carlson has indicated in the preceding paper that free fatty acids can increase myocardial oxygen consumption and work, and this has also been demonstrated by Challoner and Steinberg (1966). Abrupt increases in plasma FFA may therefore act as an undesirable drive to the hypoxic myocardium. Moreover, complete oxidation of fatty acids requires more oxygen than esterification and after acute infarction lipid oxidation in the myocardium may be retarded and triglyceride deposition stimulated—a situation which would be aggravated by very high plasma FFA levels.

SUMMARY

A study has been made of serum free fatty acid levels in 200 patients during the first 48 hours after myocardial infarction. The incidence of serious arrhythmias was significantly higher in patients with serum free fatty acid levels greater than 1,200 $\mu Eq/l$. There were also more deaths in these patients, particularly sudden deaths, two or three weeks after the onset of myocardial infarction.

High serum FFA levels are an early and valuable predictive index of serious arrhythmias and death. They may contribute to the development of arrhythmias and represent a new therapeutic challenge.

REFERENCES

CHALLONER, D. & STEINBERG, D. (1966). Effect of free fatty acid on the oxygen consumption of perfused rat heart. *Am. J. Physiol.* **210**, 280.

KURIEN, V. A. & OLIVER, M. F. (1966). Serum free fatty acids after acute myocardial infraction and cerebral vascular occlusion. *Lancet*, **2**, 122.

LAWRIE, D. M., GREENWOOD, T. W., GODDARD, M., HARVEY, A. C., DONALD, K. W., JULIAN, D. G. & OLIVER, M. F. (1967). A coronary care unit in the routine management of acute myocardial infarction. *Lancet*, **2**, 109.

MACKENZIE, G. J., TAYLOR, S. H., FLENLEY, D. C., McDONALD, A. H., STAUNTON, H. P. & DONALD, K. W. (1964). Circulatory and respiratory studies in myocardial infarction and cardiogenic shock. *Lancet*, **2**, 825.

MOSINGER, F. (1965). Photometric adaptation of Dole's microdetermination of free fatty acids. *J. Lipid Res.* **6**, 157.

SCHEUER, J. & BRACHFIELD, N. (1966). Myocardial uptake and fractional distribution of palmitate-I-C14 by the ischaemic dog heart. *Metabolism*, **15**, 945.

Addendum. The full results of this study have been published subsequently in the *Lancet* (1968), **1**, 710.

DISCUSSION

Professor Harris. There is tremendous interest at present in this problem of catecholamines and free fatty acids. It might be worth just commenting that other lipid fractions in the plasma are altered during or after myocardial infarction. There is, of course, a fall in the plasma cholesterol, phospholipids and triglycerides. I do not know of any information concerning the effects of myocardial infarction on esterfied and non-esterified cholesterol or on the individual fatty acids. But the metabolic pathways related to the production of these lipids are so diverse that it would seem likely that the common underlying factor may be diminution in circulating protein and little to do with lipid metabolism *per se*. This may tie up with Professor Shillingford's observations on the leak of albumin from the circulation and with our own work on the leak of protein out of the circulation following dextran. Of course, this does not apply to free fatty acids where it is difficult to imagine a lack of available binding sites on albumin and where, as we have heard, there is a rise in concentration after myocardial infarction. The great problem about the interpretation of free fatty acids in the plasma is the multiplicity of factors which can influence them. The ability of adrenaline or noradrenaline to increase their concentration is, as Dr Carlson reminded us, due to the activation of lipolytic enzymes in adipose tissue, which increases the hydrolysis of triglycerides. In case there is any doubt, it should be stated that this is a different enzyme from the lipoprotein lipase which appears in circulating blood following the injection of heparin, but since the net results of these two are in the same direction—namely, an increase in free fatty acid concentration—and since heparin is so commonly given in myocardial infarction—the interpretation of free fatty acid rises can become difficult. Of course, Dr Oliver has very carefully excluded this factor from his series. There are other things which will effect free fatty acid concentration. They have a very rapid turnover in the plasma; they fall precipitously in response to insulin, whether by injection or through the insulin produced endogenously in response to glucose infusion or a carbohydrate meal. With this in mind one has to think in terms of recent observations of an impaired insulin response to glucose in patients with myocardial infarction. Free fatty acids rise, as Dr Oliver has reminded us, with fasting and very considerably after exercise. They are high in patients with diabetes. There is one other problem which worries me a bit and that is the influence of the pituitary-adrenal-cortical axis. We know it is stimulated during myocardial infarction and that free fatty acids are raised by small amounts of growth hormone, and one wonders whether this perhaps might also be a factor in myocardial infarction.

It now seems reasonably established that catecholamines are raised in myocardial infarction, but there are still a number of unanswered questions and one that worries me most is really how specific this response is. We have heard some very nice data on the influence of pain on the production of catecholamines and the elevation of free fatty acids, but we are dealing here with a pain which for a long time has been recognised as carrying with it in

259

some very curious fashion a direct message of the fear of death and is it surprising that this very particular pain, which even carries its own special name, might have an effect on catecholamine release? And by the way, it would be nice to know whether patients in coronary care units excrete more catecholamines than those whose medical advisers prefer them to die a cosier and more domestic death in the bosom of their own family. Expressions which have come up time and time again in the conversations during this meeting is aggression, aggressive therapy and, my goodness me, even aggressive physicians. God help us if our patients mistake enthusiasm for aggression! Is it surprising too that a condition in which the blood pressure so often falls is associated with increased excretion of catecholamine and is it surprising that a condition in which the blood perfusing the carotid body is altered, is associated with an increase in catecholamine?

I am trying to ask how specific is this response. We know as, Dr Oliver has reminded us, that the myocardium contains high concentrations of bound noradrenaline. Does the release of this play a specific role in the production of catecholamine? If those who have investigated this think that there is no specific mechanism underlying the production of catecholamines in myocardial infarction, then do they believe that the release of catecholamines has a specific importance either for the good or the bad, as Dr Oliver was suggesting at the end of his talk. So, to start the ball rolling, I would like to say that it is important to know that catecholamines are increased in myocardial infarction, but it would be even more important to know whether this has any particular meaning for us in terms of therapy.

Dr Wallace. The points that Professor Harris has made are extremely relevant. I do not honestly know whether catecholamines are good or bad. Often the reactions which occur in the body to any acute situation can be interpreted as serving a useful purpose at the moment but their long-term effects may be detrimental. Catecholamines may play an important role in cardiogenic shock. Not only do they represent a response to a reduction in blood pressure but they may have detrimental effects and account for the rise in haematocrit. They have a detrimental effect on tissue perfusion, a picture resembling cardiogenic shock can be produced by prolonged infusion of noradrenaline; and a free fatty acid response occurs and perhaps arrhythmias also. I do not know the answer to Professor Harris' question. Perhaps we are at a stage of knowledge where we really are screening a variety of different things and we do not have the answers to these questions.

Dr Cooper. It is quite clear that the sympathetic nervous system is needed for support of the circulatory system. When we take it away or insult it, the hearts of experimental animals will not recover —unless the normal mechanisms that respond to acute stress are replaced. Changes in urinary catecholamines do not impress me greatly because they represent such a small part of the total metabolism of body catecholamines. There is no question, of course, that if the urinary catecholamines go up there has been increased activation of the sympathetic nervous system. Catecholamine metabolism is controlled by two major mechanisms—one being the immediate binding of catecholamines by a large number of structures in the body and the other being their rapid enzymatic degradation. In the absence of VMA measurements or measurements of metanephrine or nor-metanephrine, urinary concentrations are only a crude index of total activity. The effects of renal regional flow are important determinants not only of creatinine clearance but also of the total flow through the kidney and of what urinary catecholamines concentrations might be. There are many factors therefore which make it difficult very to assess the significance of urinary catecholamines. In relation to Dr Carlson's comments about fatty deposition in the myocardium there is another phenomenon, probably unrelated, which occurs in the subendocardial layers in association with high levels of catecholamines either from an endogenous source such as sympathetic cardiac nerve activity or from a shock-like state. The oxygen perfusion of the subendocardial layers of the myocardium is reduced and large areas of subendocardial necrosis occur. This is probably due to the mechanical effects of a small but forceful asychronous contraction and large areas of subendocardial necrosis occur and not only to changes in myocardial lipid. I think the answer to Professor Harris's question is that a catecholamine response is inevitable.

Dr Wallace. A recent observation made by our group may be relevant to some of the points that Dr Oliver was making concerning free fatty acids. The response to an intravenous infusion of 25 g. of glucose has been studied on the 1st, 5th and 22nd days after acute myocardial infarction.

A diabetic-type response occurred on the 1st day and this seemed to be characteristic of 75–80 per cent. of our patients with acute myocardial infarction even though many of them did not have abnormal glucose tolerance at the end, supporting Dr Allison's recent observations. The plasma insulin response on the 1st day was markedly depressed, rose to a peak on the 6th and 7th days and became more normal in the 3rd and 4th weeks. There was a very striking change and paradoxical rise in growth hormone in response to glucose loading on the 1st day whereas the normal suppression of growth hormone did not occur until the 22nd day of hospitalisation. Responses similar to this occur in patients following kidney transplantation during the stage in which the transplanted kidney is undergoing compensatory hypertrophy. We wonder if there is not a message here that the metabolic response may be appropriate to the healing process whenever tissue damage has occurred.

Dr Oliver. This question of the possibility of growth hormone being a cause of the rise in free fatty acids interested us. Although we have not measured growth hormone levels in these patients we have examined the gas chromatographic pattern of free fatty acids following their mobilisation by noradrenaline, growth hormone and a number of other stimulants. The pattern with growth hormone is essentially the same as with noradrenaline, with thyroid, with fasting, and with myocardial infarction. The principal elevation occurs in the mono-unsaturated acids, in other words, in oleate—as one would expect as a result of direct mobilisation from adipose tissue—and stearate and palmitate decrease.

Dr Carlson. I really would not like to comment on the complexity of all the factors involved in mobilisation of free fatty acids but would only mention one additional drug. Salicylates also have a very profound effect on free fatty acid levels. One interesting point mentioned by Professor Harris is the decrease in lipoproteins as measured by a decrease in cholesterol after acute trauma. This is seen also in burned patients, and we have seen over a period of about 20 days a linear correlation between the albumin concentration and the cholesterol concentration which supports the idea put forward by Professor Harris that changes in protein metabolism may be responsible for some of the changes in lipid levels. Dr Oliver asked what do these high levels of free fatty acids mean; are they due to an increase of mobilisation or a decrease in utilisation? We have measured levels of free glycerol in some patients with acute myocardial infarction. Free glycerol is liberated from adipose tissue when triglycerides are subjected to hydrolysis and we have found elevated glycerol levels in plasma. This suggests that the free fatty acid rise is due to increased mobilisation. There is also experimental evidence to show that the myocardium is fairly rich in lipoprotein lipase and after acute myocardial infarction lipoprotein lipase appears in the plasma. Have you looked at that specifically?

Dr Oliver. No, we have not.

Dr Carlson. We have, so you need not worry! There is no rise in lipoprotein lipase. Finally, it is an interesting idea that depletion of catecholamines in the myocardium would be enough to cause the elevated free fatty acid levels. I have made some rough calculations from data we have from infusing catecholamines intravenously and have tried to relate them to the same levels after myocardial infarction. I have arrived at the figure that one would need about 200 to 500 μg. of noradrenaline during one hour to have a free fatty acid level of about 1,200 μEq/l. The catecholamine content in the myocardium is about 1–1·5 μg. per g.

Dr Oliver. In other words, a 400 g. heart has about 400–600 μg. of catecholamines and it is within the range of possibility for one hour. The depletion may be initiated as a function of hypoxia but I would not like to suggest that the depletion of the myocardium of even 75 per cent. or 50 per cent. of its catecholamine is responsible for the rise of free fatty acids for long. But it may be the initiating part and then may be supplemented by more general releases from the sympathetic nerve endings.

Dr Rossi. Could the relationship between high levels of free fatty acids and serious arrhythmias result from free fatty acids blocking the insulin effect on cell membranes, glucose exchange, and also the movement in and out of the cell of potassium?

Dr Oliver. This relationship would tend to favour the passage of potassium into the cell and presumably protect against arrhythmias.

Dr Dalle. How well does insulin lower free fatty acids? Does the polarising solution do so? If so, why is it inefficient in preventing arrhythmias?

Dr Oliver. I think this is a very important question because insulin does lower free fatty acids but I do not know if this is so after acute infarction. You are obviously thinking that a physiological way of controlling high free fatty acid levels would be to give glucose presuming that glucose operates in the same way as it does when acute myocardial infarction has not occurred—when there is a rise in FFA for another reason—and this might be supplemented by giving insulin in order to drive glucose into the cell and take potassium along with it. You ask 'why has the insulin-glucose-potassium solution been shown to be so ineffective?' Well, I would hate to enter into that debate, but there is one point that I would like to make. You recall that only one-quarter of our total group with acute myocardial infarction had very high free fatty acid levels, and not everyone of those had a serious arrhythmia. Now it is not impossible that the rather poorly designed studies that have been conducted with glucose-potassium-insulin, have in fact had an effect within the group that one would expect to be responsive, but this has been submerged by the three-quarters, or something of this order, of the total in whom one would not expect a response. It may be that there is a case to be developed for re-examining the effect of glucose-insulin solutions in people who have initially very high free fatty acid levels.

Dr Dalle. Pursuing the same idea of the potential danger of high fatty acid levels, would you use heparin?

Dr Oliver. No. We particularly do not use heparin, partly because we have been impressed by the work of Dr Enger, and partly because I feel rather strongly about heparin in relationship to the rise in FFA we have reported.

Dr Dalle. Does isoproterenol also raise free fatty acid levels?

Dr Oliver. In rats it does. I do not know about man.

Dr Carlson. I do not think so.

Professor Shillingford. I was very pleased to hear Professor Harris mention the patient. If you observe patients who have high and maintained high catecholamine excretion they are almost without exception apprehensive; they are feeling ill, they do not know exactly what is wrong with them but they are not feeling right; they mostly have a fast heart rate, although some of them have a well maintained blood pressure. In 2 of our 20 patients the catecholamine excretion remained high, and they died suddenly, one at the end of three weeks and one at the end of four weeks. It seems that a maintained high output of catecholamines makes the patient feel apprehensive and ill, and may have been coincident with sudden death.

Dr Oliver. On that point you might like to know that we have not seen any patient with a high free fatty acid levels after five days but we will have to examine this more closely.

Professor Shillingford. I think that catecholamines are probably somewhat more sensitive than FFA levels. Their excretion rises to a high level at the second and third day and then falls off slowly.

Dr Oliver. Perhaps, but catecholamine levels may not be so crucial. A rise of free fatty acids initially and, as I have said, an increase oxygen consumption may sensitise the heart in some way, so that later on when the patient smokes his first cigarette or when he gets out of bed and begins to move his skeletal muscles, a further big flux of free fatty acids is deleterious.

Dr McDonald. Your lack of correlation between enzymes and free fatty acid levels suggests, if your thesis about hypoxia is correct, that free fatty acid should occur in coronary insufficiency patients. Is this the case? The second question concerns lipoprotein lipase. We have very clear evidence that there is a deficiency of lipoprotein lipase in this disease and this is genetically determined. It might be very interesting to see if the rise in free fatty acid rise relates to the basic level of lipoprotein lipase after the event.

Dr Oliver. Yes, we have looked at patients with acute coronary insufficiency because of this question of pain. Pain of myocardial origin, when no infarct had occurred, is associated with a rise in free fatty acids up to the order of about 900 or 1,000 μEq/l. This occurs on the first day and is less than after an acute infarct. When the pain passes, the free fatty acid rise in acute coronary insufficiency disappears immediately, whereas in infarction it is not only higher but more prolonged. We reported this earlier and the difference between these groups is statistically significant. Your second point is most interesting. I do not know the answer.

Dr Wallace. Is there any evidence that the infusion of free fatty acids to produce levels comparable to those you have measured in your patients will induce arrhythmias in the setting of experimental myocardial infarction?

Dr Oliver. I do not know if this has been done. It will have to be done.

Dr Nixon. There is one point. We examined free fatty acids during sleep about $2\frac{1}{2}$ years ago, with indwelling venous lines. Immediately after sleep was induced there was a fall and after two hours the free fatty acids rose. Two of our six men had rotatory eye movements, at least they were having some form of cerebration, and their free fatty acids went very high at these times, then came down again.

Dr Cooper. There is an increase in the excretion of catecholamine levels during dreams and, of course, angina, ST depression and even arrhythmias can occur.

THE ENZYME RESPONSE OF THE MYOCARDIUM TO ISCHAEMIA AND INFARCTION

GORDON WHITBY

Department of Clinical Chemistry, The Royal Infirmary,
Edinburgh, Scotland

THE myocardium is completely dependent upon an uninterrupted supply of oxygenated blood. Only under carefully controlled experimental conditions can the isolated mammalian heart be maintained for some hours with normal contractility when perfused with artificial oxygenated media. When the blood supply to the myocardium is interrupted, distal to the occlusion the processes of oxidative metabolism are arrested almost at once. Disruption of the enzymes of the respiratory chain drastically reduces the supply of A.T.P., and the integrity of the affected area of the myocardium and its continued ability to contract are immediately placed in jeopardy. Intracellular structures disintegrate and cellular permeability alters with the onset of cell necrosis. Although theoretically the myocardium could maintain itself by switching acutely from oxidative to anaerobic metabolism, the efficiency of the glycolytic pathway in providing A.T.P. is much less, per molecule of glucose metabolised, than the series of reactions involved in the full oxidative metabolism of glucose and fatty acids. Also, the circumstances which demand this transfer from oxidative to anaerobic metabolism are necessarily accompanied by an impaired ability to remove the products of metabolism. This means that occlusion of the blood supply to an area of the myocardium not only interferes with the normal processes of oxidative metabolism but leads to a rapid local build up in the concentration of products of anaerobic metabolism, lactic acid predominantly, and the inability to remove lactic acid efficiently leads to local acid-base disturbances which themselves contribute to the disruptive processes affecting cellular integrity brought on by the interference with oxidative metabolism.

Interference with myocardial integrity results in a release of intracellular enzymes into the circulation, and at least 10 enzymes have been investigated in serum as a measure of cardiac muscle damage (Table I). The activity of these enzymes per unit weight of myocardium far exceeds the activity normally demonstrable in serum, and their release from damaged tissue can be expected to

Table I. *Examples of enzymes that may show increased activity in serum after myocardial infarction*

Creatine kinase (CK)	Phosphohexose isomerase
Aspartate aminotransferase or glutamic oxaloacetic transaminase (GOT)	Pyruvate kinase
Lactate dehydrogenase (LD) and its isoenzymes	Enolase
Malate dehydrogenase	Glucose 6-phosphate dehydrogenase
Aldolase	Phosphoglucomutase

provide a sensitive index of altered cellular integrity. Most of these enzymes, being important catalysts in the steps which make up intermediary metabolic processes, are not restricted to the myocardium, and data about the activities of the aminotransferases and lactate dehydrogenase (LD) in different tissues relative to their activity normally demonstrable in serum (Wroblewski, 1958; Wilkinson, 1962) explain why alterations in serum enzyme activities by themselves may not provide clear-cut evidence for identifying the tissue from which the enzymes came; serum enzyme investigations require to be interpreted in the light of clinical and other evidence.

With the recognition of the existence of multiple forms of enzymes having the same catalytic activity, i.e., isoenzymes, interest centred on how to improve the specificity of serum enzyme tests, and most work in this field has been carried out on lactate dehydrogenase. Marked differences have been reported between individual observations on the percentage distribution of activity among the lactate dehydrogenase isoenzymes in human myocardium, these differences being ascribed partly to variations in technique, partly to differences due to autolytic change occurring post mortem, and partly to variable losses on storage of the more labile isoenzymes LD_4 and LD_5 prior to the electrophoretic examination (Wilkinson, 1965).

Kaplan and his colleagues (Cahn *et al.*, 1962) suggested that the electrophoretically fast and slow isoenzymes of lactate dehydrogenase might have different metabolic roles, and this suggestion deserves consideration in relation to the myocardial response to ischaemia and infarction. Lactate dehydrogenase of human heart muscle is inhibited by much lower concentrations of pyruvate than the enzyme obtained from hepatic tissue; it has been suggested that tissues which contain predominantly LD_1 allow pyruvate to accumulate, and that this accumulation of pyruvate leads on to

267

activation of the Krebs cycle for the oxidative metabolism of pyruvate. By contrast, it has been suggested that tissues containing mainly LD_5 preferentially convert pyruvate to lactate because insufficient pyruvate accumulates to inhibit the lactate dehydrogenase. Several groups of workers (for review see Latner, 1967) have obtained evidence to support this theory, but Vesell and Pool (1966) have questioned its validity, and the possible physiological roles of individual lactate dehydrogenase isoenzymes remain to be established.

It is not possible to investigate the response of the myocardium in man to ischaemia and infarction under controlled conditions. This is because direct access to tissue *in vivo* for enzyme studies is practically out of the question, and it is equally unethical to devise and apply experiments involving the production of controlled levels of anoxia so as to study their effects upon the human myocardium. In animals, however, this kind of study has been carried out, and the findings with few exceptions conform to the general statement that there is no significant alteration in serum enzyme activity detectable as a result of release from cardiac muscle unless there is also pathological evidence of tissue necrosis. Ruegsegger *et al.* (1959) induced reversible ischaemia of the myocardium in dogs that was sufficiently severe to produce clear evidence of ischaemic changes on the ECG, and they maintained these conditions for 45 minutes without inducing detectable alterations in aspartate aminotransferase (G.O.T.) activity. In other studies, Agress *et al.* (1955) injected plastic spheres of various sizes into the coronary arteries of dogs and detected a significant rise in G.O.T. when as little as 5 per cent. of the myocardium had been infarcted. Many groups of workers have shown a close correlation in animals between the maximum increase in serum enzyme activity and the extent of myocardial infarction, and loss of enzyme activity from the infarcted myocardium has been compared with the increases in serum enzyme activity brought about by the infarction (Hess, 1963).

Any damage to a cell leading to an increase in the permeability of its membrane will allow intracellular contents to escape. If the change in permeability is sufficiently great, macromolecules such as enzyme proteins will escape. Following their release into the circulation, intracellular enzymes are removed by catabolism, and excretion in bile or urine sometimes plays a part. Another method of elimination is by inactivation of the enzyme, and a good example of rapid removal of an intracellular cardiac enzyme by inactivation following its release into the circulation is provided by the NADP-dependent isocitrate dehydrogenase (I.C.D.) of heart muscle (Campbell & Moss, 1962). Although heart muscle contains large amounts of this isoenzyme of I.C.D., serum I.C.D. measurements have never proved of value in the investigation of suspected myocardial infarction because the enzyme is rapidly inactivated at 37° C. By contrast, the main hepatic isoenzyme of I.C.D. is much more thermostable and has proved a valuable investigation for detecting hepatocellular damage.

Detailed knowledge of the mechanisms which affect the release of enzymes from damaged tissues is surprisingly poor. Schmidt & Schmidt (1967) have investigated some of the possible factors by perfusing the isolated rat liver with a cell-free medium under conditions which resulted in a definite hypoxia although cell necrosis was not produced. They investigated the release of 17 different intracellular enzymes into the perfusing medium, and their main conclusions are summarised in Table II. Most of these

Table II. *Release of intracellular enzymes into the circulation*

(From Schmidt & Schmidt, 1967)

1. The rate of release is proportional to the gradient between the intracellular and serum activities of an enzyme.
2. The rate of relase is inversely proportional to the molecular weight of the enzyme.
3. The rate of release is influenced by the intracellular location of the enzyme, e.g., it is slower for a mitochondrial than for a cytoplasmic enzyme.

enzymes were predominantly cytoplasmic in their distribution, and for these enzymes the inverse relationship between molecular weight and rate of release was clearly demonstrated. Malate dehydrogenase and G.O.T., which are partly mitochondrial and partly cytoplasmic in their distribution, obeyed the relationship as far as their cytoplasmic components were concerned, but the molecular weights of the mitochondrial enzymes studied were not known and the factors controlling their rate of release were not so fully investigated. Ottaway (1967) has shown that the release of intracellular enzymes may not be as simple as Table II suggests, since he has obtained evidence that cytoplasmic creatine kinase (CK) is not always free in solution inside muscle cells but may instead be bound sometimes to the myofibrils.

Table III shows data collected from a number of sources (Wroblewski, 1958; Wilkinson, 1962; Dixon & Webb, 1964; Smith, personal communication) about molecular weights and relative activities in heart muscle and serum for four of the enzyme

Table III. *Factors influencing the pattern of serum enzyme response following myocardial infarction*

	Gradient of activity*	Molecular weight
Creatine kinase	200,000 : 1	81,000
Aspartate aminotransferase	8,000 : 1	110,000
2-hydroxybutyrate dehydrogenase . . .	1,000 : 1	135,000
Lactate dehydrogenase	700 : 1	135,000

* The gradient is the approximate value for the ratio of intracellular to serum activity for the enzyme in normal individuals.

determinations most frequently performed in the investigation of heart disease in man. These data help to explain the pattern of serum enzyme activity seen after myocardial infarction (Smith, 1967) and particularly the greater sensitivity of CK as an index of myocardial infarction and its relatively more rapid rise in the serum than is seen with other enzymes following ischaemic release from heart muscle. The maximum serum enzyme level observed after cardiac infarction provides an index of prognosis (Smith, 1967) when the data obtained from a series of patients are considered collectively. In addition during this Symposium, Dr Lawson McDonald has stated his belief that serial measurements of enzyme and isoenzyme activities in serum can have prognostic value for *individual* patients after a cardiac infarction. This is not altogether true. Whilst a high peak of serum enzyme activity carries a bad prognosis, the converse does not necessarily hold for the *individual patient*; a small myocardial infarction with slight tissue necrosis and a small rise in enzyme activities in the serum does not necessarily mean that the patient has a good prognosis (Wroblewski, 1958; Wilkinson, 1962). These data require to be considered in relation to the site of the infarct, and the possibility of complications arising from shortcomings in the pathological process of organisation and fibrosis of the infarcted area which cannot be predicted. It is considered unlikely that it will ever be possible always to make definite predictions about prognosis in individual patients who have sustained a myocardial infarction on the basis of serum enzyme or isoenzyme measurements.

This review has considered some of the factors which underlie the selection of enzyme activity measurements for the investigation of myocardial infarction. Within the limits of the title, it did not seem appropriate to consider the effects of prolonged tachycardia (Runde & Dale, 1966) or of complications such as congestive cardiac failure on the release of enzymes into the serum from other organs, e.g., the liver, lungs or kidneys (*Circulation*, 1967). Enzyme investigations have so far proved of limited help with the difficult clinical problem of having to decide when ischaemia ends and infarction of the myocardium commences, but their place in helping to confirm the diagnosis of myocardial infarction is well established.

REFERENCES

AGRESS, C. M., JACOBS, H. I., GLASSNER, H. F., LEDERER, M. A., CLARK, W. G., WROBLEWSKI, F., KARMEN, A. & LADUE, J. S. (1955). Serum transaminase levels in experimental myocardial infarction. *Circulation*, 11, 711.

CAHN, R. D., KAPLAN, N. O., LEVINE, L. & ZWILLING, E. (1962). Nature and development of lactic dehydrogenase. *Science*, 136, 962.

CAMPBELL, D. M. & MOSS, D. W. (1962). Some properties of human isocitric dehydrogenase isoenzymes. *Proc. Ass. clin. Biochem.* 2, 10.

Circulation (1967). Enzymes in acute myocardial infarction, 35, 427.

DIXON, M. & WEBB, E. C. (1964). *Enzymes*, 2nd ed., p. 454. London: Longmans.

HESS, B. (1963). *Enzymes in Blood Plasma*, p. 68. New York: Academic Press.

LATNER, A. L. (1967). Isoenzymes. In *Advances in Clinical Chemistry*, vol. 9, p. 69. Ed. Sobotka, H. & Stewart, C. P. New York: Academic Press.

OTTAWAY, J. H. (1967). Evidence for binding of cytoplasmic creatine kinase to structural elements in heart muscle. *Nature, Lond.* 215, 521.

RUEGSEGGER, P., NYDICK, I., FREIMAN, A. & LADUE, J. S. (1959). Serum activity patterns of glutamic oxaloacetic transaminase, glutamic pyruvic transaminase and lactic dehydrogenase following graded myocardial infarction in dogs. *Circulation Res.* 7, 4.

RUNDE, I. & DALE, J. (1966). Serum enzymes in acute tachycardia. *Acta med. scand.* 179, 535.

SCHMIDT, E. & SCHMIDT, F. W. (1967). Release of enzymes from the liver *Nature, Lond.* 213, 1125.

SMITH, A. F. (1967). Diagnostic value of serum-creatine-kinase in a coronary care unit. *Lancet*, 2, 178.

VESELL, E. & POOL, P. E. (1966). Lactate and pyruvate concentrations in exercised ischemic canine muscle: relationship of tissue substrate level to lactate dehydrogenase isozyme pattern. *Proc. natn. Acad. Sci.* 55, 756.

WILKINSON, J. H. (1962). *An Introduction to Diagnostic Enzymology*. London: Arnold.

WILKINSON, J. H. (1965). *Isoenzymes*, p. 44. London: Spon.

WROBLEWSKI, F. (1958). The clinical significance of alterations in transaminase activities of serum and other body fluids. In *Advances in Clinical Chemistry*, vol. 1, p. 313. Ed. Sobotka, H. & Stewart, C. P. New York: Academic Press.

DISCUSSION

Dr Carlson. Dr Lown has pointed out the difficulty in assessing the time of onset of acute myocardial infarction. I would like to ask Professor Whitby if he thinks that it might be more useful to relate the timing of acute myocardial infarction to enzyme levels.

If one could have a continuous enzyme curve, could this be a more precise technique from which to judge the onset of acute myocardial infarction?

Professor Whitby. Theoretically this might be the case but you would have the difficulty in the majority of the patients since they do not have their myocardial infarctions in hospital. If you could start base-line observations before the infarction commenced, and have them available for serial investigation after the incident has developed, then it is very probable that enzymes, particularly creatine kinase, would be particularly sensitive indices of the first onset of infarction. One could, in these circumstances, begin more closely to correlate peak enzyme activities with the extent of myocardial damage, but such conditions are not available.

Dr Carlson. You do not think the shape of descending slope of the curve would be sufficient?

Dr Whitby. No, I don't think the descending slope is very reliable.

Dr Oliver. It might be possible to make a mathematical model from which you could extrapolate from the shape of the descending slope towards the point of time when the infarct occurred.

Professor Whitby. This would assume that the peak activity was occurring over a very narrow time range.

Dr McDonald. We should be clear what we are measuring. Many pathologists consider that it is difficult to identify cardiac infarction for some hours.

Dr Lown. I would say that the observation that there is no pathological microscopic evidence of infarction merely reflects the inadequacy of present methods of microscopic assessment of what is initially a physiological and enzymologic derangement. I would like to pose a question to Professor Whitby. Initially rare metals were shown to be released. This was one of the earliest studies about identifying myocardial infarction; has there been further pursuit of this very area?

Professor Whitby. I am not aware of any further pursuits, but with the introduction of atomic absorption spectroscopy, this might well be worth looking into.

Professor Donald. Does anybody know the minimal size of infarct, whether it be fresh or necrosed, which will produce changes in the peripheral blood? Can there be a known infarct without important changes in the enzymes? I think many clinicians would like this point clarified.

Professor Whitby. Perhaps a partial answer is that somewhere in the region of 5 per cent. of the patients studied in coronary care units have no detectable abnormality. I did mention 5 per cent. of the dog myocardium resulting in significant detectable elevations in the glutamic oxaloacetic transaminase which is not the most sensitive enzyme for detecting myocardial damage. I don't know whether similar observations have been made for creatine kinase.

Dr Lown. We have found that in 10 per cent. of patients, in whom the admission is early and electrocardiographic changes are present, there are no changes in the stable fraction of L.D.H. which presumably approximate to LD, fraction or the rapid moving fraction, S.G.O.T. or creatine kinase. That is it works out to be 90 per cent. for L.D.H. and 88 per cent. for S.G.O.T.

Dr Lawrie. Dr McDonald mentioned that his patients who suffered V.F. had very high levels of enzymes. We agree, but only after the episode of V.F. Frequently our patients did not have extraordinarily high enzyme levels before V.F. I wonder if the effects of defibrillation cause marked enzyme release.

Dr McDonald. There is very frequently an enzyme rise after elective defibrillation.

Dr Lown. We have had patients who have not had myocardial infarction and have heart block. With normal enzyme levels and after an episode of ventricular fibrillation, their enzymes go very high. Also with defibrillation there is release of enzymes from skeletal muscle. In cardioversion a small percentage, maybe 20 or 30 per cent., will have elevated enzyme levels if multiple and high energy shocks are employed.

Dr Cooper. How and where are the enzymes cleared?

Professor Whitby. I think they are mostly removed by protein catabolism and in the case of isocitric dehydrogenase, by inactivation followed by catabolism. There is very little work on urinary excretion of enzymes. Urinary lactic dehydrogenase mostly arises from the renal tract and I think the same applies to urinary alkaline phosphatase. There is also biliary excretion of enzymes—of alkaline phosphatase and of lactic dehydrogenase. I have no information on the excretion of enzymes through the lung.

273

PROBLEMS OF MANAGEMENT

Chairman: M. F. OLIVER

SHORT-TERM ANTICOAGULANT THERAPY AFTER ACUTE MYOCARDIAL INFARCTION

CHRISTOPHER BJERKELUND

Rikshospitalet, Oslo, Norway

ANTICOAGULANT therapy in acute myocardial infarction has been given with three main purposes.

1. To prevent venous thrombosis and the associated risk of pulmonary embolism.

2. To prevent the development of mural thrombi and the associated risk of systemic embolisation.

3. To prevent appositional growth of the coronary thrombus with resulting extension of the infarcted area.

The principle of this treatment is rational from a theoretical point of view. We know that the risk of developing venous thrombosis is increased in connection with an acute infarct, particularly when strict bedrest is considered a necessary part of the regime. From the autopsy table we also know that an extensive transmural myocardial infarct is frequently associated with a mural thrombus and sometimes systemic emboli. Less well documented on a pathological and experimental basis is the importance of an appositional growth of the coronary thrombus itself. I will return to that later.

Although anticoagulants have now been recommended and extensively used for more than 20 years in the treatment of acute myocardial infarction, there is still no agreement as to their effectiveness and their indication.

The first reports in the mid-forties were all encouraging. When the result of the American co-operative study was published by Wright and his colleagues (1954), and soon supported by a number of publications, including Tulloch and Gilchrist's (1950) careful clinical trial from Edinburgh, the value of this therapy seemed well established. Even if some workers were still sceptical or antagonistic, the general view was that anticoagulants were beneficial in acute myocardial infarction. Accordingly the practice in most medical departments was to give this treatment in all cases.

Largely the administration of this therapy has been carried out in two main ways:

1. By giving oral anticoagulants only.

2. By giving these drugs with the addition of initial heparin

277

therapy for the first few days until oral anticoagulants have reduced the prothrombin values to an effective therapeutic level.

Let us at once take a quick look at initial heparinisation.

It should be emphasised that the main reason for giving this treatment is to achieve effective anticoagulation as soon as treatment is started. In this connection it is of interest to note that venous thrombosis and pulmonary embolism, as well as mural thrombosis and systemic embolisation, are very rare before the end of the first week after an acute coronary occlusion. These complications therefore hardly represent indications for initial heparin treatment.

The hope of preventing appositional growth of the coronary thrombus itself consequently constitutes the only indication for aiming at an early anticoagulant effect in connection with acute myocardial infarction. I have never been convinced by this indication.

Firstly, it is not supported by pathological or anatomical findings. The coronary thrombus is usually short, $\frac{1}{2}$–2 cm. in length, and does not extend into the branches of the coronary arteries. Secondly, no statistical evidence has been produced for a beneficial effect of initial heparin therapy on the clinical course and prognosis of acute myocardial infarction. On the contrary, two well-controlled clinical trials carried out to elucidate the value of this treatment failed to show any benefit (Table I). The first of these was published by Enger *et al.* in Oslo (1963) and the second by Brown and McMillan from Toronto (1965).

Table I. *Effect of short-term oral anticoagulant therapy— with and without initial heparin—on mortality in acute myocardial infarction*

	Mortality (%)	
	Oral anticoagulants (only)	Oral anticoagulants with initial heparin
Enger *et al.*, 1963 . . .	37	43·8
Brown & MacMillan, 1965 . .	28	30

Both these trials showed that in patients with myocardial infarction treated with oral anticoagulants initial heparin is without effect in preventing thrombosis and embolism and deaths from

278

these complications. In both studies the total mortality was insignificantly higher in the heparin group than in the control group. Heparin also increased the risk of hemorrhagic complications. Moreover, in the heparinised patients who died, the level of transaminase was somewhat higher than in the control series in both studies. Brown and MacMillan point out that these observations suggest that in patients receiving heparin greater destruction of the heart muscle cells has occurred.

Another possible detrimental effect of early heparinisation is that it may increase intimal bleeding which is known in a few cases to be the cause of the coronary thrombosis and myocardial infarction. On the other hand, it has been postulated that prompt administration of heparin reduces sludging and the anoxic consequences of shock and may, on this basis, have a favourable influence on the early course of the acute infarct. There is, however, no evidence to support this hypothesis.

Finally, the fact that the administration of heparin, even in small doses, causes a release of tissue lipoprotein lipase into the blood should be mentioned. This enzyme promotes the lipolysis of triglycerides present in the very low density lipoproteins and produces an enormous, temporary rise in the level of free fatty acids in the plasma.* In an unknown way these changes in the blood lipids may possibly also influence oxygen consumption and myocardial work. Dr Oliver has already enlarged on this point.

My conclusion is that with our present knowledge initial heparin therapy is not indicated in acute myocardial infarction.

When the report of the American co-operative study had been published, short-term anticoagulant therapy became, as already mentioned, almost universally accepted. So it remained until the result of the Copenhagen trial (Hilden et al., 1961) appeared more than 10 years later. The reason for the disagreement and the emotional discussions following this trial was, I think, more a result of these authors' conclusion than of their findings.

The principal difference (Table II) between the results of Wright et al. (1954) and Hilden et al. (1961) was that the Americans found a significant reduction of the total mortality, whereas the Danes did not. This is explained, at least in part, by the fact that secondary thrombo-embolic complications were seen less frequently in the Danish than in the American patients.

On the other hand, Hilden et al. (1961), have clearly shown that

* This is of interest because free fatty acids have in recent years engaged increasing attention in the relationship of lipids and thrombosis (Connor et al., 1966).

Table II. *Effect of short-term anticoagulant therapy in acute myocardial infarction on total mortality*

	No. of patients		Mortality	
	Treated	Control	Treated	Control
Wright *et al.*, 1954	589	442	16·0	23·4
Hilden *et al.*, 1961	371	425	22·9	25·4

anticoagulants have a significant prophylactic effect against the secondary thrombo-embolic complications of acute myocardial infarction (Table III). All the differences between the treated and control group shown in Table III are statistically significant.

Table III. *Effect of short-term anticoagulant therapy in acute myocardial infarction on thrombo-embolic complications* (Hilden *et al.*, 1961)

	Treated (%)	Control (%)
Clinical + autopsy findings:		
Thrombo-embolic complications . . .	15	25
Autopsy findings:		
Pulmonary—infarction embolism thrombosis	5	28
Mural thrombosis	24	58
Deaths from thrombo-embolic complications .	1·4	4·0

These findings are also in agreement with the results of almost all clinical and pathological-anatomical studies on this topic.

We may conclude, therefore, that anticoagulant therapy in acute myocardial infarction has a significant prophylactic effect against the secondary thrombo-embolic complications. For the sake of clarity, it should perhaps be added that this treatment has of course no direct prophylactic or therapeutic effect against shock, arrhythmias or heart failure.

Consequently, if, with early ambulation and other modern therapy of acute myocardial infarction, thrombosis and embolism

280

are considered to be of no importance, anticoagulants are not indicated. In patients with serious infarcts, arrhythmias, shock, and excessive weight (poor risk patients), in whom thrombo-embolic complications represent a significant hazard, prophylaxis with oral anticoagulants is clearly indicated.

This conclusion, in my opinion, will be correct as long as we believe that anticoagulants have an antithrombotic effect, and I doubt that anyone will be able to show conclusively that they have not.

However, one point must be emphasised in this connection, namely the importance of really intensive treatment. If we want to give anticoagulant therapy, we have to give it in a correct manner.

When we are assessing short-term anticoagulant therapy after acute myocardial infarction, the complications and side-effects of this therapy also have to be considered.

Haemorrhage is the most serious hazard and it may be fatal. It should be pointed out in this connection that dosage and control of oral anticoagulants is much more difficult in patients who are seriously ill with shock, heart failure, etc., and for that reason have unstable liver function, than in ambulant patients. The importance of haemorrhagic complications will depend upon the intensity of the treatment, the laboratory control and the experience and skill of the physician in charge of the dosage. In my opinion, bleeding complications do not, however, amount to a serious contra-indication against short-term anticoagulant therapy.

The belief that the use of anticoagulants could provoke an increase tendency to rupture of the heart has been examined, but is not conclusively established.

Side-effects of oral anticoagulants are rare and have been almost exclusively caused by phenindione. The most serious reactions are renal damage, agranulocytosis, interstitial myocarditis, haemorrhagic colitis and exfoliative dermatitis. In the literature 15 deaths due to phenindione therapy have been reported. In Norway we therefore no longer start new patients on this drug.

I have the feeling that anticoagulant therapy in coronary artery disease has already to a great extent found its way into medical history. Very briefly this history is told in the series of editorials written in the *Lancet* on this subject (1967). Two conclusions in the last of these, published three weeks ago, are typical of today's attitude to anticoagulant therapy:

' There seems little doubt that we have got as far as we can in assessing the value of anticoagulant treatment by present methods, and further laboriously collected series are unlikely to alter the pattern of conclusions.'

And finally:

' If results are to be improved, we must now concentrate on the complications—shock, cardiac arrest, and ventricular fibrillation—that cause death in the first few days after infarction. These complications demand the facilities of the specialised cardiac intensive care unit. . . .'

Perhaps the most important thing we can learn from this history of anticoagulant therapy is to realise the very great difficulties so frequently connected with the evaluation of a new therapy. I believe this also applies to the intensive coronary care unit.

REFERENCES

BROWN, K. W. G. & MACMILLAN, R. L. (1965). A critical evaluation of initial heparin therapy in acute myocardial infarction. In *Anticoagulant Therapy in Ischemic Heart Disease*, p. 70. Ed. Nichol, E. S. New York : Grune & Stratton.

CONNOR, W. E., HOAK, J. C. & WARNER, E. D. (1966). The role of lipids in thrombosis. In *Pathogenesis and Treatment of Thromboembolic Diseases including Coronary, Cerebral and Peripheral Thrombosis*, p. 193. International Symposium. Stuttgart: Schattauer-Verlag.

Lancet (1967). Anticoagulant treatment for myocardial infarction, **2**, 405.

ENGER, E., JULSRUD, A. C. & KIRKEBY, K. (1963). Initial heparin therapy as a supplement to peroral anticoagulants in acute myocardial infraction. *Acta med. scand.* Suppl. 397, 49.

HILDEN, T., IVERSEN, K. & RAASCHOU, F. & SCHWARTZ, M. (1961). Anticoagulants in acute myocardial infarction. *Lancet*, **2**, 327.

TULLOCH, J. A. & GILCHRIST, A. R. (1950). Anticoagulants in treatment of coronary thrombosis. *Br. med. J.* **2**, 965.

WRIGHT, I. S., MARPLE, C. D. & BECK, D. F. (1948). Report of the committee for the evaluation of anticoagulants in the treatment of coronary thrombosis with myocardial infarction. *Am. Heart J.* **36**, 801.

WRIGHT, I. S., MARPLE, C. D. & BECK, D. F. (1954). *Myocardial Infarction its Clinical Manifestations and Treatment with Anticoagulants. A study of 1031 cases.* New York: Grune & Stratton.

DISCUSSION

Dr Fejfar (Geneva). It would be interesting to hear of experiences using fibrinolytic enzymes in the treatment of acute myocardial infarction.

Professor Chazov. In our country we use heparin and fibrinolytic enzymes during the first hours after myocardial infarction. The value of heparin and fibrinolytic preparations depends upon the time between the onset of the infarction and the time of administration. When started early and carried out for a sufficiently long time—up to 5–6 days—this therapy markedly improves the course of myocardial infarction.

We have used fibrinolytic drugs and heparin in one group of patients and heparin only in another group. The effect of fibrinolytic therapy is not only on the principal thrombus but also through the spasmolytic properties of heparin and fibrinolytic enzymes on the so-called secondary thrombus. In experimented animals, the vessels surrounding the zone of necrosis open up and the area of necrosis is restricted.

Although the value of fibrinolytic enzyme therapy is still disputed, our experience indicates that prognosis is improved and there are fewer complications.

Taking into consideration that thrombogenesis is increased after myocardial infarction and natural anticoagulation reduced, heparin should be given for at least 8–10 days and fibrinolytic enzymes for 3–4 days. There is no necessity for administering fibrinolysins twice a day, since one injection brings about stable and prolonged activity.

Dr Oliver. I would like to obtain the privilege of the Chairman for a moment to say that it is extremely important that carefully designed trials, using a random system for allocating to treatment and control groups, are conducted to test the value of fibrinolytic enzymes. We must not fall into the same trap that we have been in for 10 years with regard to anticoagulant therapy. It is quite easy to show an improvement in prognosis after acute myocardial infarction with a variety of treatments which theoretically might be expected to improve the outlook when small numbers are selectively treated. It is incumbent and essential for anybody putting forward a new form of treatment to outline the design, selection, randomisation system and conduct of their trials.

Professor Chazov. Yes, we have very good control studies.

Dr Ruda (Moscow). The two groups comprised patients with confirmed acute myocardial infarction. Both consisted of 500 patients and they were selected in alternate order—one treated, one control, one treated, one control.

Dr Cross. I would like to ask Dr Bjerkelund two questions. He stated that thrombo-embolic complications are rare during the first week. I wondered whether he would make the same comment, in view of Dr Russek's earlier work, with regard to patients with varicose veins, congestive failure and arrhythmias. Are they not more prone to develop early thrombo-embolic complications than the ones who were without these complications? Secondly, I would like to know in his series how he matched his patients on admission and what classification was used to get rid of selection bias?

Dr Bjerkelund. Poor risk patients certainly have more chance of secondary thrombo-embolic complications—poor risk in the sense described by Dr Russek—but I think most studies have in fact shown that secondary thrombo-embolic complications do not occur in the first few days but come more at the end of the first week.

I think that you were enquiring about my own trials in this field. While I have studied long-term anticoagulants, I have never made any control trial of short-term effects. I was speaking only of the experiences of others.

Dr Cross. I was asking about the work of Enger that you quoted.

Dr Bjerkelund. I think that was one of the best studies which has been done. They had 300 patients, 146 in one group and 154 in the other. There was a high mortality, about 40 per cent., even although they excluded the first 24 hours in the evaluation of heparin therapy. I do not agree with this and I have included the mortality in the first 24 hours in the data presented here because this was done by Brown and Macmillan.

Dr Pisa (Copenhagen). We must be clear what we expect fibrinolytic treatment to achieve. The time interval is most important if we want to dissolve a thrombus. We did some experiments studying the return of contractility to the ischaemic area of the heart muscle in dogs. Previously it had been suggested that, if the occlusion is over 45 minutes, the loss of contractility is irreversible. We have shown that after 1 hour of occlusion, the contractility returns to the ischaemic area in approximately 30 minutes. This is also true after two hours of occlusion if the arteries are open and enough time is allowed for a good perfusion. After two hours, it took between four to seven days for contractility to return to the previously ischaemic area. Now we are investigating the effect of a three-hour interval and it takes about 20 days to get contractility back with normal perfusion. We certainly can open the arteries and dissolve the thrombi in the affected area but the question is when to start with fibrinolytic treatment to get the best effect.

THE CIRCULATORY EFFECTS OF ANALGESICS IN MYOCARDIAL INFARCTION

ALEXANDER MUIR

Royal Infirmary, Edinburgh

ALTHOUGH the pain experienced by patients after acute myocardial infarction may vary considerably in intensity, in the majority it is severe and requires potent analgesics. In 1930, Moor prescribed intravenous morphine, and over the years, this drug has become standard therapy in both hospital and general practice. In 1965, Thomas and his colleagues drew attention to the serious haemodynamic changes that can occur in some patients following the use of morphine. The most important of these, they found, was a fall in the systemic arterial pressure. The *British Medical Journal* (1966a) commented on these results and concluded that, despite its disadvantages, morphine was likely to retain its important place in the treatment of myocardial infarction. Nevertheless, the same journal a few months later (*British Medical Journal,* 1966b), whilst discussing cardiogenic shock, recommended that heroin should be used in the severely ill, but quoted no evidence to support this statement.

Many physicians in this country have used heroin for relief of severe pain but where the pain has been less severe, pethidine has been used as an alternative analgesic. However, the effects of these drugs on the circulation in patients with recent myocardial infarction have not been assessed.

We report now the circulatory changes following the administration of heroin and pethidine; in addition, we have also conducted further observations on the haemodynamic effects of morphine. Some of our data has been published earlier this year (McDonald *et al.*, 1967).

METHOD

We studied 22 patients all of whom had sustained a myocardial infarct, as judged by history and electrocardiographic and enzyme changes, within the previous 48 hours. Ten patients were given 5 mg. of heroin, eight patients were given 100 mg. of pethidine and four patients were given 10 mg. of morphine. These dosages are generally reckoned to be equi-analgesic (Foldes *et al.*, 1964) and are those used in clinical practice.

At the start of the study, five of the ten patients who received heroin, two of the seven patients who received pethidine and two of the four patients who received morphine, had ischaemic chest pain.

The studies were carried out with the patients in their own beds in a specially adapted side-room of a general medical ward. Control observations were made for 20 minutes. Observations were then made for a further 50 minutes following the injection of the analgesic drug.

The ECG was monitored continuously throughout the period. Recordings of aortic, pulmonary arterial, and right atrial pressure were interrupted only for the sampling of arterial and mixed venous blood. Cardiac output, as measured by the dye dilution technique using indocyanine green, was recorded at five-minute intervals during the control period, at 2·5 minutes and five minutes after the start of drug injection and at five-minute intervals thereafter. Details of our techniques have been described elsewhere (McDonald *et al.*, 1967).

RESULTS

Clinical observations

Of the ten patients who were given heroin, eight fell asleep and remained so for the rest of the study. The other two felt pleasantly drowsy. One patient who had complained of severe nausea during the control period fell asleep and on waking at the end of the investigation felt completely well.

Four of the eight patients who received pethidine felt drowsy and slept intermittently. The other four patients complained of dizziness and nausea and sweated profusely. These unpleasant symptoms gradually disappeared after 20–30 minutes but one patient vomited four minutes after the injection and the nausea persisted to the end of the study.

Of the four patients who received morphine, one fell asleep whilst the others became drowsy. No unpleasant side-effects were experienced.

In each group, the analgesic effect of the opiate was adequate in those patients with chest pain.

Circulatory changes
Heroin. The mean changes of the ten patients who received heroin are illustrated in Figure 1.

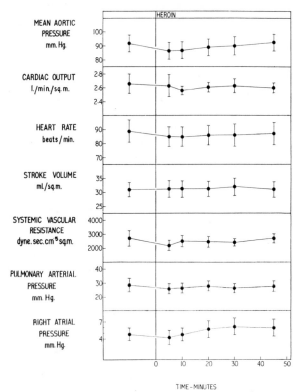

FIG. 1. Mean changes following 5 mg. intravenous heroin injection in ten patients with acute myocardial infarction.

For the group there was a fall in the mean aortic pressure of 5 mm.Hg five minutes after the start of the injection. Thereafter, the pressures returned to and remained at normal levels. This was a consistent trend except in one patient in whom the pressure continued to decline for 30 minutes before returning to control values. The lowest level in this patient was 16 mm.Hg below the control observations. No significant trend in cardiac output was observed after the administration of heroin. Maximum changes from control levels were in one patient a fall of 0·5 litres per minute per sq.m. and in another a rise of 0·56 litre per minute per sq.m.

There was no significant change in heart rate, stroke volume, systemic vascular resistance, mean pulmonary arterial pressure or right atrial pressure.

287

Pethidine. The mean changes of the eight patients who received pethidine are illustrated in Figure 2.

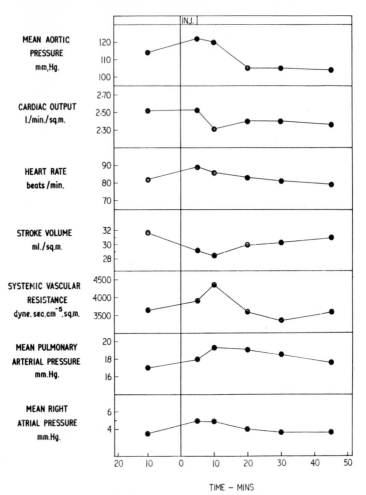

FIG. 2. Mean changes following 100 mg. intravenous injection of pethidine in eight patients with acute myocardial infarction.

In seven patients, there was an increase of 2–21 mm.Hg (mean 12 mm.Hg) in the mean aortic pressure, lasting for 10–15 minutes after the start of the injection. In the remaining patient, the mean aortic pressure decreased at once and by the tenth minute after the start of the injection was 22 mm.Hg below the control level (the average increase in pressure at the tenth minute was significant, P < 0·05). By the 20th minute, the mean aortic pressure in all eight patients had fallen below the control levels, from the 30th minute until the end of the study, the average decrease of 10 mm.Hg (range 6–20 mm.Hg) was highly significant (P < 0·001).

The changes in cardiac output following the injection were variable. In five patients the cardiac output fell, the fall being greatest between the 10th and 20th minute. In two patients, the cardiac output initially rose before falling by the 30th minute. In one patient, the cardiac output rose and remained higher than the control period. As a result of variation in individual response, the mean change for the group was not significant.

The heart rate increased within five minutes of the administration of pethidine by an average of 9 beats/min. (range 2–24 beats/min., P < 0·05). The stroke volume decreased by an average of 3·5 ml./sq.m. (P < 0·01). Thereafter both heart rate and stroke volume tended to return to control levels.

The systemic vascular resistance was increased in all patients in the first 10 minutes after the injection (P < 0·05). Thereafter in all patients, the systemic vascular resistance fell and in six of the eight the levels became lower than in the control period.

The changes in mean pulmonary arterial pressure and mean right atrial pressure were variable and showed no consistent trend.

Morphine. The mean changes of the four patients who received morphine are illustrated in Figure 3. The mean aortic pressure fell in all four patients, although in three of the patients the decrease was small. In the fourth patient, the fall was of 17 mm.Hg. at the fifth minute after the start of the injection and in this patient the maximal decrease was of 23 mm.Hg at the fifteenth minute.

Cardiac output increased in all patients, the range being between 0·25 and 0·5 l./min./sq.m. The greatest increase occurred in the patient who had the large fall in aortic pressure. Heart rate increased minimally in all four patients and stroke volume was also increased. In two of the patients the initial increase in stroke volume was followed by a fall below control levels. In all four patients there was an initial decrease in systemic vascular resistance.

In all four patients there was a rise in mean pulmonary arterial pressures ranging from 1–7 mm.Hg. The changes were maximal at 10 minutes but persisted throughout the study period. Changes in right atrial pressure were small and variable.

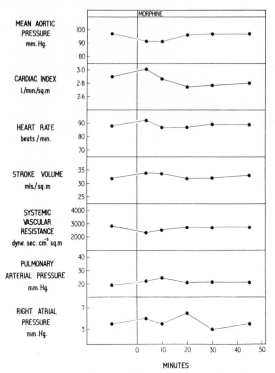

FIG. 3. Mean changes following 10 mg. intravenous morphine in four patients with acute myocardial infarction.

Pulmonary arterial pressure

Although in response to individual drugs the changes in pulmonary arterial pressure were variable when the readings for all 22 patients were examined, a consistent trend became apparent. In those patients with high pulmonary arterial pressure there was a fall in pressure and, conversely, a rise in pressure occurred in those patients with normal pulmonary arterial pressures.

DISCUSSION

These studies were carried out as a practical assessment rather than a pharmacological study. They do, however, illustrate that these drugs cause a differing circulatory response.

Heroin has no dramatic effect on the circulation; the only

consistent finding is a small fall in mean aortic pressure. This contrasts with our observations on the circulatory changes following pethidine and morphine.

Pethidine would seem to produce a dual action on the circulation. Initially, there is a ' stimulatory ' phase lasting 10–15 minutes, during which mean aortic pressure is increased. This is followed by a gradual decrease in mean aortic pressure, cardiac output, heart rate and systemic vascular resistance. This initial rise in mean aortic pressure following pethidine has been reported in normal subjects (Prescott *et al.*, 1949) and in obstetric patients (Gallen & Prescott, 1944). The mechanism of this biphasic response to pethidine is not clear. Sapru (1966) observed a similar change after a bolus injection of morphine; this he postulated was due to histamine release.

The changes following the administration of morphine were small in three of the patients but the fall in mean aortic pressure in the fourth patient was similar to that described by Thomas and his colleagues (1965) in patients with myocardial infarction, and by Sapru (1966) in patients with left ventricular failure.

Whilst our patient numbers are necessarily small, our experience with side-effects was similar to those described by Dundee *et al.* (1967). When they compared the cumulative total of side-effects of opiates, heroin had a much lower score than morphine or pethidine.

In conclusion, therefore, it would appear that pethidine and morphine produce more circulatory disturbance, and in this small series, pethidine produced more side-effects than heroin.

At present, we would suggest that heroin is a suitable analgesic for use in the relief of pain following myocardial infarction and that where the dose of 5 mg. is considered too great for mild pain a smaller dose is preferable to the potential upset of pethidine or morphine.

REFERENCES

British Medical Journal (1966a). Pain relief in myocardial infarction, **2**, 3.
British Medical Journal (1966b). Cardiogenic shock, **2**, 481.
DUNDEE, J. W., CLARKE, R. S. J. & LOAN, W. B. (1967). Comparative toxicity of diamorphine, morphine and methadone. *Lancet*, **2**, 221.
FOLDES, F. F., SWERDLOW, M. & SIKER, E. S. (1964). *Narcotics and Narcotic Antagonists*. Springfield, Illinois: Thomas.
GALLEN, B. & PRESCOTT, F. (1944). Pethidine as an obstetric analgesic. *Br. med. J.* **1**, 176.
MCDONALD, H. R., REES, H. A., MUIR, A. L., LAWRIE, D. M., BURTON, J. L. & DONALD, K. W. (1967). Circulatory effects of heroin in patients with myocardial infarction. *Lancet*, **1**, 1070.
MOOR, F. (1930). Intravenous morphine in coronary thrombosis. *Lancet*, **2**, 959.

PRESCOTT, F., RANSOM, S. G., THORP, R. H. & WILSON, A. (1949). Effects of analgesics on respiratory response to carbon dioxide in man. *Lancet*, **1**, 340.

SAPRU, R. P. (1966). *The effect of some physiological factors and pharmacological agents on left ventricular failure in man.* Ph.D. Thesis, University of Edinburgh.

THOMAS, M., MALMCRONA, R., FILLMORE, S., SHILLINGFORD, J. (1965). Haemodynamic effects of morphine in patients with acute myocardial infarction. *Br. Heart J.* **27**, 863.

DISCUSSION

Professor Shillingford. First of all I would like to congratulate Dr Muir on this very important work. I think it is essential that we should thoroughly understand the pharmacological action of all the drugs—even the very simple ones—that we are using in the treatment of myocardial infarction and, in fact, in other diseases. Up till now we have not known what happens to the circulation following these drugs. The results with morphine are very similar to those of Thomas working in our unit. However, we found that of a large number of patients receiving morphia, there are some in whom the morphia will fire off a vasovagal attack. This occurs in those in whom morphia induces nausea and vomiting and in whom there is sweating. The patients look ill and their blood pressure falls. I want to report to you the original observation which led us to examine more fully the haemodynamics associated with morphia. The patient had had an anterior infarction. The blood pressure was 150/80 with a heart rate of 85. He had fairly severe pain and so he had a very small amount of morphia intravenously into the catheter, without any extravenous punctures or anything like that, and we were interested to see—or rather exercised to see—a considerable fall of pressure. At the end of six minutes it was something like 30/10. We asked him how he felt, and he said he felt fine, and promptly became unconscious. With the slowing of the heart, we thought it was the vasovagal syndrome so we raised his legs in the air and tilted up the end of the bed and the pressure returned. Now, we did not know at that time whether this effect was a sensitivity to morphia itself, or whether it was also a vasovagal attack. There was no significant alteration of the heart rate at first, and yet there was a fall of pressure. This is difficult to explain on the basis of a vasovagal effect. Perhaps there was a considerable initial release of venous tone with pooling. Later, there was severe bradycardia and all the signs of the vasovagal syndrome. This experience led us on to examining a whole series of patients and our results were very similar to those of Dr Muir with some fall of pressure in most of them. I would like to ask Dr Muir whether he made his observations with the patient lying flat, sitting up or standing, as I think the results would be very different in each case. In the past we have sat patients up following an infarct and given them a quarter or a half a grain of morphia; the patient appeared to have a good night's sleep but in the morning we would find that he had died in the night. I have seen this hypotensive reaction in about 10 per cent. of patients receiving morphia. We had exactly the same results with pethidine, with a slowing of the heart and vaso-vagal effects. As a result, we are strongly in favour now of using heroin. The patients themselves seem to find it a very satisfactory drug indeed, and it would seem to be the safest of all of them in not potentiating bradycardia. Perhaps if we used morphine and the heart rate is not fast, we should always use atropine at the same time.

On the whole, I think it might be desirable to withhold all drugs as far as one is able to, but one has to use them with severe pain. Very often in the past these powerful analgesics have been given to make patients sleep or when they have got slight pain, and perhaps we should be somewhat more cautious in their use. The circulatory effects are very involved. It is not easy to see exactly what is happening and the effects vary considerably depending on venous and arterial tone. A patient with venous constriction and associated heart failure will have a different reaction as far as the pressure around the circuit is concerned, from one with normal arterial tone. I was trying to work out why in some of your patients the pulmonary arterial pressure rose, whilst in others it fell. I think it is probably something connected with the degree of failure and associated venous and arterial pressure. If I had an infarction, I would like heroin.

Dr Muir. In fact all our patients were studied as far as possible flat, but to make them comfortable they were allowed, as soon as required, one or two pillows. We became rather cocky with heroin and we tilted two patients to some 12 degrees—the bed was tilted, they were not sat up—and we had no adverse haemodynamic effects at all.

Professor Donald. Dr Sapru, who was formerly working with us found in a study of morphine in left ventricular failure that all his cases developed quite severe hypertension if they were allowed to sit up, within the next hour or so. He found the same in some normal controls. They were not the fittest of the normals, but they nevertheless were normals. In the left ventricular failure patients, there was an extremely marked fall in practically all cases and they had to be kept lying flat afterwards.

Dr Sloman. I agree with Professor Shillingford regarding the use of atropine with morphia. It used to be the fashion in the old days in our country always to give atropine with morphia and I think perhaps this should be a routine. Secondly, I would like to ask Dr Muir regarding the route of administration. While realising that in pharmacological studies it is necessary to use the drug intravenously, this is not the normal method of use in general practice or, for that matter, in our hospitals. I wonder if he has information on the haemodynamic effects of intramuscular administration—particularly of morphia but perhaps of the other drugs as well?

Dr Muir. We gave all the drugs only intravenously. They were given through one of the lumens of the catheter. We have no information on intramuscular use. I might come back on this, as some of the general practitioners here do use quite large doses of morphia intravenously. It is thought, I think mainly by the surgeons, that if you are going to give drugs, you should give them intravenously for the best effects. It is therefore not altogether uncommon for our patients to have intravenous therapy.

Dr Kirby. Amongst 10 normal subjects in our department in whom we were giving morphine to study the respiratory effects, we noted a fall in blood pressure in a perfectly normal young subject whose systolic pressure was 105 when we started and within minutes of giving him intravenous morphine 10 mg., the systolic pressure had fallen to 60. This was an alarming experience in a perfectly normal subject. He was lying down but when we raised the foot of the couch, his blood pressure returned to 95. We would also add that 8 out of the 10 normal subjects vomited and proceeded to do so for a number of hours.

Dr Fejfar. When we studied the effects of intravenous morphine on patients with mitral stenosis, we showed quite the same results as Dr Muir. There were mixed changes in cardiac output but the most marked were on pulmonary arterial pressure. It decreased if it was high, but increased if it was low. Did you at the same time investigate ventilatory function and the difference between the various drugs in this respect?

Dr Muir. In fact the blood gas changes were similar with all three analgesic drugs.

Dr McNicol. Can you give us the mean figures of the control and five minutes after?

Dr Muir. They were 38·6 and 42 mm.Hg. with heroin. Our experience with morphine and pethidine was very similar. PO_2 fell very slightly.

Dr Meltzer. I did not understand whether these patients had had an infarction or not.

Dr Muir. Oh yes. All of these had infarction within 12 and 14 hours.

Dr Meltzer. Well, I can presume that they behaved like other patients with infarction—about 80 per cent. of them had arrhythmias when you did this. Is that right?

Dr Muir. No, in fact there was only one person with an arrhythmia which shows that we had a selected group.

Dr Meltzer. Well, that is my point exactly because it makes such a tremendous difference whether the patient is arrhythmic or not when you do this. If you selected patients who had passed the arrhythmic period you would get very misleading results. We, for instance, have found that there is a good correlation between pain and the rhythm of the heart at the time of admission. One of the best ways to stop pain is simply to control the rhythm. If you have somebody in bigeminy and control the bigeminy you can very frequently get rid of the pain without morphine. Dr Sowton showed an interesting slide yesterday of turning up the pacemaker and when the tension time index went up he was able to create angina. This is very similar to situations which you see clinically. Now, as you were studying patients without arrhythmias, I wonder if this is at all comparable to what you see clinically in 80 per cent. of the people.

Dr Muir. I think we can say that some of our patients had pain but only one of them had an arrhythmia during the acute drug studies. They were monitored continuously throughout the period of study. I will say they had a few extrasystoles as we put the catheter in, but we did not have more than extrasystoles.

Dr Dalle. I am wondering whether the disadvantage of morphine—namely reducing venoconstriction which has been called pharmacodynamic phlebotomy—may not be an advantage in the treatment of pulmonary oedema in which it has very good reputation.

Dr Lown. We have used morphine almost exclusively with atropine. The incidence of vasovagal reaction is 1 per cent., so it is not a sizeable problem. You must realise that most of our patients are sitting, but they are sitting only part of the time. We never use analgesic drugs except when they have pain, at which time they become recumbent or in the reversed Trendelenburg. Furthermore, the drug is not given intravenously when it can be avoided, because as with many other drugs the circulatory effects are much greater when the drug is given this way. We prefer morphine for the very reason that Dr Dalle has mentioned. We do not like to use demerol (pethidine) because it has a tendency to create tachycardia especially when atrial fibrillation or flutter occurs. Its vagolytic effect tends to accelerate the heart unduly and causes serious consequences.

Dr Lassers. Are you suggesting, Dr Meltzer, that all patients with pain from infarction are having arrhythmias?

Dr Meltzer. No. Not all but there is a high correlation. If you take all people on admission and divide them into two categories—those with pain and those without pain, then those with pain have a much higher incidence of arrhythmias.

Dr Lassers. But then surely that does not apply to what Dr Muir has shown.

Dr Meltzer. No, but it is quite different if you take a group which is not having arrhythmias at the onset. I think the whole situation is different in people who do not have arrhythmias.

Dr McDonald. I agree with what Dr Lown has said regarding morphine and the incidence of the type of reaction that Shiilingford has described. In our experience it is actually less than 1 per cent.

Professor Shillingford. I think there is a very important practical consideration that comes out of this. Suppose a patient has a myocardial infarction in his home and his doctor sees him in severe pain. Often in our country he gives 30 mg. morphine, the ambulance man arrives to take the patient to hospital, puts him on a stretcher or sitting up in a chair, takes him down the stairs, and at the bottom of the stairs he is unconscious. This happened to a very good colleague of ours. Perhaps the ambulance men should be taught to sit patients in a chair and tilt it back or have some arrangement to hold them flat. With regard to the use of atropine with morphia, I think it is very helpful unless the heart rate is fast and then you may speed it up too much.

CORONARY CARE UNITS
AND THE COMMUNITY

Chairman: D. G. JULIAN

EDINBURGH COMMUNITY STUDY OF ACUTE CORONARY DISEASE

ANDREW ARMSTRONG

Royal Infirmary, Edinburgh

' If clinical research is to be used to get the full picture of disease it must equip itself to carry observations beyond the hospitals ' (Sir James Spence).

WITH the establishment of the Coronary Care Unit as a therapeutic instrument in the management of patients with acute coronary disease, we are now in a position to consider its place in the community, and whether intensive care of coronary patients can be extended to all who would benefit.

The Royal Infirmary of Edinburgh is the principal community hospital of the city and the landward area around, and so is in the line of first referral of acutely ill patients by general practitioners and the emergency services. Thus, the Coronary Care Unit in this hospital provides primarily a community service taking the majority of patients with myocardial infarction. With this experience, the basis of a hospital programme for the management of acute coronary disease has been created.

Complementary with this experience, we must gain knowledge of the disease as it presents in the community, with respect to its total incidence, its early mortality and the pattern of the acute attack. We must seek to know how many patients are treated outside hospital; why delays occur in the admission of patients; if hospital admission itself constitutes a risk. With this knowledge we should be in a position to plan the most economic service to the optimum benefit of the community.

In the Edinburgh Community Study of Acute Coronary Disease we are gathering data to provide the basis of satisfactory community care. Our primary aims are to discover the total incidence of acute coronary disease in Edinburgh and to determine the early pattern of the acute attack.

The principal community of our enquiry is a section of the Edinburgh population who are the registered patients of 171 general practitioners and who are under the age of 70 years. Each of these doctors has agreed to notify us of their cases of suspected or actual acute coronary disease whether patients are managed at home or in

299

hospital or present with sudden death. We introduced the Community study personally to each practice and have met with an excellent response and continued co-operation.

Hospital cases are observed during their in-patient period and are documented on admission and at the time of discharge from the ward and again six months after the initial event. Domiciliary cases are visited for the recording of an ECG and the taking of blood for serum enzyme levels. The clinical data are supplied by the general practitioners. In cases of sudden death we obtain details of previous history and of the circumstances of death either from the general practitioner or from the police surgeon.

The rest of the Edinburgh population, that registered with the remaining 92 general practitioners and under the age of 70 years, is studied with respect to hospital and sudden death cases. The third category studied concerns the patients who come from outside Edinburgh into the city hospitals.

We have a system of checks to make sure that notification is as complete as possible and also to pick up cases of those general practitioners not in the Study proper.

The Community Study is designed to involve each general practitioner for one year and to achieve this we arranged a staggered start and termination. We are at present about half-way through the Study and our preliminary analysis covers incidents from mid-January to mid-June 1967. This analysis involves relatively small numbers and any conclusions must be tentative and should await confirmation of the whole Study when complete.

During the period up to mid-June 1967 we studied and documented 666 incidents comprising 448 hospital, 97 domiciliary and 121 sudden death cases. These figures have no comparative value as they are drawn from different groups in varying proportions, but from these totals we can isolate firstly all hospital cases and secondly the domiciliary and hospital cases of general practitioners collaborating in the Community Study.

CORONARY CARE UNITS AND THE CORONARY LOAD

In Edinburgh there are two coronary care units, one of six beds at the Royal Infirmary, and a four-bedded unit at the Western General Hospital for male patients only. In addition to these two major community hospitals there are another nine hospitals which share the load of acute medical admissions.

If we agree that the optimum in clinical management is an initial period in the intensive care area for every patient with acute

300

myocardial infarction, we must gauge the adequacy of our arrangements by the proportion of patients so treated.

Table I illustrates the hospital distribution of all our observed cases of acute myocardial infarction. Two diagnostic categories,

Table I. *The distribution of patients with acute myocardial infarction (including the category ' insufficient data ') according to the type of initial hospital treatment, for all Edinburgh hospitals*

Unit	Delay from onset to admission		Total
	< 48 hr.	48 hr. +	
Royal Infirmary: CCU	100	7	107
Royal Infirmary: Conventional	68	7	75
Western General Hospital: CCU	48	5	53
Western General Hospital: Conventional	12	2	14
Other hospitals: Conventional	36	4	40

that of myocardial infarction and the category labelled insufficient data, have been combined. The great majority of the ' insufficient data ' patients died before the diagnosis could be substantiated by ECG and serum enzyme levels, but the clinical history was strongly in favour of the diagnosis.

Of the Royal Infirmary admissions, 107 out of 182 patients were given an initial period of observation and treatment in the Coronary Care Unit, that is less than 60 per cent. of the hospital's load of acute myocardial infarction. Considering the hospital intake for Edinburgh, the two Units provided initial care for 55 per cent. It would appear that the present number of intensive care beds

301

would have to be doubled to cope with the whole acute coronary load unless some form of selection can be introduced for patients admitted or a difference made in the duration of stay within the Unit.

The influence on mortality of the coronary care units cannot yet be measured. The mortality figures in the Royal Infirmary show a striking difference between intensive and conventional care, 10·5 per cent. of 107 CCU patients and 25·5 per cent. of 85 conventionally managed patients. This difference cannot, however, be wholly ascribed to intensive care as the distribution of age, delay before admission and the initial grading of severity all favoured a higher mortality in the conventional category.

DOMICILIARY CARE

We have studied domiciliary care as it is currently undertaken in Edinburgh by our Community Study general practitioners. We are interested in why patients with acute myocardial infarction are managed at home. The general practitioners have been asked this question with respect to each case studied and the most common reason was ' doubt about diagnosis '. This is borne out by Table II where the hospital and domiciliary patients are compared with respect to diagnosis. The middle column are those patients who go directly to hospital without previous consultation with the general practitioner who therefore cannot exercise the option of home or hospital treatment. The first and third columns represent patients who are referred to hospital and are retained at home respectively. The diagnostic category of myocardial infarction preponderates in the hospital patients, 58 to 25 per cent. in those managed at home. The diagnostic categories of ' ischaemia ' and ' other diagnoses ' feature largely in the domiciliary patients.

Lack of disturbance was the second most frequently quoted reason for domiciliary care. This is confirmed on comparing the grading of severity based on the general practitioner's initial examination in both the hospital and domiciliary cases. Table III shows the preponderance of mild cases in the home-treated patients and a considerable proportion of those with early complications in the hospital group.

CONCLUSIONS

Our present intensive care arrangements in Edinburgh fall short of providing a complete community service.

Table II. *The diagnostic categories of patients registered with the Community Study general practitioners according to the place of initial care and whether referred or directly admitted*

Diagnosis	Hospital				Domiciliary	
	referred by G.P.		admitted direct			
	Number	(%)	Number	(%)	Number	(%)
Myocardial infarction .	159	58	23	59	24	25
Probable myocardial infarction . . .	11	4	2	5	4	4
Myocardial ischaemia .	56	20	8	20	29	30
Insufficient data . .	9	3	2	5	8	8
Other . . .	40	15	4	10	31	32
Total	275		39		96	

Table III. *The initial grading of severity based on the general practitioner's examination in those patients with acute myocardial infarction referred to hospital and those cared for at home*

Grading of severity	Hospital	Domiciliary
Mild	76	18
Cardiac failure	23	1
Shock	3	0
Cardiac failure and shock	7	0
Insufficient data for grading	50	5
Total	159	24

The effect on the community mortality is not yet defined and stress will have to be laid on the various other factors which influence the outcome of the acute coronary attack in assessing results.

Domiciliary care appears principally to be motivated by doubt about the clinical diagnosis and the lack of physical disturbance in the patient.

Discussion. See p. 309.

ACUTE MYOCARDIAL INFARCTION IN A BRITISH GENERAL PRACTICE
Experience during 20 years

JOHN FRY

Beckenham, England

THE approach of the general practitioner to acute myocardial infarction, and in fact to disease in general, is different from that of the hospital-based specialist.

The reasons are fairly obvious. The general practitioner and his equivalent in U.S.A. and in U.S.S.R. derive their experience from the patterns of disease that occur in a relatively small and static population of 2,000–3,000 persons. The numbers of cases of myocardial infarction will be very much fewer than those seen by the specialist, and, since there is usually no pre-selection, the clinical spectrum will show a relative preponderance of the less serious cases.

On the other hand the hospital specialist will, in the United Kingdom, be dealing with cases of myocardial infarction from a population that may be 100 times that of the general practitioner and in consequence he will see many more cases with a greater proportion of the more serious grades.

Special Features of British General Practice

The British general practitioner still works in the traditional ways of his predecessors. He is the single and only portal-of-entry to the medical care services to the 2,500–3,000 persons in his practice. They have direct and free access to him at all times. There is no such free access to hospital specialists; all those requiring hospital and specialist care are referred there by the general practitioner.

304

The British general practitioner thus provides long-term continuing care over 20, 30 or 40 years to ' his ' patients.

He is still a ' generalist ' who does not restrict his work to any special age or sex groups, nor to any special clinical conditions.

He provides comprehensive care in the community for expectant mothers, children and the aged and for the whole range of the ' common diseases that commonly occur and for the rare diseases that rarely happen '—but he has no access to hospital beds.

CORONARY HEART DISEASE IN GENERAL PRACTICE— A PROFILE IN MINIATURE

Bearing in mind the features of British general practice, and because all his patients are ' registered ' with him and attend no other doctors without a record report to the general practitioner, it is possible for the doctor, so inclined, to study the true patterns of coronary heart disease.

In my practice over 20 years coronary heart disease was diagnosed in 400 persons, an *annual incidence rate* of 4 per 1,000. (We have our own ECG machine and we also have records of hospital investigations and autopsy reports).

This incidence increased progressively from the age of 40 onwards and was three times greater in males than in females.

With an incidence such as this, the general practitioner with an average practice of 2,500 may expect to have 8–12 new cases of coronary heart disease each year.

The *clinical mode of presentation* of the initial attack was as follows in my own practice:

Sudden death	. . .	20 per cent.
Clinically severe myocardial infarction .	. . .	13 per cent.
Clinically moderate myocardial infarction .	. . .	35 per cent.
Clinically mild myocardial infarction .	. . .	12 per cent.
Angina on effort	. . .	20 per cent.

(Sudden death through Clinically mild myocardial infarction) }80 per cent.

We have good facilities for *diagnosis and management* of our patients with coronary heart disease in their own homes and we have admitted to hospital only one-third of acute myocardial infarctions.

In spite of the strong case that can be made for admitting all cases of acute myocardial infarction to intensive care units, there are good reasons also for keeping the less severe grades at home.

305

The problem is how to select those who can be managed safely at home and those who require urgent admission to an intensive care unit.

The *outcome* in patients followed up for 10 years or longer was death in 60 per cent. (45 per cent. if ' sudden deaths ' are excluded), survival with disability in 20 per cent. and good health in 20 per cent.

Thus, in a British general practice a clinical diagnosis of myocardial infarction will be made in between 5 and 10 of his patients each year, which is about the same rate as new cancers and acute appendicitis. He will admit about two or three of these to hospital and manage the others with reasonably good results.

Acute myocardial infarction

First-day deaths. Of particular interest to our discussions on acute myocardial infarction was the fate of my 320 patients (excluding the 80 out of 400 whose initial presentation was as angina of effort) and in particular the 110 who died on the first day of the attack.

During the period of 20 years, 165 out of the 320 persons with myocardial infarction died from a cardiovascular cause (52 per cent.), and 110 (M: 88; and F: 22) of these, or two-thirds of all those who died from a cardiovascular cause, did so on the first day of their initial attack.

The periods from onset of the acute attack at which these 165 persons died was as follows:

On 1st day	.	110	66 per cent.
During 1–7 days	.	9	5 per cent.
Later	. .	46	29 per cent.
		165	

Place of death. It is of the greatest significance to note that of all the 110 first-day deaths 78 (or 70 per cent.) took place in the victim's home, 14 (or 13 per cent.) in hospital and 18 (17 per cent.) elsewhere.

The fact that 70 per cent. of these deaths occurred in the home stresses the fact that we must be prepared to take intensive care resuscitation to the home rather than await the victim's arrival in hospital.

Time of death. My experience confirms that of others, i.e., that these deaths occur very quickly and we have little time in which to act.

The time of death in the 110 persons who died from acute myocardial infarction on the first day of their attacks was as follows:

Instant deaths (or within 15 minutes)	.	56 (51%)
First-hour deaths (15–60 minutes) .	.	34 (30%)
First-day deaths (1–24 hours)	. .	20 (19%)

RESUSCITATION ' POSSIBLES '

In order to assess the proportion in whom resuscitation might have been feasible a further analysis of the 110 first-day deaths from acute myocardial infarction was made.

Excluded were 56 in whom death was instantaneous and 14 who were known to have been so frail or suffering from associated diseases that would have made any attempts at resuscitation quite unreasonable.

There were, therefore, 40 ' possibles ' in whom resuscitation would have been reasonable with a chance of success.

Instant death	.	56 (51%)
Unfit for resuscitation . . .	.	14 (13%)
' Possibles '	.	40 (36%)

———

110

———

Thus, in over a third (36 per cent.) of those dying on the first day from an acute myocardial infarction, resuscitation might have been attempted. To put it another way, out of all the 320 cases of acute myocardial infarction some 40 who died might have been saved by modern intensive care techniques.

Who were these ' possibles '?

There were relatively more males who died on the first day (40 per cent.) compared with females (18 per cent.), and as might be expected the feasibility of resuscitation decreased with age. Resuscitation was considered to have been feasible in 60 per cent. of those who died aged 69 or less and in only 10 per cent. of those aged 70 or more.

The great majority (29 out of 40 or 72 per cent.) of these ' possibles ' *died in their own homes* and most *died quickly, within the first hour* (32 out of 40 or 80 per cent.).

SOME IMPLICATIONS

What tentative guide lines can be drawn from these findings? The first point to stress is that most of my patients with acute myocardial infarction died in their own homes and died quickly.

Second, that if the aged and the frail and the instant deaths are excluded, there still remained more than a third of the persons who died on the first day and in whom modern resuscitation might have been successful.

It is reasonable, therefore, to reconsider our approach to the intensive care of patients with acute myocardial infarction. If lives are to be saved then intensive care facilities be must taken to the patient's home as quickly as possible.

Based on my figures a service for the whole of the United Kingdom would have to be prepared to undertake resuscitation in some 24,000 out of the annual 115,000 deaths from acute myocardial infarctions.

Translated to a district hospital serving a population of 250,000 a mobile intensive care cardiac unit may expect some 120 calls a year or two to three each week.

In a general practice group of four partners there may be four such emergency situations each year.

In terms of lives saved, even if only a 10 per cent. success rate is achieved, 2,500 lives may be saved each year.

This situation presents a challenge to us all—from the administrators and planners who have to decide on priorities, to cardiologists who have to organise the mobile units, to general practitioners who have to be prepared to set the plan in motion and to the public who have to take the first steps in seeking aid in times of need.

SUMMARY

1. In a British general practice providing total and comprehensive care for an average of 2,500 patients, 400 persons with coronary heart disease have been observed and followed-up over 20 years.

2. The annual incidence rate was 4 per 1,000. The most usual clinical presentations were sudden death in 20 per cent.; severe myocardial infarction in 13 per cent.; moderate myocardial infarction in 35 per cent.; mild myocardial infarction in 12 per cent.; and angina in 20 per cent.

The outcome was that 60 per cent. died, 20 per cent. are disabled, and 20 per cent. are well at 10-year follow-up.

3. In 320 patients with acute myocardial infarction, 66 per cent. of all deaths from cardiovascular causes occurred on the first day, 5 per cent. in the first week (1–7 days) and 29 per cent. later.

4. Of the 110 first-day deaths, 70 per cent. occurred in the patient's home, 13 per cent. in hospital and 17 per cent. elsewhere. Deaths on the first day occurred instantaneously in 51 per cent., in the first hour in 30 per cent. and between 1 and 24 hours in 19 per cent.

5. It has been estimated that in 40 out of 110 (36 per cent.) first-day deaths resuscitation would have been feasible. In these ' possibles ', death occurred at home in 72 per cent. and within the first hour in 80 per cent.

6. A plea is made for the development of mobile intensive care cardiac units that may save up to 2,500 lives a year in the United Kingdom.

DISCUSSION

Dr Frommer. Dr Armstrong has called attention to the dismal lack of detailed information that we have upon a problem which we have really recognised for decades as being a leading cause of death and disability. In the process of developing these statistics, he is giving great attention to the difficulties that he had encountered, and all will continue to encounter in collecting this kind of information. I think perhaps some time ago we were justifiably therapeutic nihilists, but on the basis of the experience that we have listened to in the past few days it is appropriate to say that while all the answers are not in, there are methods of therapy which are promising, which are important and which really must be delivered to the people. We are really left with two major sorts of research to be pursued. One is new ways of therapy and better understanding of the disease process, and the other is additional and more effective ways of delivering this kind of medical care to patients who are afflicted with myocardial infarction. I think that the speakers have called attention to the very great importance of focusing upon the patient as well as the disease process and the recognition of the fact that the vast majority of patients are seen outside the academic institutions from which most of us come, and the fact that probably a half or more of the patients die of myocardial infarction before they get to the hospital. I would ask a question of Dr Armstrong. In discussing the data of the patients treated at home compared with patients treated in the hospital, would it be possible to give an account of those patients who were initially treated at home and whose subsequent course caused them to be hospitalised? I did not get a clear understanding as to how these were handled in the statistics. In Dr Fry's paper, it was not clear at what point the mortality occurred. For example, the patients with angina had a 40–50 per cent. mortality. In what space of time?

Dr Armstrong. We define our domicilary cases as those which are initially treated at home, and the numbers which I showed latterly were in fact those who had initial treatment at home. This did not preclude subsequent referral to hospital. In fact, of the 24 with myocardial infarction who were treated at home, eight were subsequently referred to hospital and one of these died. Of the eight who were referred to hospital, this was done after we made the diagnosis and it was on the basis of this diagnosis that they were referred. This emphasises the point that doubtful diagnosis is the main factor in keeping the patient at home.

Dr Julian. There has, in fact, been quite a change as far as I can see in the pattern of admission of patients in the last year. It would appear that in the year before the opening of the Coronary Care Unit we admitted approximately 380 patients who fulfilled our criteria for routine admission. In the first year of the Coronary Care Unit there were nearly 500 patients who fulfilled these criteria.

Dr Fry. I have been interested mainly in the natural history of these diseases. What happened with the angina patients was that often they had a myocardial infarction later on. I am not trying to sell anything, but I have produced a book called *Profiles of Disease* where all this is tabulated. I cannot answer exactly when the angina presentations died, but they did not die within a short time. I would say probably over years rather than months or weeks.

Dr Frommer. But how promptly did the 10 per cent. whose symptoms were considered mild die?

Dr Fry. Well, very few of them died and they certainly did not die early. Perhaps I was under an illusion, but I used to believe that I could pick out the ones that I could deal with at home, but I am not so sure now. This visit has not done me much good.

Dr Julian. I'm glad about that! As I understand it, many of the mild cases were not first-day cases?

Dr Fry. In fact, this is one of the definitions. They came back two or three days later with 'indigestion' still there.

Dr Julian. It is a little different then from what we call a mild case at the time of onset.

Dr Fry. Incidentally, the chap who is best at retrospective diagnosis is the Coroner's officer. He is the person who goes and sees the wife or the relative after the death but before the postmortem. The one that we have in my area is right in about 90 per cent. of the cases when he says this is a coronary death. I think we have to look at the Coroner's pathologist material a lot more carefully. I never really realised until I talked to the Coroner's officers, who are usually policemen, that they are the ones who, just by listening to people, to wives giving their story, are able to pick out the answer a lot better than I can.

Dr Kirby. With regard to the problem of anxiety, a psychiatrist at our hospital has looked at just over 50 of the first group of patients admitted to our coronary unit which is in a district and not a teaching hospital. These were men who had their first myocardial infarction and were below the age of 60. He has found so far no adverse effects of being put into a coronary care unit. Those patients who developed anxiety afterwards were those who had a personality which engendered this feeling of anxiety. Furthermore, in the past three years we have been interested in cardiac resuscitation and we looked at some 20 patients whom we followed up over a period of time. We have not found any great anxiety except in the people who could not return to work.

Dr Julian. I think that is a very important point, Dr Kirby. If a coronary care unit is producing anxiety, it is not providing coronary care.

Dr Fry. There is just one point and that is that men who get coronaries are anxious men. In fact what Dr Kirby has said is that if they were anxious before, they will be more anxious after.

Dr McNicol. We have looked at the effect of coronary care as opposed to general ward care, and the coronary care atmosphere has been, by and large, reassuring to the average patient. The point of maximal emotional trauma has been at the time of transfer to ordinary care.

Dr Oliver. I think this question of coronary care unit neurosis is very important. I really want to make a point to Dr Fry who has indicated correctly, I believe, that many of them are anxious men. It is for this particular reason that I think the staff of coronary care units should give a very clear and careful explanation on admission of what the unit is all about. We think we have two clear reactions. The first reaction is one of confidence. The feeling that having come into the unit, they are secure and are being watched and with a sensible and not too elaborate explanation they relax. The second reaction is also one of confidence when they leave the unit, when they are transferred to the medical ward, because they then feel that the immediate reason for being in the unit has passed. I would have thought that if cardiac neurosis develops, as it does to some extent in all coronary patients, it is independent of the advent of coronary care units and as it used to be in general medical wards. The system of rehabilitation is also important. In some hospitals, as we have heard in the W.H.O. course, patients are kept in bed for nearly two months. Personally I get most patients up after about 10 days and out of hospital after three weeks, and they have usually walked up a flight of stairs before they go out.

Dr Fry. There is just one other point. There is a need for a third wave of confidence when they come out of hospital to home. These patients, who are 10 miles away from the teaching hospital where they were under treatment and feel as though their arms have got cut off, with every little ache they want to be back in their hospital.

Dr Fejfar. What I have learned from these papers is the difficulty of comparing one area with another. One has to study the rate of coronary disease in a given community.

Dr Lown. I would like to call attention to the remarkable coincidence of Dr Fry's figures with those that have been gathered in the United States, specifically the Baltimore study that has already been referred to, by Kuller and co-workers. In this large community study after one year the figures are almost the same as those of Dr Fry—namely 67 per cent. as compared with 65 per cent. who are dead within the first day. Of these deaths in Dr Fry's series 83 per cent. were dead within one hour. Of course this raises very critical questions. Where do we go beyond coronary care? Because certainly pre-coronary care with flying squads cannot encompass this problem and therefore we are in a staging area for a further advance. I think Dr Fry's contribution is important insofar as the general practitioner invariably brings our focus most precisely on the problem because he is the infantry man. I think the problem right now is that we have to start thinking how to identify the individual who is going to die and to arrange telemetering for those who are most susceptible.

FIRST AID IN MYOCARDIAL INFARCTION

E. I. CHAZOV

Institute of Therapy, Moscow

THIS report describes the main principles applied in the U.S.S.R. in the treatment of myocardial infarction, permitting reduction of mortality by one-third during the last 15 years. Mortality from myocardial infarction, and the gravity of the disease, are largely determined by complications occurring during the first hours after the onset and are due to shock, acute cardiac failure with oedema of the lungs, rhythm disturbances, etc. At present a number of effective methods have been developed for the treatment of these complications. One of our main problems is to apply these methods at the earliest time after the onset of myocardial infarction and its complications. We held, and this has been later confirmed, that the immediate prognosis of the disease depends on the interval between the onset of the disease and the doctor's arrival at the patient's bedside, and also on the time of the institution of treatment after the infarction: this was especially true for the treatment of shock and the use of anticoagulants and fibrinolytic preparations.

Proceeding from these data we have developed a particular organisation for the treatment of myocardial infarction. This consists of special medical teams visiting patients at home in special cars and rendering highly qualified immediate aid. Emphasis is placed on early hospitalisation of all myocardial infarction cases.

There are two types of medical ambulance squads. The first category, staffed by a physician and a nurse, is intended for rendering first aid to a patient with uncomplicated myocardial infarction. The physician has a portable apparatus for administration of nitrous oxide; he may use heparin, administer strophanthin or cordiamin to treat cardiac incompetence, and give mesaton for shock, etc. In grave, complicated cases of myocardial infarction a special ambulance squad arrives, staffed also by a physician and paramedical personnel and an orderly. This squad has at its disposal all the necessary apparatus and drugs for management at home at the level of modern standards and for safe transportation of the patient to hospital.

TREATMENT OF PAIN SYNDROME

The first symptom encountered in the majority of patients with myocardial infarction is prolonged and grave pain. Pain should

313

be rapidly controlled since it may promote shock. Various methods of anaesthesia are widely used at present—potentiated anaesthesia, complex administration of mild synthetic hypnotics with neuroplegic preparations, etc.

We mostly use nitrous oxide anaesthesia with simultaneous neuroendocrine block using chlorpromazine or promethazine in the presence of normal arterial pressure. Nitrous oxide is devoid of any side-effects and it is given with oxygen in a proportion of 80 : 20 for the first 15 minutes, and later in a proportion of 50 : 50. In the absence of nitrous oxide administration, trimeperidine promethazine is widely used with hydrochloride. Taking into consideration the side-effects (intestinal paresis, stimulation of emetic centre, changes of the acid-base balance) we limit as far as possible the use of opium preparations. A marked anaesthetic effect can also be achieved by the administration of heparin with fibrinolytic preparations.

TREATMENT WITH ANTICOAGULANTS AND FIBRINOLYTIC PREPARATIONS

In the absence of contraindications 10–15,000 I.U. of heparin are given at home as soon as the special squad arrives, to each patient suspected of myocardial infarction. Fibrinolytic therapy (fibrinolysin, streptokinase) is started within the first hours after the onset of the disease. This treatment is derived from the fact that thrombosis of the coronary arteries is revealed in 70–80 per cent. of myocardial infarction cases. Besides, before anticoagulants were introduced into the therapy, almost 25 per cent. of the patients developed thrombo-embolic complications. When started early, and carried out for a sufficiently long time (5–6 days), this therapy leads to marked improvement in the course of myocardial infarction —rapid control of pain, less cardiac failure, less rise of blood transaminase and more rapid signs of ECG healing. The effect of therapy is associated not only with the action of the preparations on the principal thrombus, but also with the spasmolytic properties of heparin and fibrinolytic enzymes. In addition, the effect on the so-called secondary thrombi is of great significance in reducing the area of ischaemia and necrosis.

TREATMENT OF RHYTHM DISTURBANCES

These are recorded by continuous ECG monitoring and occur in about 85 per cent. of patients with myocardial infarction. Treatment consists primarily of prophylaxis of cardiac insufficiency and of ventricular fibrillation. Agents used by the ambulance squad in myocardial infarction include novocainamide (procaine amide), cocarboxylase and potassium. Each team possesses a defibrillator but this method of treatment produces a satisfactory effect only in cases of paroxysmal ventricular tachycardia, and seldom in atrial fibrillation. Atrial fibrillation is best controlled by administration of cardiac glycosides (strophanthin or corglycon). The early intravenous administration of an insulin-glucose-potassium mixture, is considered to be of importance in preventing disturbances of rhythm.

SHOCK THERAPY

The principle of early high grade treatment is especially important in the therapy of shock. Physicians in the ambulances have at their disposal all the modern facilities for treating acute cardiovascular incompetence. Proceeding from the concept that cardiac shock is a process involving not only haemodynamic disturbances but also metabolic and hormonal shifts, disturbing the regulation of the vascular system, we institute complex therapy, including an intravenous drip containing strophanthin, noradrenaline and steroids. It should, however, be emphasised that there exists a group (about 25–30 per cent. of the so-called areactive forms of collapse) in which modern methods give no effect. At present a method of counterpulsation is being checked, expanding our therapeutic possibilities, without, however, solving the cause.

The effective and immediate *treatment of acute cardiac incompetence* largely determines the prognosis. Left ventricular failure, usual in such cases, is mostly expressed in oedema of the lungs. This condition requires urgent medical aid. Undoubtedly, the leading treatment is intravenous injection of cardiac glycosides. Their administration may be combined with diuretics—novurite, lasix, or urea. It should be pointed out that the mechanism of urea action in oedema of the lungs is more complicated than the diuretic action alone. A mixture of oxygen with antifoamsilan, a silicon preparation serving as foam extinguisher, is a good symptomatic means for controlling foam formation in the respiratory tracts. Its use considerably improves the patient's respiration and consequently his state.

PATIENT'S TRANSPORTATION

Proceeding from the main principle in the treatment of patients with myocardial infarction—that of early hospitalisation—in such

315

large cities in the U.S.S.R. as Moscow, Leningrad, Kiev, Sverdlovsk, Rostov, Tbilisi and many others, patients are transported to the hospital within the first hour after the onset of the disease.

As a rule, patients are admitted to specific departments, especially equipped, and attended by expertly trained personnel. Transportation itself has in no way influenced the course of myocardial infarction. For instance, in Moscow, only 4 of over 4,000 patients transported to the hospital died in the ambulance, and in Sverdlovsk not a single one of 6,000 patients died during transportation.

Observations have demonstrated that early hospitalisation reduced mortality in myocardial infarction. For instance, in one of the Moscow districts, the mortality rate among hospitalised patients was 2·5 times less in comparison with those treated at home. It should be emphasised that the course of the disease was identical in character in both of these groups.

Discussion. See p. 318.

FLYING SQUAD SERVICES

FRANK PANTRIDGE

Royal Victoria Hospital, Belfast

STUDIES by Yater *et al.* (1948) and Bainton & Peterson (1963) showed that 60 per cent. of deaths from coronary thrombosis occurred within one hour and some 80 per cent. within 12 hours of the onset of symptoms. Mittra (1965), in an investigation confined to patients with coronary thrombosis admitted within 48 hours of the onset of symptoms, found that the average interval between onset and admission was 11·6 hours. If therefore the great majority of deaths occur before the patient reaches hospital, intensive coronary care units can have but a very limited effect on the mortality.

A prospective study by the University Department of Social Medicine, Belfast, confirmed this proposition. In the year studied which ended in August 1965, there were 998 deaths among the City's population of a half a million. Only 414 of these patients reached hospital and of these, 102 were dead on arrival. The median time between onset of symptoms and ward admission of those who survived to be admitted was 8 hours 15 minutes. Many factors are concerned in this delay. The patient may not immediately seek medical help. The practitioner may not be aware of the high risk of sudden and preventable death. An ambulance may not be able to deal with the call immediately. The patient may have to wait his turn among other ill patients in a casualty department. Delay in the patient notifying his doctor is not a major factor since 50 per cent. of male patients notified their doctors within 1 hour and 17 minutes of the onset of symptoms.

It was reasoned that if the practitioners were made aware of the high early mortality and if a mobile unit carried intensive care to the patient, then the major causes of delay in the patient getting intensive care might be eliminated. The Royal Victoria Hospital seemed geographically well placed for the operation of a mobile intensive care unit since it is near the centre of the City. The initial stages in organising the unit were:

1. The practitioners were acquainted with the facts regarding the early high mortality.

2. A training scheme in the technique of resuscitation was arranged for those family doctors who were interested.

3. A signal system was arranged for the rapid activation of the duty houseman or registrar and activation of the ambulance control.

Family doctors were given a special number. This got absolute priority at the telephone exchange. The unit can be on its way within two minutes of the signal from the doctor arriving at the Central Hospital Telephone exchange.

It is now possible to reach 85 per cent. of patients within 15 minutes and 50 per cent. within 10 minutes.

In the past 20 months, 469 patients have been admitted to the Unit. Forty-nine per cent. had proven infarction, 29 per cent. were classified as acute coronary insufficiency, 11 per cent. had prolonged chest pain, thought to be ischaemic but with a normal cardiogram, and 3 per cent. of the calls were thought to be unjustified.

Fifty per cent. of patients now come under intensive care within two hours.

While the primary object of the scheme was to get patients under intensive care quickly and so prevent ventricular fibrillation, it has been found possible to correct ventricular fibrillation occurring in various situations outside hospital. The first patient resuscitated outside hospital was of interest. When defibrillation was achieved in the patient's own home, complete AV block and profound hypotension were apparent. Pacing by catheter was required in the patient's home before he was fit to transfer to hospital. His AV block was transitory and he was quite well after admission, but unfortunately died three weeks later from recurrent fibrillation.

Fifteen patients who developed ventricular fibrillation outside hospital have been resuscitated. Of these 10 survived their stay in hospital and 9 are still alive. Four of these patients developed ventricular fibrillation during transit in the mobile unit. One individual developed ventricular fibrillation in his own home just as his doctor arrived; one collapsed in a doctor's surgery; one man ' dropped dead ' in a garage and one ' dropped dead ' in a busy street.

The mobile unit has removed the risk of transit to hospital. It has been mentioned that in the survey carried out by the Department of Social and Preventive Medicine 102 of 414 patients brought to hospital were dead on arrival. In a 20-month period during which 469 patients were brought to hospital there has not been a single death during transit.

REFERENCES

BAINTON, C. R. & PETERSON, D. R. (1963). Deaths from coronary heart disease in persons fifty years of age and younger. *New Engl. J. Med.* **268,** 569.
MITTRA, B. (1965). Potassium, glucose, and insulin in treatment of myocardial infarction. *Lancet* **2,** 607.
YATER, W. M., TRAUM, A. H., BROWN, W. G., FITZGERALD, R. P., GEISLER, M. A. & WILCOX, B. B. (1948). Coronary artery disease in men 18 to 39 years of age. *Am. Heart J.* **36,** 334, 481, 683.

DISCUSSION

Dr Julian. This is a very exciting paper, Dr Pantridge. May I take the privilege of questioning your figures of deaths in the ambulance? It appears to me both from our experience and also from that of others, that the proportion of deaths occurring in ambulances is much lower than you report. Dr Armstrong, can you give us the Edinburgh figures of death in transit?

Dr Armstrong. It is somewhere in the region of 1–2 per cent.

Dr Nixon. I have the figures for the North London Borough of Camden. Of 100 consecutive deaths from coronary disease, 47 died before the ambulance reached them, 13 died in the ambulance and 40 within the first 24 hours of arriving in hospital. So the figures in London are very close to those in Belfast.

Professor Shillingford. Were the patients alive when they were put into the ambulance?

Dr Nixon. Yes. Thirteen died in the ambulance.

Dr Pantridge. Out of 414 people who reached hospital, 102 were dead on admission. Now, whether these people died in the ambulance or were dead when the ambulance people picked them up we do not know, but I do not think they would have been put in the ambulance if they had been dead.

Dr McKendrick. These figures are critical but they are difficult to obtain. In Liverpool in two successive years 900 and 1,000 patients were taken to hospital and were dead on arrival. If the ambulance personnel think these people are undoubtedly dead, they take them to the city mortuary and not to the hospital. They are taken to the hospital if they have a hope of life. In the first two months of this year, 58 patients in January and 60 in February were dead on arrival at hospital from coronary disease. It was terribly difficult without embarrassing the ambulance drivers to get any further with this, but as far as I can guess, approximately 20 of the Jnauary cases were thought to be alive when put into the ambulance.

Dr Julian. The differences reported may relate to the length of time people have to spend in ambulances. Can Dr Pantridge give any idea of what the average length of time in Belfast was?

Dr Pantridge. The median time between the onset of disease and ward admission was 8 hours and 15 minutes, and only a small amount of that was due to delay in the patient getting the doctor. Quite obviously there must have been a lot of time lost getting the ambulance there and getting the patients in. How long they spent in the ambulance, I do not know.

Dr Sloman. Can I focus attention on the psychological factors in all this? In the first six months of this year, we had 56 cardiac arrests outside our coronary care ward at the hospital. Of these, 13 occurred in our casualty department or admitting room. Of these 13, 9 had acute myocardial infarction and only 2 were re-suscitated. I suggest that the management they received in the ambulance and the management they receive in the casualty department is pretty crucial and critical and gets back to the psychological problems. We must back up the system in the home, in the ambulance and immediately on arrival in hospital.

Dr Oliver. I have been most impressed by Dr Pantridge's communication. There are four points I would like to make. Firstly, are we producing deaths by rushing people into hospital—as one very prominent physician in this country has said ' bundling them into ambulances '—and are we therefore producing a false incidence of arrhythmias and mortality on arrival in hospital? Next, I think it is extremely important when discussing flying squad services to be clear into what type of intensive care area the patient is going to be transmitted. It is not the slightest bit of good having a highly efficient flying squad service and landing the patient up in a rather understaffed unsatisfactory intensive care area. It has got to be a high-grade area because all the resuscitation measures

319

cannot be done in an ambulance; they have to be continued after-wards in the type of units which we have been discussing.

The third point, to some extent relates to that, because I think that travelling distances have to be considered. Obviously Dr Pantridge has got a highly organised system and the distances which his ambulances have to travel are probably not very great—they cannot be in view of the speed of admission that he has. The problem that the general practitioner has is 'When do I transfer a patient to hospital?' This depends very much on how far away the general practitioner is from the hospital, what system of trans-port there is, and again to what area the patient is transported. Are we saying then that these flying squads are only of value if they can get to a nearby hospital or are we extrapolating and wondering whether they could transport a patient for a period of an hour, or over 40 miles? Fourthly, relating to the economy of these am-bulances, Dr Pantridge gave us a figure which I have no doubt is realistic and I am not going to argue with it. But it would appear that you have approximately one call per day on average, or one and a half maybe, and for this you have standing by pretty highly trained personnel all the 24 hours.

Dr Pantridge. With regard to your first point about bundling people into ambulances, this is exactly what we do not do. There is speed in order to get the patient under intensive care, but the team may spend some considerable time before the patient is considered fit to move. We have not had a single death in the ambulances and I think only one within one hour.

My whole argument is this. I do not know whether it is right to keep people at home or to bring them into hospital, but if you are going to bring patients into hospital, then you should bring them in at a time when the risk is maximal, but you should first make sure that they are fit to travel.

Dr Lown. When you say 15 minutes, Dr Pantridge, is that from the time of call?

Dr Pantridge. From the moment the call for the doctor arrives from the telephone exchange.

Dr Lown. After observing patients in a coronary care unit for 24 hours or more, it is frequently difficult to say whether the patient has acute myocardial infarction and this must be exponentially more difficult earlier on. Our major problem is, how do you diagnose acute myocardial infarction even with all the help we do have? Many of the discussions of the last few days have been focussed as though acute myocardial infarction was a catastrophic event—that it is so positively unique it can be recognised readily.

I wish you would communicate to me how this is done, because this would be the most important information I could take back to the United States! In the earlier stages of infarction the general practitioner is faced with a most difficult problem. The time delay is created first of all by the factor of the patient denying his symptoms, and, secondly, the general practitioner may encourage delay in order to find out exactly what is going on. These are the primary areas of delay rather than the call and the transport.

Dr Oliver. I do not really believe that you are bundling patients into hospital, Dr Pantridge. I am merely posing the question because I feel it should be posed. In fact, I would agree with you that it is improbable that you are.

Dr Meltzer. What Professor Chazov is doing makes very good sense to me. Sending a team to treat somebody is a different idea from sending an ambulance—the ambulance is irrelevant. What he is really doing is moving care to the patient. Now, I gather this is not what you are doing, Dr Pantridge, is that right?

Dr Pantridge. That is exactly what I am doing.

Dr Meltzer. Well, I did not understand that in the same sense. Is your ambulance equipped in the same way to treat everything or are you simply bringing personnel to the home?

Dr Pantridge. It is a mobile intensive care unit.

Dr Lown. If you send out one ambulance driver, how is he equipped to cope with the medical situation?

Dr Pantridge. I send out a junior doctor, a nurse and usually add a third pair of hands—a medical student. I did point out in one case that a junior doctor successfully carried out pacing in the patient's home.

Dr Killip. One thing Dr Oliver said which I think we should challenge is that speed of admission depends upon distance. In Belfast and in Edinburgh this may be so but it is certainly not so in New York City. It depends upon density. It may take one as long as an hour or an hour and a half to do a mile, at certain times of the day. I would like to re-emphasise what Dr Lown said about this problem of diagnosis. I was pleased to see that Dr Pantridge had a 29 per cent. incidence of what he called major ischaemic attacks without evidence of infarction. In our own experience in this group of patients in whom, as Dr Lown correctly said, one is uncertain about whether a major necrosis has occurred or not, the mortality is very low, but you have to treat it initially as though it were an established acute myocardial infarction. This is the sort of thing that I would suspect that Dr Armstrong and co-workers are going to have to consider very carefully in the final analysis of their data. Incidentally, in New York City 30 per cent. of our practising physicians do not have any hospital affiliations whatsoever. I think it would be very difficult to have any documentation at all to help you decide whether a patient with chest pains did or did not have myocardial infarction, if he were treated at home throughout the episode. One final point I think is worth making is that of the three different types of study which we have heard, only one could really be done at the present time in the United States—and that is an evaluation of the flying squad concept. Our medical system is set up so that it would not be meaningful for a general practitioner to present his experience since it relates to a closed community. A community study, because of the nature of our medical system, would be almost impossible.

Dr Wallace. If I have made a correct interpretation of the difference between Dr Chazov's flying squad and Dr Pantridge's, it seems to me very important. Professor Chazov's responds to emergency calls by the patient but in Dr Pantridge's case presumably the doctor always either talks to the patient or goes to see the patient first.

Dr Pantridge. In replying to Dr Lown may I say that the diagnostic accuracy is quite bad in fact, probably worse than yours; 49 per cent. had transmural myocardial infarction and I think 29 per cent. had prolonged chest pain and abnormal electro-cardiograms, but without enzyme or QRS changes which would indicate definite myocardial infarction. You cannot say that is a very good diagnostic performance. With regard to the time factor, I do not believe that you will ever get very many of these people in the first hour, simply because it is unlikely that the public will get into contact with the doctor much quicker than they do at the present time—a mean of 1 hour 15 minutes.

Dr Marquis. There is an enormous enthusiasm for Dr Pantridge's type of service in the community we deal with, it is important to realise that it is valuable as a research project, but in my opinion it is much less valuable as a potential community service without the total coverage they have in Moscow. This is supported by figures given so ably by Dr Fox. Now I think that we have got to recognise two things. Firstly, not all these patients can be saved. There is going to be an inevitable mortality from immediate death, either electrical or from cardiac rupture. The cardiac rupture incidence in the coroner's service is very high compared with the hospital service. Secondly, economically we cannot provide this service to every member of the community and we must therefore consider the effects on the patient who cannot get the service either because of distance or density or for some other reason. He may be adversely affected by anxiety, fear of death and so on, and we must take this into account when looking at the total community. For the man who can get the service it is excellent, but it is going to have a deleterious effect on that part of the community which cannot possibly ever get it.

Professor Shillingford. I wonder if everybody who had an infarction at home were given a shot of lignocaine, it would not achieve the same thing as a cardiac ambulance?

Dr Lown. If you take animals that have had coronary ligation, you can interdict those arrhythmias that develop late on with lidocaine or other antiarrhythmic measures like dilantin or procaine amide. Arrhythmias that develop early in the course after ligation are less readily prevented by drugs. This may also operate at the earliest stage of acute myocardial infarction and requires separate study.

Dr Wilson (London). I am very interested in Dr Pantridge's scheme from the point of view of looking towards community services. I wonder whether we could get a little further towards seeing how far away Belfast is from providing a community service. As I see it, with a population around half a million, one would expect about 1,500 infarcts a year. Now assuming that one tried to get all the patients into hospital what extra effort would be required? I wonder if Dr Pantridge could give us a hint on this and perhaps tell us what proportion of patients are treated at home and how many go to other hospitals? In discussing staffing did he take into full account all the extra personnel, which is the most costly part of the service, or is he riding a bit on the personnel of the teaching unit, who would not be available generally in a non-teaching centre?

Dr Pantridge. The total increase in establishment was one ambulance driver and one registrar. I think you have made a good point and I doubt if it would be quite as easy to arrange a roster in a hospital that was not as well staffed. It is true that we operate from a teaching hospital and probably have more staff than is otherwise available.

THE ROLE OF THE ADMINISTRATION IN THE EVALUATION OF CORONARY CARE

MICHAEL HEASMAN

Scottish Department of Home and Health, Edinburgh

OF all the experts who have gathered in Edinburgh to discuss coronary care none is less expert than I and, as the only hope of a non-expert in an expert community is to generalise, I shall be seeking generalisation which I hope will enable me not to reveal too profound an ignorance of your subject. Thus what I have to say concerns not only the evaluation of coronary care, but with the change of a few words, could apply equally to the evaluation of any other technological development in medicine. Please note that I shall not be concerned except marginally with the implementation of policy.

Naturally, I shall be discussing this problem from a British viewpoint, for I know no other, and I shall be rather more concerned with central administration. However I hope that what I have to say will not be irrelevant to those of you who come from overseas although the precise role of the central as opposed to the local administration may be considerably altered.

My own answer to the question as to what role the administration has in the evaluation of coronary care can be given quite shortly. It is: ' None ', except to see that it is evaluated in such a way that the health service problems are posed and answered and to help wherever they can to obtain these answers.

This evaluation is relevant at two levels—the first within the specialty concerned and the second in the general health service context. The first level of evaluation is normally undertaken initially by the clinicians concerned, often with the help of the epidemiologist. The second is a matter for the administration with the advice not only of clinicians in the cardiological field, but from other specialties as well.

I would like to deal with this second and general level of evaluation first, because we know so little about it. As yet we have no means of evaluating the contribution that coronary care can make and what priority it should have in the health service as a whole. At the moment the decisions that we should make, must of necessity, be based largely on subjective opinion rather than on objective data. The administration's role is to weigh the case for the

324

establishment of coronary care units against all the other priorities with which they are faced. They have to restrain the natural enthusiasm of the protagonists of coronary care, and try to balance their need against that, say, of the geriatrician who is appealing for better provision to meet his particular interests. I can only hope that we do not always give way to the group who shout the loudest, but at the present, shout you must if you are to be heard but your shouting must be backed by well-documented data.

The plain fact is that we have no means of weighing objectively the advantage of a life saved in a coronary care unit against the advantages of a number of patients being enabled to end their days in greater comfort rather than ' sans everything ' (to quote the title of a recent book published in this country).

With technology advancing at an ever increasing rate and with more and more expensive devices doing bigger and better things, this is becoming more of a problem. If there is an answer, there is little doubt that it will rely upon some sort of cost-benefit techniques where much of the benefit must be measured in social rather than financial terms. These techniques are as yet undiscovered.

Before leaving this topic, I should perhaps make the point that problems of assessment of coronary care in relation to the general health service picture is not only one of cost. We have to consider questions such as staffing priorities as well. It is little use providing Dr Fox with his 46,000 nurses, if to do so we have to denude other areas of badly needed personnel.

I would like now to return to the first type of evaluation that I mentioned, that is evaluation within the specialty concerned.

When a new procedure (or indeed a new drug) is introduced I think it is probably fair to say that in most countries of the world the administration, be it medical or lay, would not normally become involved provided that the cost, in the broadest sense of the word, is little different from that of the procedure (or drug) it is purported to supplant. As far as drugs are concerned, clinical trials are usually held and the efficacy of the new procedure established sufficiently for the clinician using it to be aware of the risks and of the benefits.

However, when cost becomes an important item administration must become interested, not because they are unwilling to spend money on a particular development but because in most communities in the world today, the amount that can be spent on health is both insufficient for all purposes and relatively stable, so that the amount free for the financing of new developments is comparatively small. Thus, the administration has to be provided with some means of evaluating the benefit likely to accrue against the costs and comparing this either with the present system or with some other worthwhile alternative.

The administration is entitled to ask if the technique is of proven benefit, not only in relation to the hospital patient but in relation to the community. Does the moving to hospital of a patient with a relatively minor attack precipitate a second and more serious episode? Does resuscitation in a coronary care unit result in a worthwhile prolongation of useful life? They are entitled to ask for an evaluation of the new procedure in relation to any alternatives.

These sort of questions raise the topic of clinical trials. This is a subject which I do not want to discuss in any detail here except to say that, if it is ethically possible, then trials should be mounted to study the value of domiciliary versus intensive coronary care, and of various hospital treatment procedures versus the care given in a coronary care unit. Even if perfection in the design is not possible, I believe that it is essential that an attempt should be made with the best that is feasible under the prevailing circumstances.

The role that the central administration plays here is a very important one. Either with its own epidemiological and statistical experts or with outside help the administration can bring together those in the van of these developments and organise and co-ordinate multi-centre trials which they can also finance.

While development is taking place and perhaps before sufficient equipment to meet all needs are available, it should be possible for the administration to ensure that in the first instance the equipment goes to those people most able to use it; but more than this, I think it is perfectly proper to make it a condition of supply to an individual hospital that the doctor in charge should undertake an evaluation in accordance with an agreed programme.

While techniques are being developed and trials of their efficacy being held, administration should be asking questions about the size of the problem were it decided that the technique was of proven benefit for national introduction. To do this, incidence studies must be held in the community in detail sufficient to allow an estimate to be made of the number of patients who would benefit from the techniques under different treatment policies. This, of course, is the primary purpose of the Edinburgh Community Study which Dr Armstrong told you about earlier.

The administration must also consider the siting of the new units and the logistic problems involved. Evaluation is needed of units in large regional centres, compared with smaller units in the periphery perhaps with less well-trained staff. We need to know something of the role that the ambulance can play.

Before administration can give guidance on training requirements it should have some assessment of the level of skill required to perform the respective procedures.

One can go on almost indefinitely. Many of the problems that I have posed from an administrative viewpoint in relation to coronary care have been dealt with in this conference and are either answered or are being studied. Others require considerable work if objective evidence is to be available on which administrative decisions can be based.

In his advisory capacity, the administrator has to look at coronary care as part of a very much larger picture than the clinician normally sees. He has a role as an epidemiologist. He is concerned with the mass aspects of a disease rather than with the individual patient, and it will be noticed that many of the points that I have made have, in fact, been epidemiological ones. This epidemiological role shades off into a managerial one and it is in this latter connection he has a possible part to play in assisting the formation of clinical policy. In view of what I have just said about the care needed not to venture into areas of clinical responsibility this may come as a surprise. However, I believe that a new technique such as intensive coronary care, which operates in a restricted field offers great possibilities for the use of the new administrative or management techniques involved in mathematical operations analysis. Dr Killip mentioned the need for quality control and I would just like to develop this a little further. The clinical policies in force in most coronary care units in this country have been arrived at empirically and cover such aspects as age limits for patients, and a minimum and/or maximum length of time that the uncomplicated case remains in the unit. If complete data are available on cases rejected as well as those accepted by the unit, and with other data such as those on timing of onset of attacks, arrival at, and departure from the unit and of episodes of ventricular fibrillation, one is presented with material which is amenable to mathematical operational analysis. This can present the clinicians with a set of alternative policies with some indication of the likely effect such policies will have. These can assist in determining factors such as the optimum size of the unit, the increase in the number of cases that would result if the length of stay were reduced and what cost this might have in extra complications. I wish to emphasise that the operational analyst is not going to interfere with clinical policies. He would be using advanced statistical techniques to present the

327

clinician with alternatives from which he (the clinician) will select the most efficient. Such techniques at all times allow the clinician to apply his judgment for the treatment of the individual patient.

Apart from this last point, I have been talking mostly about the interest that we administrators have in your techniques, and I have mentioned some of the questions that we want answered. We cannot and must not impede progress. Somehow we have to draw the line between the restraining of natural enthusiasm while answers are being found and the need to push ahead as fast as possible. Whether we in Britain have achieved this balance is not for me to say. Of one thing I am certain, this conference has gone a long way towards showing exactly where we stand today.

Discussion. See p. 335.

POLICY AND FUTURE OF INTENSIVE CORONARY CARE

SAMUEL M. FOX, III, M.D.

Heart Disease Control Program, Public Health Service Washington, D.C.

THERE are many directions that one could follow under such a title, having heard this excellent Symposium concerning what we know and what we do not yet have firmly established in the way of concepts, practices and opportunities for improved coronary care.

It is my impression that most participants at this conference believe coronary care units have a useful place in the management of patients suspected of having acute myocardial infarction or related circumstances of major cardiovascular hazard. In the United States of America the value of coronary care units is widely accepted, even though we do not have the type of statistical data that our appropriately sceptical colleagues demand as part of valid scientific proof. Admitting the inadequacy of much of the available data on this subject, it is my personal belief that it would be worthwhile, even at this late date, to undertake properly designed studies (using random allocation and other techniques) to assure that the difference in observed results of coronary care are direct consequences of the application of the new knowledge by specially trained staff. Certainly, we do not yet have a proper accounting of the costs that are involved in achieving the apparent benefits—an important element needed for present-day medical planning.

At the moment in the United States, we have at least 350 coronary care units that specifically restrict their patient populations to those considered to have myocardial infarction, definite or suspected, as the prime diagnosis. Most of these units are operating with difficulty because of the shortage of properly trained personnel. As I have mentioned previously, it is not our proposition that we should try to enlist 40,000 or 50,000 nurses for this effort; I think it is unrealistic to attempt this under present circumstances with nurses being needed in so many other areas. It seems more appropriate to try to generate a new cadre of individuals (' clinical physiologists ') in addition to an attempt to increase the number of specially trained physicians and nurses in the new concepts and practical details of coronary care.

It would be presumptuous, I believe, to try to project into the future regarding the many drugs, mechanical assistance devices, and other new and promising approaches on which we have had excellent specific commentary from highly qualified workers during this Symposium. It may, however, be of interest to try to approach the extension of coronary care services along lines of what has been referred to in the United States as a ' systems analytic approach '.

A schematic diagram of this approach is depicted in Figure 1. First let us consider the box designated ' Preventive Programs ' to be found on the right side of the diagram. This aspect of the

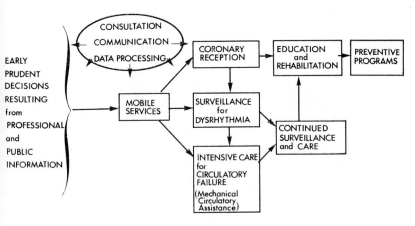

FIG. 1. A ' systems approach ' to coronary care.

' output ' end of the system seems a most important component of an expanded concept of coronary care. As patients proceed through the other elements of the system it would seem of great importance that survivors would be aided in their efforts to reduce the risk of recurrent attacks and to overcome the pessimism that often occurs. It is hoped that the personal experiences of the patients progressing through graduated steps of care would prompt them to undertake prudent programmes aimed at preventing the recurrence of episodes which caused their initial admission. If we do not include a preventive programme in our overall approach, I believe we are losing an excellent opportunity to live up to the higher ideals of preventing disease as well as adequately handling it once it has become clinically obvious. At the moment we have no proven preventive measures, but many modifications in living habits seem prudent.

Dr Wallace has discussed the necessity of looking into some of the aspects of rehabilitation and particularly has raised the important question of the appropriate time at which to undertake active rehabilitation. He has pointed out the need both of increasing physiological capacity through the physical activity of walking about and taking care of one's self, and of the rehabilitation of a person's self-confidence and optimistic approach to living. Within the area indicated by the next box to the left (' Education and Rehabilitation ') is an excellent opportunity for education concerning what we know about the nature of coronary disease and, perhaps, what we do not know but consider to be prudent relative to avoiding complications and recurrences.

In the diagram directly below ' Education and Rehabilitation '', we note a box entitled ' Continued Surveillance and Care ' representing a less intensive form of observation and treatment. This is a relatively unexplored but important element in our projected total system. If I remember correctly, Dr Meltzer has stated that his experience indicates that one-third of all hospital deaths of acute coronary patients deaths occurred *after* 96 hours in hospital.

Others have reported similar experience, perhaps due to the saving of lives in the units. It is quite possible that our current experience will change as we get earlier patient admission into the system, about which I will speak shortly, but even so it is important to recognise that late deaths do occur. It seems clear that a real yield of survivors, able to take an active place in society, can be achieved through continued less intense monitoring outside of the unit that will make available the benefits both of resuscitation services and of prevention or early management of complications.

330

In the United States there has been a sizeable effort to try to find the place for radio-telemetry of electrocardiographic and other analogue-type signals for patients under observation. It would appear that the continued surveillance and early ambulation phases would lend themselves well to the application of these newer telemetric techniques. In spite of much enthusiasm for its application to more critically ill patients, radio-telemetry has not yet seemed especially advantageous for those confined to bed. Certainly, much more research into progressive care, rehabilitation and secondary prevention is indicated and should be rewarding.

In the middle of our scheme we find the entity which now is the centre of the coronary care effort in many parts of the United States. It is in the ' Surveillance for Dysrhythmias ' area that the greatest savings in lives has taken place and in connection with which the new ' aggressive prophylaxis ' approach to complications has been most applicable. Directly below this is a separate entity titled ' Intensive Care for Circulatory Failure ' which would also provide for patients with the ' shock syndrome '. In some American hospitals these activities are undertaken in an architecturally separate area, adjacent to the ' surveillance ' area, in an attempt to reduce noise and anxiety for those with more adequate heart muscle function. Personnel may serve both areas concurrently, however.

As the techniques for the mechanical assistance of the circulation become of proven value, a more sophisticated place for their application might be needed, either adjacent to or separate from the other areas for coronary patients. At the moment it appears that the application of pharmacological and other techniques, such as rotating tourniquets for the congestive failure and shock syndromes, usually can be undertaken almost anywhere in the hospital. The specially trained nursing and other staff are likely to be more effectively grouped in a specific area of coronary care facilities, emergency rooms and/or post-surgical recovery rooms than if these facilities are spread diffusely throughout the general hospital. To conserve personnel most effectively, combined facilities have much to recommend them.

Thus far in this development of a coronary care system there is little new—nor much that has not been considered by most of us.

A major opportunity that commands our attention is how to extend coronary care services out into the community and how to expedite the application of these services earlier in the individual coronary episode. Of the reported 580,000 annual deaths attributed to coronary heart disease in the U.S.A., over half are alleged to occur outside of hospitals or nursing homes. These 300,000 deaths of a total population of approximately 200 million probably include many elderly individuals who, for one reason or another, will prefer to pass from this life in the warmth of their homes after all modern therapy has been applied: nevertheless, we must provide a more effective system for the remaining large majority.

It is calculated that over one-third of all male deaths in the U.S.A. that occur between the ages of 35 and 64 are due to coronary disease, presumably in individuals whose heart muscle has or could be conditioned into having a reasonable reserve capacity.

What can we do to get these individuals into protected circumstances earlier in the course of the disease or a particular coronary episode? Drs Pantridge and Chazov have reported on their pioneer approaches to the provision of mobile services. Others have indicated the extended period of time that frequently occurs between the onset of coronary symptoms and hospital admission.

It is of particular interest that Dr Pantridge's report emphasised the movement of the coronary care services to the patient and, specifically, it is important that the patient is seldom moved until corrective and/or preventive therapy is applied ' on site ' as indicated. This should allay the concern of many individuals that the ambulance would swoop down on the patient and pluck him out of a setting that may be acceptable for excellent temporary care. Of course at some future time mechanical assistance devices, useable only in hospital, may provide a rationale for more immediate removal.

Without going further regarding these creative efforts to provide mobile services, let us look at the last box on our diagram, labelled ' Coronary Reception '.

At first I considered the terms ' Coronary Care Atrium ' and 'Coronary Triage Area' but, due to the probable lack of familiarity of many people with these words I have settled on 'Coronary Reception Area ', although with considerable continuing dissatisfaction.

The provision of such a reception area hopefully would serve to reduce some of the major factors that impede hospital admission early in the course of the coronary episode—factors that elevate the ' input impedance '. Some of these factors include the length of time persons think is involved in getting forms and records filled out, in the U.S.A. the need for documentation of third party or individual financial ability to support the hospitalisation, and the need to identify a specific bed—a situation that often requires a call from the patient's physician.

Also of great importance, but not directly related to these considerations, is the lack of sufficient ambulances or equivalent facilities for the provision of competent and prompt service with minimum aggravation of the patient's anxiety.

Another factor felt to contribute to the reluctance of many persons to enter a hospital is their unwillingness to be removed for even a few days from the important activities of their normal life. Although a ' systems approach ' to *any* hospitalisation should emphasise methods of reducing unnecessary time in the hospital; it is of paramount importance to analyse the possibly unique time equation that relates to coronary episodes. Thus there is also a need to lower the ' output impedance ' as a part of factors delaying the decision to get into the protected environment of coronary care. People must be assured they will be able to go back into the main stream of life as soon as medical circumstances permit.

In short, we are faced with a major question that deserves careful consideration: do we gain more in total human values through the reduction of these apparent impediments that make people reluctant to avail themselves of coronary care when we include taking reasonable chances in discharging those considered good risks before the complete resolution of the episode? The possibilities seem sufficient to justify evaluation of different approaches to developing an attractive system which provides early admission and prompt discharge when the probabilities seem acceptably low that further difficulties will not be encountered.

What, then, do we picture in the way of a coronary reception area? Perhaps, in terms of the physical arrangements, we could start with a large room containing several dual-purpose, mobile reclining lounge chairs that would elevate the legs and recline the back. The chairs could be levelled for emergency therapy, which would take place in an adjacent ' treatment room ' to which the patient could be promptly wheeled. Moveable noise-reducing screens could provide a measure of privacy for the ' coronary suspect '. A relative or friend of the patient might be available to provide for the patient in the way of food, drink, reading material, etc. to avoid the expense of many hospital employees. These relatives or friends would have to be very carefully selected since their own anxiety might well produce the opposite of the needed patient reassurance and support.

In order to help assure the patient that he is not entering any deeper into the total coronary care system than is necessary for his individual condition, he might remain partially dressed in his own clothing to the extent that necessary therapy can be applied

333

and monitoring devices can be used. He also might be given the freedom of using a nearby lavatory and toilet. Other restrictions on his movement might be reduced through radio-telemetric monitoring to an aerial that would convey the signal to competent personnel located in a more classical coronary or intensive care unit or emergency room—from which they could rapidly respond to the needs of those in the ' Reception Area '. As in all such efforts the personnel are the essential ingredient and the other elements are but the means to permit them to apply their talents efficiently.

A person would be transferred into the standard ' surveillance ' area or elsewhere in the hospital when certain criteria are met relative to the electrocardiogram, serum enzymes and points elicited by a careful history and physical examination that could be obtained after the ' suspect ' is settled in the ' Coronary Reception Area '. The important factor would be the ease of admission to the temporary protection of this ' harbor of refuge ' without fuss or delay.

It appears possible that some persons should be registered by their physicians as being of such high risk of dysrhythmia, infarct or other catastrophe so that they could be admitted and monitored in the Reception Area without having to make arrangements through their physician for each episode. Others could be immediately admitted from ambulances or the emergency room until their symptoms, signs and laboratory data defined their status.

Basic to the rationale of such a Reception Area is the suspicion, supported by some clinical experience (but not by a large body of data), that many persons referred to as having experienced sudden coronary deaths actually experienced prodromal symptoms and signs for a period of time adequate for a prudent decision and effective action.

Another important part of a larger system of coronary care is a communication centre or ' control point ' that conceivably could provide round-the-clock consultation from knowledgeable physicians who could discuss and advise on the problems of many persons in widely scattered facilities. Through presently available communication facilities, physiological data (ECG, plethysmographic, pulse contour, etc.) could be presented to the consultant, and various measurements and analyses could be made using computer techniques. The frequency and number of types of atypical waveforms could be enumerated and displayed with a diagnostic probability score accompanied by a list of relevant therapeutic ' action items ' worthy of consideration. This type of information and interpretive consultation might permit some mobile services and coronary care areas to operate with less ' on-site ' coverage by physician and other short-supply professional personnel.

By directing patients to those units that have open beds with ' unsaturated ' staffing at that particular time, it might be expected that the total regional coronary care effort could be more effective and economical. Indeed, it is necessary in the U.S.A.—and I suspect elsewhere—that any such proposal as this system must be justified on the basis of the increased benefits outweighing the added costs.

Special consideration should be given to the problems of providing a coronary care service in a small community hospital. Perhaps the best possible approach would be to tie such hospitals into a regional analysis and reduction centre. This would not only be economically possible, but would also provide competent consultative services to the staffs of the small hospitals. This would obviate the need for transfer of many patients to referral centres.

In closing, I hope we can maintain a continuing communication on this pleasant and stimulating international level as we all examine what is available in the way of improvements in coronary care. We should undertake general professional and lay education concerning the use of segments of the system only when the capability to provide the services is achieved. The future appears to provide even greater opportunities for stimulating and rewarding research than that which has led to the knowledge brought out so well in the Symposium.

Finally, I wish to emphasise that extending the system of coronary care forward to induce earlier prudent decisions for observation, diagnosis and care should be matched by an equal effort to provide sustained prudent preventive programming as the patient leaves the ' harbor of refuge ' to navigate on his own.

Discussion

Professor Donald. Although it must be demonstrated more objectively what the returns of coronary care are in money and in community health, there are already great benefits—a stimulation of interest in heart disease in general, the active attack on a disease which had comparatively little attention previously, and a spread of interest from coronary disease to other areas of cardiology. Again, coronary care is inevitably moving into the community and this a great need in British medicine where the hospital and the community must become more of one organisation. I would only have one word of comfort for Dr Heasman. It is likely that many of these expensive procedures and pieces of apparatus may well get cheaper. I would remind him that oxygen tents were once stored all over the country and a vast amount of money was either paid for them or paid for their rental. After a few years research into oxygen therapy, all we now need are cheap masks or nasal catheters. I am sure this type of development will occur in coronary care with increasing knowledge and techniques. With regard to operational analysis, I think I must warn Dr Heasman that there may be some dangers here. When these organisations get underway they will find that many things like coronary care units depend on men working 16 hours a day. As it is their duty to see that these men do a responsible day's work and not enough to kill themselves in a short time, they will be in difficulty!

Dr Fox. I would like to make a comment which I meant to include earlier. One of the major problems we have in the States is justifying the empty bed in a coronary care unit. In other words, if you speak to our colleagues that are operating units, you find that their administration is in difficulties during the busy winter season when people come in out of the cold as well as with real medical indications. In the States you cannot hold a bed open when the hospital could be earning anywhere from 50 to 100 dollars a day from that bed. Now this is where in a community organisation there must be an efficient secretarial staff so that a doctor dealing with mobile services knows where there is a bed, or they may have to decide that a three-bed unit will eventually reduce its personnel by one. Alternatively, it may be necessary to try to empty these beds and put more nurses off to other services or give them time off to be enlisted when needs get greater. This is a very important thing in our economics and one of the reasons why we have difficulties in getting coronary care services.

Dr Nixon. One thing that is worth emphasising is pre-coronary diagnosis. This is picking up the coronary patient at a stage even before Pantridge does. I personally believe that coronary attacks very rarely come out of the blue. In my own hospital, most of the patients with cardiac infarction have come there from their work, but surprisingly often their wives say they have been sick for days. I think that it was the Baltimore study of sudden coronary deaths which showed that about half the patients who had sudden coronary death had in fact been to their physician within the preceding week. I think there is a large part to play in educating the doctors who first encounter these patients to pay more attention to these symptoms. The thing that stops them diagnosing pre-coronary symptoms straight off is the fear of diagnosing it. When the patient comes with suspicious symptoms the doctor does not like this word ' coronary disease ' and would much rather pat the patient on the back and tell him to go away.

Dr Julian. I am sure this is a very good point but the question that arises is what do we do with these patients? I find practitioners are always asking how they should manage the patient with the recent onset of angina or an exacerbation of angina. We cannot admit them all to coronary care units.

Dr Wilson. I must say I am very baffled by Dr Fox's account of the future status of coronary care units in the States—as to how a comprehensive service can be provided in the absence of a health service. In this country the possibility of providing coronary care as a service in the whole country is but one of our dilemmas in deciding what research needs to be done and how we can best use our resources. I would like to ask whether the approach of providing general intensive care and coronary care in the same general area is acceptable. If my figures are right, we would need something like 200 or more units in England and Wales to provide this service, assuming between 5 and 10 beds each, staffing at about $2\frac{1}{2}$ nurses to each patient and a minimum of about 15 nurses per unit with medical staff to match. We are faced with this proliferation of different special units, and the question is whether we should be providing coronary care with, or as a part of, intensive care.

Dr Julian. I think there are a number of points on which we might conveniently try and get some consensus of opinion. Although we are all here committed to coronary care as a concept, do we believe that the future of coronary care lies in having the coronary care unit as an independent but adjacent part of an intensive care area? Would anybody like to agree or disagree with this?

Dr McNicol. I would like to agree with this concept. We are working in a non-teaching hospital with district hospital type staffing. It will not be possible for us to continue running separate intensive care and coronary care units. We have in fact a coronary care unit and no intensive care unit; this in some respects is unjustifiable but we are interested in coronary care and I think when the time comes when we have both they will need to be physically related.

Dr Fejfar. I believe that coronary care units are just a transitory development. In my opinion, they are useful in showing to what extent they can improve the care of these acutely sick patients. As far as the organisation is concerned, the future is going to see complete reorganisation of community and hospital services with surgical and medical emergencies all grouped together in certain areas and where you have such things as round-the-clock laboratory services. You distribute your patients on admission according to the diagnosis. Of course you will have a special medical department for diagnostic purposes, another for treatment of chronic patients, and another for rehabilitation. Then you can save personnel.

Dr Lown. I have been impressed during the last three days not by differences and diverse experiences, but by the similarity of our experience. This of course has profound implications. We are unified by a common experience and yet we do not have a nomenclature in common. For instance, the grading of myocardial infarction as mild, moderate and severe is a nebulous concept that we would reject as non-objective and primordial. In assessing the severity of myocardial infarction as a whole, I would like to make a suggestion that, through the good offices of the World Health Organization, we try to produce a unified nomenclature. This would have great significance because then we could assess the efficacy of therapy more rapidly anywhere in the world. When talking to Professor Chazov I found that mortality from shock in Moscow is exactly the same as it is in Boston and the same is true through the other gradations. The moment we understand each other there are no differences. Another point is that the CCU cannot be viewed as a monolithic structure. It is a transient phase as Dr Fejfar says. Now during this phase various gradations of care should be provided for every coronary patient. Its simplest conception perhaps is some simple device for defibrillation, which is certainly not expensive, and elementary monitoring with a nurse merely to perform resuscitation. There is a range of grades between this and more elaborate systems of monitoring and care. We have to start, as is frequently true in medicine, with our primary responsibility in treating patients, and often after initiating treatment we subsequently learn the rationale for it. This has been true in the experience of Withering and many others. I think its possible right now to assess, as Professor Shillingford suggested earlier, the efficacy of lidocaine or other anti-arrhythmic drugs in the home situation and see if they can prevail as a prophylactic measure and so dispense with the need for rapid transport. Lastly, I wish to make this point, that I think we may be also opening a Pandora's box. All progress exacts costs. In this case we must not over-emphasise research from the point of view of the well-being of the patient as I think there cannot be such a dissociation of research and service. Our primary responsibility is service, and research must flow from the benefit to the particular patient we are studying.

Dr McDonald. I think there has been too little said about premonitory symptoms and what we should be doing about them. There is no question that the majority of patients with cardiac infarction have premonitory symptoms, and an increasing number are coming into our units, and an increasing number would come into Dr Fox's coronary reception areas. This is an extremely important clinical zone on which to concentrate now. We should try and report, in the course of time, patients of this type who come into our units as well as those with cardiac infarction. It does seem to me that we are faced in this country with the need to find more money for coronary units and allied facilities. Equally, I think it would be a fair interpretation of the happenings of the last three days to say that most clinicians in this room feel that there is very little point in admitting a patient to hospital after cardiac infarction if he does not go into a coronary unit. If we made it our policy to admit fewer patients with cardiac infarction to hospitals where there is not a coronary unit, we could have more funds for special care.

Dr Nixon. We have recently got a unit in which we have included in one suite, coronary, surgical and other intensive care cases. It was designed to give to those that need it a bit of peace and quiet but it is under one Sister and one administration.

Dr Julian. I am sure that we all agree that coronary care units have achieved something, otherwise I do not suppose we would be here. We rather doubt whether the general ward treatment does anything and we believe that the time has come to promote coronary care generally but only if we have the appropriate trained personnel. This is where we must look to the administrators to help us. As I understand it, there is no dissension from the view that coronary care units should be a transient phase whilst we are developing general intensive areas with a special coronary division. We must push for action in following up the lead of Dr Pantridge and Professor Chazov and getting into the community but we seem to agree that prophylactic therapy in the home is a more promising line of research than the provision of special ambulances. It is certainly in the premonitory or even presymptomatic phase of acute myocardial infarction that the next major advance is needed.

GLOSSARY

Alternative names of drugs:

Adrenaline	Epinephrine
Demerol	Pethidine, Meperidine
Diamorphine	Heroin
Diphenylhydantoin	Phenytoin
Epinephrine	Adrenaline
Heroin	Diamorphine
Isoprenaline	Isoproterenol
Isoproterenol	Isoprenaline
Lidocaine	Lignocaine
Lignocaine	Lidocaine
Meperidine	Demerol, Pethidine
Noradrenaline	Norepinephrine
Norepinephrine	Noradrenaline
Pethidine	Demerol, Meperidine
Phenytoin	Diphenylhydantoin

INDEX

Acidosis, 222–224
Adrenaline, 237
Ajmalin, 96
Ambulance, cardiac, 308, 315–323
  deaths in, 316–323
Analgesics, 285–295
  haemodynamic effects, 286–290
Anticoagulants, 277–284
  effect on mortality, 278
  effect on thromboembolic complications, 280
Apex cardiogram, 173–177, 209–212, 215
Arrest, cardiac, 9, 41, 97, 102, 139
Arrhythmias, 6, 9, 10, 14–17, 31, 73, 140, 295, 315
  atrial. *See* Atrial arrhythmias
  catecholamines and, 241
  classification, 15, 16, 73
  haemodynamic effects of, 140, 204
  pain and, 295
  ventricular. *See* ventricular arrhythmias
Artificial heart, 229, 232
Assisted circulation, 229, 232
Asystole, 9, 19, 26, 31, 139
Atrial arrhythmias, 73–84
  ectopic beats, 17, 73–84
  fibrillation, 17, 73–84
  flutter, 17, 73–84
  tachycardia, 17, 73–84
  with block, 178
Atrial infarction, 79, 81, 82
Atrioventricular block. *See* Block, atrioventricular
Atropine, 15, 77, 118, 153, 294

Block, atrioventricular,
  associated arrhythmias, 138, 153
  complete, 138–153, 156, 160–165
  cardiac failure and shock, 26, 140
  catecholamine excretion, 239
  drug therapy, 153
  haemodynamic effects, 140, 206
  incidence, 41, 138
  mortality, 42, 143
Bradyarrhythmias, 15, 26, 94, 138, 205
Bradycardia, sinus, 15, 74, 159, 205
Bundle branch block, 138

Cardiac output, 11, 140, 201
  in atrioventricular block, 140

Cardioversion. *See* Shock, D.C.
Catecholamines, 12, 87, 93, 237–265
Catheterisation, cardiac, 22, 23, 116, 228
Community, and coronary care, 299, 304, 331
  general practice, 304
  Study, Edinburgh, 299–304
Complete pump failure, 18–20
Computer analysis of ECG, 64, 65
Coronary Care Unit,
  administration, 27, 28, 34, 47–69, 324, 328–339
  admission times, 4, 11, 13, 29, 36
  age and admission, 13, 34
  design, 57–65, 328–339
  effectiveness, 4–6, 11, 27, 37–44
  future of, 328–339
  instrumentation, 57–69
  mortality, 5–7, 11, 18, 21, 27, 30, 36–44
  neurosis, 64, 311
  nursing, 51
  policies, 1–44
  regular care comparison, 3–6, 11, 27, 37–44
  results, 1–44
Coupled electrical stimulation, 96, 133, 135, 150–152
Creatine kinase, serum, 266–273
Crepitations, pulmonary, 12, 184, 186, 216

Death, sudden, 84, 300, 305
Defibrillation. *See* Shock, D.C.
Digitalis. *See* Glycosides, cardiac
Dilantin. *See* Phenytoin
Diuretic therapy, 12, 179–188
Dysrhythmia. *See* Arrhythmia

ECG, intracardiac, 61
Electrical instability, of the heart, 15, 84
Electric shock. *See* Shock, D.C.
Enzymes, serum, 33, 78, 266–273
  anoxia and, 268
  defibrillation and, 273
  ischaemia and, 268
  release, 269
Epinephrine. *See* Adrenaline
External percussion, of heart, 83

341

MADE AND PRINTED IN GREAT BRITAIN BY
MORRISON AND GIBB LIMITED
LONDON AND EDINBURGH